FRONTIERS IN GASTROINTESTINAL CANCER

CURRENT ONCOLOGY

Nathaniel I. Berlin, *Series Editor-in-Chief*

TITLES IN CURRENT ONCOLOGY

FRONTIERS IN GASTROINTESTINAL CANCER

Bernard Levin and Robert H. Riddell, *Editors-in-Chief*

FRONTIERS IN GASTROINTESTINAL CANCER

Edited by

BERNARD LEVIN, M.D.
Formerly: Associate Professor, Department of Medicine
Director, Gastrointestinal Oncology Service
University of Chicago Hospitals and Clinics
Present address: Professor, University of Texas
Section of Digestive Diseases and Gastrointestinal Oncology
Division of Medicine, M.D. Anderson Hospital, Houston

ROBERT H. RIDDELL, M.D.
Formerly: Associate Professor of Pathology
University of Chicago Hospitals and Clinics
Present address: Professor, Department of Pathology
McMaster University, Hamilton, Ontario

ELSEVIER
New York • Amsterdam • Oxford

Elsevier Science Publishing Co., Inc.
52 Vanderbilt Avenue, New York, New York 10017

Distributors outside the United States and Canada

Elsevier Science Publishers B.V.
P.O. Box 211, 1000 AE Amsterdam, The Netherlands

ISBN 0-444-00852-7

ISSN 0743-930X

Manufactured in the United States of America

CONTENTS

PREFACE

Gastrointestinal cancer continues to be a significant factor in much human suffering. Unknown causes, changing epidemiological patterns, the difficulty of early diagnosis, and the apparent resistance of some malignancies to chemotherapeutic agents all serve to heighten the immense clinical and scientific challenges faced by the investigator and practicing physician.

The critical reader may well consider the term "frontiers" to be rather presumptuous. However, we feel that this volume does present a selection of important topics that convey some of the exciting scientific and clinical advances in this field. Distinguished investigators responded enthusiastically to our invitation to contribute manuscripts. We specifically requested them to discuss their own work in the context of the overall area. These "minireviews" cover topics ranging from etiology, pathogenesis, histopathology, and experimental carcinogenesis to therapy. We believe that our authors have succeeded admirably but will leave to the reader the ultimate judgment of our failure or success. At the very least, we hope we have been able to stimulate interest and controversy in this important area.

CONTRIBUTORS

Editors

BERNARD LEVIN, M.D.
Formerly: Associate Professor, Department of Medicine and Director of the Gastrointestinal Oncology Service, University of Chicago Hospitals and Clinics
Present address: Professor, University of Texas, Section of Digestive Diseases and Gastrointestinal Oncology, Division of Medicine, M.D. Anderson Hospital, Houston

ROBERT H. RIDDELL, M.D.
Formerly: Associate Professor of Pathology, University of Chicago Hospitals and Clinics
Present address: Professor, Department of Pathology, McMaster University, Hamilton, Ontario

Chapter Authors

VINCENT G. ALLFREY, PH.D.
Laboratory of Cell Biology, Rockefeller University, New York, New York

JEANNIE CHAMBERS, R.N.
Department of Radiation Oncology, The Johns Hopkins Hospital, Baltimore, Maryland

GARY M. CLARK, PH.D.
Department of Medicine, Division of Oncology, University of Texas Health Science Center at San Antonio

WILLIAM D. DEWYS, M.D.
From the Prevention Program, Division of Cancer Prevention and Control, National Cancer Institute, Bethesda, Maryland

DANIEL E. DOSORETZ, M.D.
Assistant Professor, Department of Radiation Therapy, Massachusetts General Hospital and Harvard Medical School, Boston, Massachusetts

KAMBIZ DOWLATSHAHI, M.D., F.R.C.S.
Assistant Professor, Department of Surgery, University of Chicago

DAVID M. EDDY, M.D., PH.D.
Director, Center for Health Policy Reseach and Education, Duke University, Durham, North Carolina

SUSAN S. ELLENBERG, PH.D.
Cancer Therapy Evaluation Program, Division of Cancer Treatment, National Cancer Institute, Bethesda, Maryland

WILLIAM D. ENSMINGER, M.D., PH.D.
Professor, Departments of Internal Medicine and Pharmacology, University of Michigan, Ann Arbor

DAVID S. ETTINGER, M.D.
Department of Medical Oncology, The Johns Hopkins Hospital, Baltimore, Maryland

J. GEBOERS
Licensee in Mathematics, Assistant, Division of Epidemiology, University of Louvain, Belgium

LEONARD L. GUNDERSON, M.D., M.S.
Associate Professor in Oncology, Mayo Clinic, Rochester, Minnesota

JOHN W. GYVES, M.D.
Instructor, Department of Internal Medicine, University of Michigan, Ann Arbor

FREDDIE ANN HOFFMAN, M.D.
Clinical Investigations Branch, Cancer Therapy Evaluation Program, Division of Cancer Treatment, National Cancer Institute, Bethesda, Maryland

R. BRUCE HOSKINS, M.D.
Clinical Assistant Professor in Radiology, Southern Illinois University Medical School; Radiotherapist, St. Johns Hospital, Springfield, Illinois

JANET A. HOUGHTON, PH.D.
Department of Biochemical and Clinical Pharmacology, St. Jude Children's Research Hospital, Memphis, Tennessee

PETER J. HOUGHTON, PH.D.
Department of Biochemical and Clinical Pharmacology, St. Jude Children's Research Hospital, Memphis, Tennessee

J. V. JOOSSENS, M.D.
Professor of Medicine, Head, Division of Epidemiology, University of Louvain, Belgium

LEONARD B. KAHN, M.B., B.CH., M.MED.PATH., M.R.C.PATH.
Chaairman, Department of Laboratories, Long Island Jewish—Hillside Medical Center; Professor of Pathology, State University of New York at Stony Brook

JOHN Y. KILLEN, Jr., M.D.
Cancer Therapy Evaluation Program, Division of Cancer Treatment, National Cancer Institute, Bethesda, Maryland

JERRY L. KLEIN, Ph.D.
Department of Radiation Oncology, The Johns Hopkins Hospital, Baltimore, Maryland

GENE KOPELSON, M.D.
Assistant Professor in Therapeutic Radiology, Tufts New England Medical Center, Boston, Massachusetts

KEN KOPHER, B.S.
Department of Radiation Oncology, The Johns Hopkins Hospital, Baltimore, Maryland

STEVEN LANGE, M.D.
Division of Medical Oncology, Vincent T. Lombardi Cancer Research Center, Georgetown University, Washington, D.C.

TERENCE A. LAWSON, Ph.D.
The Eppley Institute for Research in Cancer and the Department of Pathology and Laboratory Medicine, University of Nebraska Medical Center, Omaha

PETER K. LEICHNER, Ph.D.
Department of Radiation Oncology, The Johns Hopkins Hospital, Baltimore, Maryland

BERNARD LEVIN, M.D.
Formerly: Associate Professor, Department of Medicine, and Director of the Gastrointestinal Oncology Service, University of Chicago Hospitals and Clinics
Present address: Professor, University of Texas, Section of Digestive Diseases and Gastrointestinal Oncology, Division of Medicine, M.D. Anderson Hospital, Houston

DAVID M. LOESCH, M.D.
Department of Medicine, Division of Oncology, University of Texas Health Science Center at San Antonio. Present address: Wright-Patterson Air Force Base, Dayton, Ohio

ALAIN P. MASKENS, M.D.
Groupe de Recherche Alimentation et Cancer, Brussels, Belgium

RABIA MIR, M.D.
Attending Pathologist, Long Island Jewish-Hillside Medical Center; Assistant Professor in Pathology, State University of New York at Stony Brook

SOHRAB MOBARHAN, M.D.
Associate Professor, Department of Medicine, Section of Gastroenterology, University of Illinois, Chicago

RICHARD C. NAIRN, M.D.
Professor and Chairman, Department of Pathology and Immunology, Monash University, and Alfred Hospital, Melbourne, Australia

STANLEY E. ORDER, M.D., Sc.D.
Director of Radiation Oncology, The Johns Hopkins Hospital, Baltimore, Maryland

ERIC PIHL, M.D.
Associate Professor, Department of Pathology and Immunology, Monash University, and Alfred Hospital, Melbourne, Australia

MORRIS POLLARD, D.V.M., PH.D.
Lobund Laboratory, University of Notre Dame, Notre Dame, Indiana

PARVIZ M. POUR, M.D.
The Eppley Institute for Research in Cancer and the Department of Pathology and Laboratory Medicine, University of Nebraska Medical Center, Omaha

AMELIA REICHMANN, M.D.
Melamid Cytogenetics Laboratory, Section of Gastroenterology, Department of Medicine, University of Chicago

ROBERT H. RIDDELL, M.D.
Formerly: Associate Professor of Pathology, University of Chicago Hospitals and Clinics
Present address: Professor, Department of Pathology, McMaster University, Hamilton, Ontario

TYVIN A. RICH, M.D.
Assistant Professor, Joint Center for Radiation Therapy, Harvard Medical School, Boston, Massachusetts

PHILIP S. SCHEIN, M.D., F.A.C.P.
Division of Medical Oncology, Vincent T. Lombardi Cancer Research Center, Georgetown University, Washington, D.C.

HELMUT SCHMIDT, M.D.
Department of Medicine, University of Erlangen, Erlangen, West Germany

STANLEY S. SIEGELMAN, M.D.
Department of Diagnostic Radiation, The Johns Hopkins Hospital, Baltimore, Maryland

ROBERT SILGALS, M.D.
Division of Medical Oncology, Vincent T. Lombardi Cancer Research Center, Georgetown University, Washington, D.C.

FREDERICK P. SMITH, M.D., F.A.C.P.
Division of Medical Oncology, Vincent T. Lombardi Cancer Research Center, Georgetown University, Washington, D.C.

I. C. TALBOT, M.D., F.R.C.PATH.
Department of Pathology, University of Leicester, United Kingdom

JOEL E. TEPPER, M.D.
Assistant Professor in Radiation Therapy, Massachusetts General Hospital and Harvard Medical School, Boston, Massachusetts

DANIEL D. VON HOFF, M.D.
Department of Medicine, Division of Oncology, University of Texas Health Science Center at San Antonio

MOODY D. WHARAM, M.D.
Department of Radiation Oncology, The Johns Hopkins Hospital, Baltimore, Maryland

ARIE J. ZUCKERMAN, M.D., D.Sc., F.R.C.P., F.R.C.Path
Department of Medical Microbiology, and WHO Collaborating Centre for Reference and Research on Viral Hepatitis, London School of Hygiene and Tropical Medicine (University of London)

DIET AND ENVIRONMENT IN THE ETIOLOGY OF ESOPHAGEAL CARCINOMA

KAMBIZ DOWLATSHAHI, M.D., F.R.C.S., AND SOHRAB MOBARHAN, M.D.

In most parts of the world, carcinoma of the esophagus is a rare disease. The incidence in the United States and Europe is 3 to 4 per 100,000 population per annum (Cutler and Young, 1975; Doll et al., 1970). In certain other areas, this rate increases more than twentyfold to almost 100 new cases per 100,000 population per annum, and esophageal cancer becomes the most frequently occurring neoplasm in the community (see Figures 1 and 2).

GEOGRAPHIC INCIDENCE

The sharp geographic demarcation between regions of high incidence of esophageal cancer and relatively close neighboring areas with a much lower incidence, such as in northeast Iran, has given rise to a great deal of scientific debate regarding the role of nutritional deficiencies and environmental carcinogens and their possible reciprocal interaction in the development of esophageal cancer. In recent years, a significant body of epidemiologic and biologic studies has accumulated suggesting that dietary factors, particularly micronutrients such as trace elements and vitamins, could influence carcinogenesis. These may act by modifying the activity of either carcinogens or host protective mechanisms against cancer. Esophageal cancer has a strong association with malnutrition secondary to poor economic conditions, special dietary habits, and/or alcoholism.

In our discussion, we will distinguish the predisposing factors, such as the nutritional status, from the promoting factors or carcinogens that act directly on the esophageal mucosa.

From the Department of Surgery, University of Chicago; and the Department of Medicine, Section of Gastroenterology, University of Illinois, Chicago.

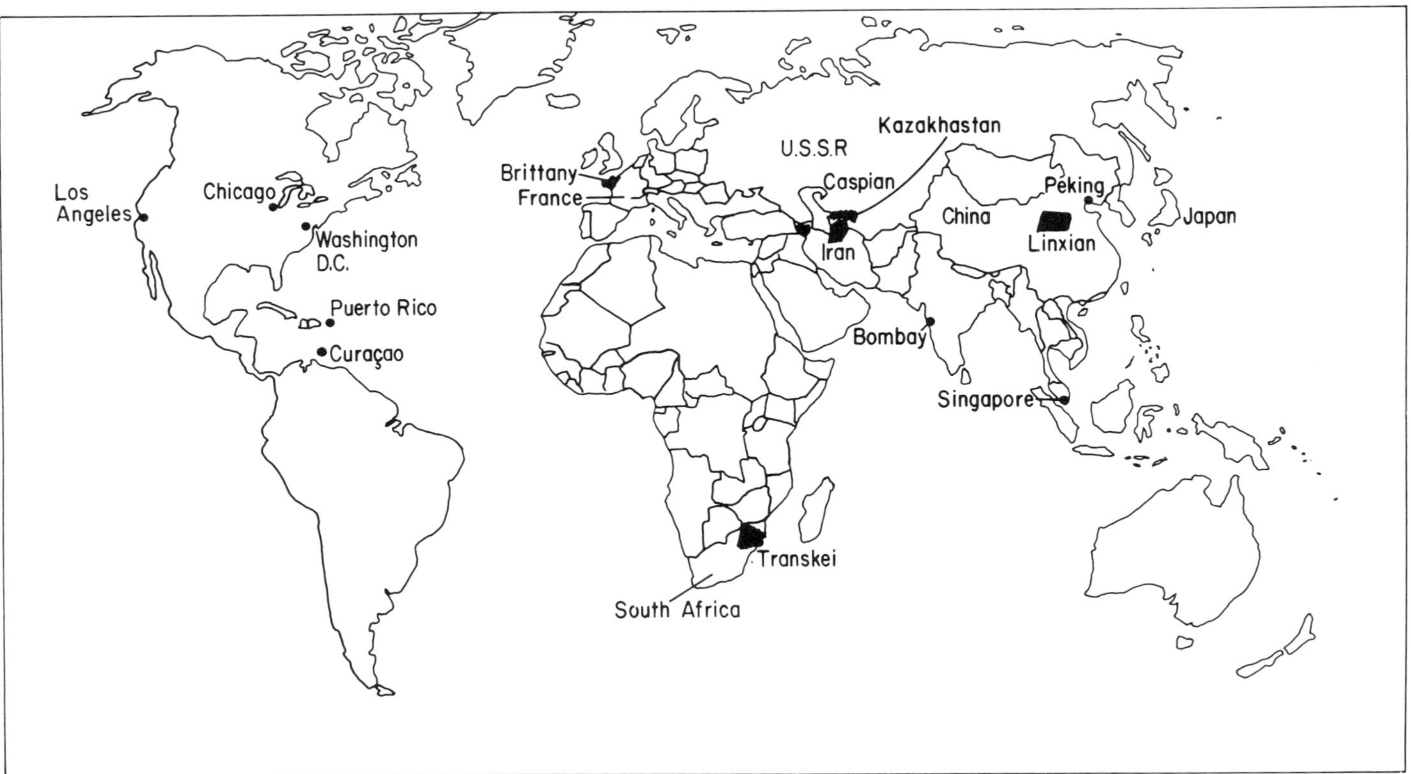

FIGURE 1. World map. Reported areas of high esophageal cancer incidence are shaded and labeled.

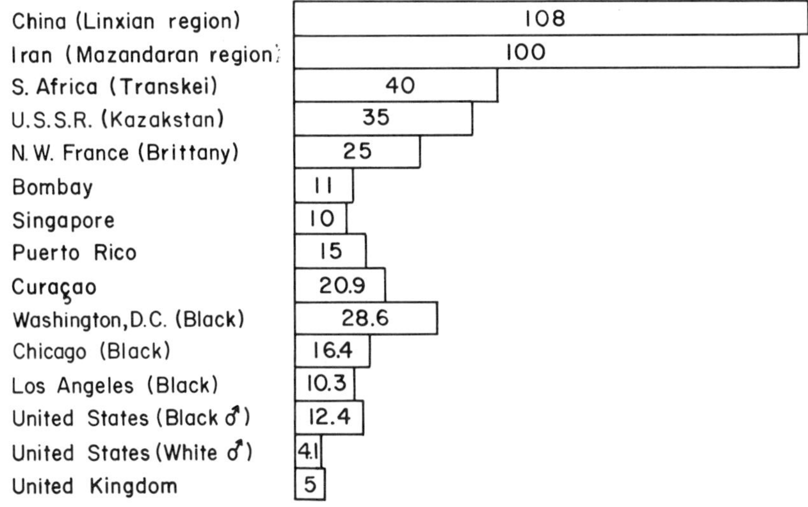

FIGURE 2. Annual incidence of esophageal carcinoma per 100,000 population compiled from regional published reports. Numbers include both sexes unless otherwise specified.

China

Formal registration of esophageal cancer in northern China since 1959 has revealed a high incidence of this carcinoma in three provinces south of the Taihang Mountain, situated southwest of Peking. In the Linxian (Linhsien) county of Henan, for example, the adjusted average incidence rate during the period from 1959 to 1970 was 108/100,000 population per annum (Coordinating Group, 1975).

People of this region live on farms and are generally of low income. Their diet consists mainly of rice, millet, sweet potato, corn, wheat, and seasonal vegetables. The inhabitants of the high incidence area were found to consume a good deal of pickled vegetables (Yang, 1980).

Possible carcinogens, such as secondary amines, nitrites, and a variety of fungi, particularly *Geotrichum candidum,* were found in pickled food samples from the region. These samples were also found to be mutagenic to *Salmonella typhimurium,* strains TA98 and TA100, and extracts caused gastric cancer in rats (Yang, 1980).

Measurements of various trace elements, especially zinc, molybdenum, and magnesium, in water and food samples from areas with high and low risk of esophageal cancer have shown an increase in correlation between mortality and the level of such trace elements. Molybdenum and zinc have been studied extensively. The absence of molybdenum in the soil contributes to the accumulation of nitrites and nitrates in the plants and vegetables. These compounds, together with secondary amines from the decomposition of moldy foods, form methylbenzylnitrosamines (Yang, 1980). Nitrosamines were also found to be present when bread was inoculated with the fungus *Fusaria verticilliodes* and incubated with small quantities of sodium nitrite.

Further studies have shown that the use of molybdenum fertilizer induces reduction of nitrate and nitrite and, interestingly, increases the ascorbic acid content of vegetables (Yang, 1980). The role of zinc deficiency in the genesis of esophageal cancer and its possible interaction with vitamin A, alcohol, and carcinogens will be discussed in detail in the following sections. It appears that a low content of trace elements induces deficiency of such elements in tissues. Lower levels of molybdenum in hair, urine, and serum in the population of high incidence areas as compared with the areas with low incidence have been reported. Similarly, zinc deficiency (as determined by measurement of zinc content of hair) of such populations and also patients with esophageal cancer are noted (Yang, 1980). Dietary evaluations have shown that total calorie and protein intake of a population with high risk of cancer were about 90% of the recommended dietary standards. However, only 0.5% of the protein and 9% of the fat were from animal sources. Preliminary nutritional studies showed widespread incidence of riboflavin deficiency and possible seasonal deficiencies of vitamins A and C. A recent study from the same area of 58 men and 53 women with premalignant lesions of the esophagus showed deficiencies of riboflavin in 97% and vitamin A in 5%. In addition, 24% of these subjects also had low levels of plasma zinc (Thurnham et al., 1982).

Further evidence of a relationship between local diet and esophageal cancer in China comes from the observation that chickens, which are fed food scraps, develop gullet cancer, which is unknown in the low incidence regions of China (Yang, 1980).

Vitamin A and riboflavin are essential for growth and maintenance of esophageal mucosal integrity, and vitamin C is important in metabolism of nitrates. As we shall see later, there are significant animal experimental data to suggest that vitamin A deficiency could play an important role in the pathogenesis of esophageal cancer.

Iran

In 1972, a high incidence of cancer of the esophagus was reported along the southern shores of the Caspian Sea, with considerable local fluctuations. Incidences of more than 100/100,000 per annum were recorded among the villages of northeast as well as northwest Iran, while the intervening region, which has a rainy climate and an abundance of vegetation, had only a baseline rate of 5/100,000 (Mahboubi et al., 1973). The basic diet of the Turkomans and Mazandaranis in the high incidence area is bread, tea, and some smoked fish, but little meat. In contrast, the staple diet of the low incidence population is rice, fresh fish, seasonal vegetables, and citrus fruit, which are available locally and cheaply.

Documented cases of esophageal cancer showed that nearly all patients were from the poorest stratum of rural society with low income and large families to support (Joint Iran–IARC, 1977). The average consumption of meat was limited to once a week. Many of these farm workers had access to fresh dairy products and raised cattle and poultry, but they consumed little themselves, instead using these products more as a source of income than for nourishment.

Although only a mild degree of iron deficiency anemia was found among the patients with cancer of the esophagus, the population of three villages in the high incidence area showed a significant degree of zinc deficiency in the hair samples tested (Mobarhan et al., 1979) as compared with populations with low risk cancer in Iran and the United States. Such a degree of zinc deficiency could be secondary to the high fiber content of bread consumed in this area. Other nutritional studies among the Turkoman population of this region have shown that the daily intake of vitamin A, riboflavin, and vitamin C is low. However, serum or tissue levels of these micronutrients were not measured.

Researchers in the area have advanced many theories regarding carcinogenic substances in the region that have recently been supported by laboratory evidence. Turkomans and Mazandaranis, on the average, consume 1 L of tea per capita daily, but no carcinogenic substance has been found in the tea drunk in this region. The temperature of the tea has also been a matter of lengthy debate, particularly because the Turkomans drink their tea fast and hot. The actual intraesophageal temperature of people in the high incidence region, measured by using a thermocouple, was not significantly different from that of a group of university students in a low incidence group (Mobarhan et al., 1979). A recent study has demonstrated that the flour from the wheat grown in the area contains a needle-shaped mineral fiber measuring 50–150 μm in length and causing increased fibroblastic activity in tissue culture, suggesting it to be carcinogenic, similar to the asbestos fibers that cause mesothelioma (O'Neill et al., 1980).

Another possibility lies with the use of opium and its pyrolytic compounds among the local inhabitants. Although its use was banned in Iran three decades ago, opium is smoked and eaten extensively for various bodily aches, insomnia, and diarrhea. In a series of 127 cases of esophageal cancer, studied by the authors between 1974 and 1976, 61% of the male and 24% of the females gave a history of opium use for 5 to 20 years prior to the onset of dysphagia. During the examination of the patients by means of endoscopy, opium was frequently smelled and brown particles were seen attached to the mucosa. Such widespread use was confirmed by other investigators making informal inquiries and analyzing the morphine content of urine samples from the inhabitants in the high incidence area.

Hewer and collaborators (1978) demonstrated that pyrolytic products of opium (sukhteh) displayed mutagenic activity in *Salmonella typhimurium* strains TA98 and TA100 activated by rat liver microsomes. Further investigations suggest that heterocyclic aromatic hydrocarbons and primary aromatic amines are the major active principals of the displayed mutagenicity (Malavielle et al., 1982). More evidence in support of opium playing a role in promotion of cancer comes from a clinical study conducted in Shiraz, Iran, where a high incidence of bladder cancer was reported among opium addicts (Sadeghi et al., 1979). It is hypothesized that opium, through its pharmacologic properties, diminishes esophageal peristalsis and inhibits lower esophageal sphincter relaxation, therefore augmenting contraction of the pyloric sphincter and thus providing a longer period of contact of carcinogen with the mucosa (Dowlatshahi and Miller, in press).

South Africa

In 1962, Burrell reported a significant increase in the number of Bantu patients from Transkei with esophageal cancer admitted to East London hospitals, South Africa. A review of 85 consecutive autopsy examinations of blacks in East London, who died from causes other than cancer of the esophagus, showed carcinoma in situ or esophagitis (Rose, 1981). More than one half of these patients were classified as having lived below poverty level. Inspection of the hospital autopsy records and interviews with Bantu community peers revealed that such prevalence did not exist 25 years earlier. Sociologic studies confirmed that, after World War II, a large number of young men had migrated from their rural homes to industrial centers, such as Johannesburg, in search of prosperity. Women were left behind to live on small plots of land known as "gardens." The differential rate of cancer of the esophagus between men and women among urban Bantu was 26 to one, which seems to reflect this migrational tendency (Burrell et al., 1966).

These studies led to the postulate that the susceptible Bantu men were exposed to carcinogens in their new environment. One such carcinogen was thought to be in the alcohol illicitly distilled in barrels that were previously used for storage of tar and other petrochemical residues. Burrell and his colleagues studied the primary environment of these patients and noted that the greatest clustering of cases were found on the central South Transkei plains. This area is characterized by very little rainfall, and its inhabitants subsist mainly on maize and wheat. Riboflavin was found to be deficient, and skin abnormalities, general infection, and pellegra were more marked as compared with the inhabitants of the low incidence area to the north. Serum vitamin A was normal, but the carotene level was significantly low (Rose, 1981). Hewer and collaborators (1978) found that the homegrown tobacco pipe residues of people from the same high incidence area displayed mutagenic activity in activated *Salmonella typhimurium.*

The plants in the "gardens" showed a deficiency of the trace elements molybdenum, zinc, copper, iron, and manganese. The foliage of these plants, mainly maize and pumpkins, had withered leaves that responded to molybdenum treatment. The trace elements just mentioned appear to be necessary for the production of protein from nitrites in plants (Burrell et al., 1966).

France

Brittany is an economically poor and agriculturally underdeveloped region in the northwest of France. The population of the region is slightly older than average due to the high rate of migration of the younger family members to the industrial centers of France (Tuyns and Masse, 1973). Inspection of death certificates between 1958 and 1966 revealed an overall mortality rate from esophageal cancer of 21.4 per 100,000 population per annum, with a peak of 50 per 100,000 in the central region and a male preponderance of 17:1.

A case control study of the diet of patients with cancer of the esophagus revealed that they ate smoked fish, butter, potato, and offal and that the food of the area, though not analyzed, appeared to be rich in vitamins (Tuyns et al., 1979).

The high rate of alcoholism among the people of the area is implicated as an etiologic facor in esophageal cancer. Cirrhosis was common among the population; in a separate autopsy study of 111 patients with cancer of the esophagus, Mandard and coworkers (1981) reported 18% of these patients to have concomitant cirrhosis. The drinking pattern of the people of Brittany is said to differ from that in other areas of France in that more cider and wine is imbibed. However, experimental work on Wistar rats failed to show that the alcoholic beverages consumed locally had any carcinogenic effect on the esophagus (Mandard et al., 1981).

In contrast, a study by Tuyns and coworkers concluded that the only major difference between esophageal cancer patients and a control group was the excessive consumption of alcoholic beverages and tobacco smoking and that the effects of these two factors were multiplicative (Tuyns et al., 1979).

Other Regions with an Increased Incidence of Cancer of the Esophagus

In parts of India, the habit of chewing betel quid is common. Cancer of the esophagus is also prevalent, the rate being 11 per 100,000 per annum. In a recent report from Bombay, the betel quid ingredients (catechu betel nut, betel leaf, lime, and tobacco) were tested singly or in combination for their carcinogenicity on the golden Syrian hamster cheek pouch, the mucosa of which closely resembles the human esophageal mucosa histologically. Dimethylbenzylamine application was used as the standard carcinogen on the cheek pouch of a control group of animals (Ranadive et al., 1979). Ranadive and coworkers also reported that tobacco and lime enhanced the carcinogenic effect of the betel nut. The polyphenolic fraction of the betel nut tannin was said to be a particularly potent carcinogen causing cancer and precancerous lesions in the majority of the oral, as well as the gastric, mucosa of hamsters.

In the United States, data from the Third National Cancer Survey indicate an age-adjusted mortality rate from esophageal cancer of 12.4 per 100,000 per annum for black males as compared with 4.1 for white males. For females, these figures fall to 2.6 among blacks and 1.0 among whites. Pottern et al. (1981) conducted a case control study among blacks in Washington, D.C. They noted that the esophageal cancer mortality rate among black males as recorded by the National Center for Health Statistics was 28.6/100,000 per annum in Washington, D.C. compared with 16.4 in Chicago and 10.3 in Los Angeles. This study showed that the major risk factor was ethanol consumption, which was estimated to be causally associated with 80% of the esophageal cancer cases. The relative risk seems to have increased with the amount of alcohol used. Evidence of the high consumption of alcoholic beverages in Washington, D.C. is obtained from the liquor sales tax revenues, which are substantially higher than the national average. These investigators also noted that in the years 1965–1971, cirrhosis among Washington, D.C. blacks was found to be about 2.5 times higher than in black males nationally. When other factors were studied, dietary analysis showed that patients with cancer of the esophagus ate less meat, dairy products, fresh vegetables, and fruit. Cigarette smoking did not seem to enhance the risk of esophageal cancer development in the study mentioned here, although there is some evidence that this may not be the case elsewhwere.

NUTRITIONAL FACTORS

Among various nutritional factors involved in the pathogenesis of esophageal cancer in the United States and the rest of the Western world are zinc, vitamin A, and riboflavin. Their possible interaction with alcohol has received significant attention during the past two decades. The following is an outline describing the relationship between these nutrients and alcohol in the development of esophageal cancer.

Zinc Deficiency

The total body content of zinc in adult humans is 2 to 3 g, and it is the most abundant trace element after iron. Zinc participates as a component of many metalloenzymes and plays an essential role in cell replication, protein synthesis, and normal development of all animal species (Sandstead and Rinaldi, 1968; Sandstead, 1973; Solomons, 1980). Many dietary factors influence the bioavailability of zinc. For instance, copper and iron as bivalent cations share the same absorptive pathways and compete with zinc for intestinal absorption. The primary route of zinc excretion is through the feces; urine is usually a minor excretory pathway. However, under certain conditions such as chronic alcohol intake and hepatic disease, urinary loss is increased, resulting in a negative total body balance (Russell, 1980).

A review of the literature suggests that zinc deficiency has a special effect on the esophagus. Indeed, while it induces hypoplastic changes in other tissues, it produces hyperplasia and parakeratosis in the skin and esophagus. In 1955, Tucker and Salmon demonstrated that swine parakeratosis was the result of zinc deficiency and could be prevented by zinc. Follis (1966) reported parakeratosis of the esophageal mucosa in zinc-deficient animals. Similar morphologic lesions were observed in the tongue in zinc-deficient squirrel monkeys (Barney et al., 1967) and in the esophagus of rats (Barney et al., 1968). Parakeratosis consists of thickening of zinc-deficient esophageal epithelium and abnormal keratinization. Diamond and Hurley (1969) reported esophageal lesions in zinc-deficient full-term rat fetuses, showing increased cellular proliferation. Similar lesions were shown in the esophagus of adult zinc-deficient rats (Diamond et al., 1970).

In 1977, Fong and coworkers reported low levels of zinc in serum, hair, and tumor tissue in patients with esophageal cancer in Hong Kong. These investigators (1978) also reported that zinc deficiency in rats increased the incidence of and shortened the lag time for esophageal tumor induction by methylbenzylnitrosamine. In 1978, Mobarhan and coworkers studied the level of hair zinc of the normal population in northern Iran (an area with high incidence of esophageal cancer) and compared it with the two similar groups of patients with low incidence of esophageal carcinoma in Tehran and Baltimore, Maryland (Mobarhan et al., 1979). As seen in Table 1, the hair zinc level is much lower among the population of northern Iran (P = .005 and P = .001).

Many enzymes involved in protein, fat, carbohydrate, nucleic acid, and alcohol metabolism are zinc dependent. The activity of alcohol dehydrogenase, a zinc-dependent enzyme, has been shown to decrease in the esophageal

TABLE 1. Comparison of the Level of Hair Zinc in the Asymptomatic Population of a High Incidence Village for Esophageal Carcinoma in Northern Iran with the Levels of Two Control Groups

Location	Incidence of esophageal carcinoma	Number of subjects	Hair zinc (μg/mg)
Northern Iran	High	35	154 ± 28
Teheran, Iran	Low	15	270 ± 60
Baltimore, Maryland	Low	25	223 ± 90

mucosa of zinc-deficient animals (Prasad et al., 1967). A possible explanation for the effects of zinc deficiency on esophageal mucosa is that zinc deficiency leads to an abnormal regulation of nucleic acid metabolism (Sandstead and Rinaldi, 1968; Sandstead, 1973). In the normal esophagus there is a balanced and well-controlled cell differentiation and turnover. Regulation of this process is essential for the development of the various cell layers, particularly the stratum corneum. It is proposed that in zinc deficiency there is abnormal control of nucleic acid metabolism and turnover, which leads to alterations of stratum corneum (hyperkeratosis and parakeratosis).

Effects of Zinc and Ethanol on the Esophagus

In 1979, Gabrial and Newberne demonstrated that the incidence of esophageal cancer induced by methylbenzylnitrosamine was similar in two groups of rats fed with either a zinc-deficient diet or a controlled diet plus alcohol. However, the combination of alcohol and zinc deficiency in a third group of rats resulted in a much higher incidence of cancer. These results suggest that alcohol and/or zinc deficiency increase the susceptibility of the esophageal mucosa to carcinogens and that this may be due to alteration in the surface epithelium and keratin.

In recent studies Ahmed and Russell (1982) have shown that chronic alcohol intake (28 days) in rats maintained on a zinc-deficient diet (0.9 g zinc/ml of diet) induced marked negative zinc balance, significant fecal urinary zinc loss, and severe depletion of whole body zinc as compared with control animals with a zinc-deficient diet without ethanol. Histologic examination of the esophagus of these rats (Mobarhan et al., in press) showed parakeratosis of the esophagus in 77% of ethanol fed rats but only in 11% of controls. In earlier animal studies, Horie and coworkers (1965) reported that alcohol as a solvent increases the penetration of benzopyrene present in tobacco tar and 4-nitroquinoline 1-oxide into the esophageal mucosa. Alcohol may thus facilitate the induction of esophageal papillomas and even cancer of the esophagus in mice. These data suggest that alcohol could promote the onset of dysplastic and malignant changes either through a direct effect on the esophageal epithelium or indirectly by inducing zinc deficiency.

Alcoholism is frequently associated with zinc deficiency (Sandstead and Rinaldi, 1968, Sandstead, 1973, 1980; Russell 1980). However, different laboratories have shown conflicting results concerning the effect of ethanol on zinc metabolism. Sullivan and Lankford (1962, 1965) reported that ingestion of ethanol by normal people or alcoholics with or without liver diseases did not increase urinary zinc excretion. However, in 1969, Gudbjarnason and Prasad demonstrated a significant increase in urinary zinc excretion and a simultaneous decrease of serum zinc concentration in normal human subjects. Russell (1980) studied the effect of long-term alcohol ingestion (17 days) in five alcoholics without liver disease. Urinary zinc excretion was twice as high during the drinking period when compared with the nondrinking period, and serum zinc levels were decreased.

Interactions Between Zinc and Vitamin A

Zinc is probably required for vitamin A mobilization from its storage site in the liver (Russell, 1980). Zinc-deficient animals have been reported to have lower circulating vitamin A levels. This is probably secondary to impaired synthesis of retinol binding protein (RBP), which is essential for the transport of retinol from the liver to other tissues. Administration of a zinc-supplemented diet to zinc-deficient animals results in increased serum levels of vitamin A and RBP (Smith et al., 1973; Brown et al., 1976). Short-term (5 days) zinc supplementation has been shown to cause a significant rise in serum vitamin A and RBP levels in children with protein-calorie malnutrition (Shingwekar et al., 1979). It appears, therefore, that zinc plays an important role in mobilization of vitamin A from the liver. Thirty to 60% of alcoholic patients without liver disease have low serum zinc levels and vitamin A deficiency as defined by a low serum vitamin A level. In addition, abnormal dark adaptation is present in about 15% of detoxified alcoholic patients without liver disease (McClain et al., 1979; Russell, 1980).

In a recent study of vitamin A nutrition in 42 alcoholic patients without liver disease conducted by us (Nagel, Mobarhan, et al., 1982), it was noted that 19.5% had low circulating levels of vitamin A (serum retinol: mean $\pm$ 1 SD 16.75 $\pm$ 7.7 μg/dL). Indeed, 50% of the patients with low circulating levels of vitamin A did not have clinical signs of malnutrition. These results suggest that chronic alcohol ingestion even in the absence of protein-calorie malnutrition or liver disease may cause vitamin A deficiency.

Effects of Vitamin A Depletion on Mucosal Surfaces

The essential role of vitamin A in maintaining the integrity of the epithelium was described more than half a century ago by Wolbach and colleagues (1925). Epithelium in animals with vitamin A depletion loses its capacity to biosynthesize mucus, and mucus-secreting epithelial cells are replaced by keratinizing cells. In addition, mitosis and metaplastic changes increase significantly (Bollag, 1970; DeLuca et al., 1972; Moore, 1967; Wong and Buck, 1971). In epithelial cells, the retinol is phosphorylated to retinyl phosphate and its glycolate derivative, mannylretinyl phosphate. Retinyl phosphate is an integral part of the endoplasmic reticulum and participates in specific glycosylation reactions and glycoprotein biosynthesis (DeLuca, 1977; Wolf et al., 1979). In vitamin A depletion, RNA and DNA are decreased and, on treatment with vitamin A, the synthesis of RNA in epithelial cells of the small intestine is stimulated. In addition, in depleted rats transfer-RNA is depressed (Sporn et al., 1975). Vitamin A and its derivatives are able to reverse the squamous metaplastic changes induced by the vitamin A deficiency in cultured tracked epithelium of hamsters (Moore, 1967). Similar effects in tumors grown in vitro may be the result of contact dependency (Lotan and Nicholson, 1978).

In 1926, Fujimaki demonstrated that vitamin A deficiency causes spontaneous development of gastric carcinomas and marked metaplastic modification of epithelia in different experimental animals. Recently, it has been documented that retinol and retinoids could induce cellular repair of pathologic changes caused by carcinogens (Calmon, 1980; Bollag, 1976; DeLuca et al., 1980; Newberne and Rogers, 1981; Sporn et al., 1976, 1977). Vitamin A deficiency in animals has also been shown to enhance the carcinogenic activity of various substances on the respiratory tract (Harris et al., 1972), bladder (Cohen et al., 1976; Squire et al., 1977), colon (Narisawa et al., 1976), cervix (Chu and Malmgreen, 1965), prostate (Lasnitzki and Goodman, 1974), and mammary gland (Grubbs et al., 1977).

In animals with vitamin A depletion, the esophageal mucosa becomes thickened with marked keratinization (Chu and Malmgreen, 1965). Administration of retinoids and betacarotenes can prevent dyskeratosis and papilloma formation of the esophageal mucosa induced by several carcinogens (Peto et al., 1981; Schweinsberg and Schott-Kollat, 1976). Several retrospective and prospective human studies have demonstrated that there is a lower incidence of epithelial cancer in subjects with higher consumption of vitamin A or high levels of serum retinol (Basu et al., 1976; Bjelke, 1975; Atukorola et al., 1979; Wald et al., 1980). In one study it was noted that the dietary intake of vitamin A in 122 patients with esophageal cancer was significantly lower than in controls (Peto et al., 1981).

In a study of 12 patients with biopsy-proven esophageal cancer, circulating levels of vitamin A were below 20 mg/dL in three (25%) patients and below 30 mg/dL in another three patients. Anthropometric data showed normal lean body mass in one third of those patients with low circulating levels of vitamin A (Noetzel et al., 1983). These data suggest that some patients with esophageal cancer have vitamin A deficiency even in the absence of protein-calorie malnutrition.

Riboflavin and Esophageal Cancer

In riboflavin-deficient mice the earliest microscopic changes occur in the esophageal epithelium and forestomach (Wynder and Klein, 1965). In addition, it has been shown that riboflavin deficiency enhances chemically induced skin carcinogenesis. In alcoholics a high incidence of riboflavin deficiency secondary to poor intake or reduced bioavailability has been reported (Rosenthan et al., 1973; Majumdar et al., 1982). However, riboflavin deficiency in humans occurs rarely as an isolated clinical entity and it is usually associated with deficiency of other B group vitamins. Although some authors give significant importance to riboflavin deficiency in the development of esophageal cancer (Van Rensburg, 1981), specific data regarding interaction of riboflavin, carcinogens, and alcohol on esophageal mucosa are not yet available.

DISCUSSION

Without exception, in *high incidence* areas (Figure 1), carcinoma of the esophagus occurs among the "nutritionally deprived." Nutritional deprivation is a broad term defined as a state in which there is a deficiency of one or several essential elements of the diet, such as vitamins A, B-complex, and C, or such trace metals as zinc, molybdenum, magnesium, and iron. Some of these deficiencies are present in countries where this cancer is common.

If we accept the status of nutritional deprivation, which results in esophageal mucosal vulnerability, as an essential prerequisite for the development of esophageal cancer, then we can look for a carcinogenic agent that will promote tumor development. In such a setting, the Turkoman farmer who cannot afford to provide himself with more than bread and tea as a staple diet becomes just as susceptible to a carcinogenic insult as does his European or American urban counterpart who spends most of his income on alcoholic beverages and cigarettes.

In the absence of mucosal nutritional deprivation, it is unlikely that the carcinogen will cause esophageal cancer. This hypothesis will explain why in Iran, for example, where opium use is a widespread social habit among inhabitants of both high and low incidence areas of the Caspian littoral, the incidence of esophageal cancer is higher in Mazandaranis and Turkomans (high incidence) than in Guilanis. Similar contrast differences have been noted in the diet of those in the high and low cancer incidence regions of Africa (Van Rensburg, 1981). In the low incidence area, the dietary staples were sorghum, millet, cassava, yams, and peanuts, which are all rich in vitamins. In contrast, in the high incidence region, the dietary staples were corn or wheat, both of which have a poor vitamin content.

An analogy can be drawn between these precancerous states, which are reversible, and a congenital skin condition, *xeroderma pigmentosum*, where the epithelial cells cannot repair DNA damage inflicted by the ultraviolet rays of the sun because of an enzymatic deficiency. Epithelial cancer will ensue after prolonged exposure to sun. It is conceivable that such a chain of events occur in the epithelial cells of the esophageal mucosa. In the absence of one or several essential micronutrients, such as retinoids, riboflavin, zinc, or magnesium, the normal processes of cell differentiation, maturation, and repair become defective. Mutagenic agents may therefore be more effective in promoting neoplasia.

A premalignant state has been documented by us and others among the asymptomatic populations of villages in the high esophageal regions of the Caspian littoral (Dowlatshahi et al., 1978; Crespi et al., 1979). In one study, indirect (blind) cytologic brushing of the esophageal exfoliated cells revealed dysplasia in 7%. Hair zinc and dietary intake of vitamin A of these people were also shown to be low. The pyrolytic products of opium, which have been shown to be mutagenic or even carcinogenic, may therefore promote esophageal cancer in these subjects.

SUMMARY

A variety of factors predispose the esophageal mucosa to the development of carcinoma. In Asia and Africa they are specific micronutrient deficiencies secondary to financial poverty. Among U.S. urban inhabitants they are the result of lack of nutritional education and abuse of alcohol and tobacco. Once repair of esophageal mucosa is compromised, any promoting agents (nitrosamine in Linxian, pylorized opium and mineral fibers in Iran, "injonga" in Transkei, tobacco and alcohol in France and the United States, and betel nut in Bombay) will promote the neoplasm over the course of time in a dose-dependent fashion.

Until recently, much effort has been devoted with a considerable degree of success to detection of carcinogens in the diet and environment of people in the high incidence areas of the world. We believe that, in the future, the question of specific nutritional deficiencies, such as vitamins and trace elements, should be addressed with more vigor because there are large gaps in our knowledge of their roles in normal differentiation of epithelial cells. Efforts should therefore be made to screen populations at high risk for the development of esophageal carcinoma through brush cytology among asymptomatic persons. However, this may still result in refusal to accept treatment in some patients in whom abnormalities are found. Perhaps a better understanding of the nutritional defects of populations in higher risk regions and correction of such defects to promote host resistance will be more fruitful.

REFERENCES

Ahmed SB, Russell RM (1982) The effect of ethanol feeding on zinc balance and tissue zinc levels in rats maintained on zinc deficient diet. J Lab Clin Med 100:211–215.

Atukorola S, Basu TK, Dickerson JWT, et al. (1979) Vitamin A, zinc and lung cancer. Br J Cancer 40:927–931.

Barney GH, Macapinloc WN, Pearson WN, et al. 1967) Parakeratosis of the tongue—a unique histopathologic lesion in the zinc deficient squirrel monkey. J Nutr 93:511–517.

Barney GH, Orgenin-Crist MC, Macapinloc MP (1968) Genesis of esophageal parakeratosis and histologic changes in the testes of the zinc-deficient rat and their reversal by zinc repletion. J Nutr 95:526–534.

Basu TK, Donaldson D, Jenner M, et al. (1976) Plasma vitamin A in patients with bronchial carcinoma. Br J Cancer 33:119–121.

Bjelke EB (1975) Dietary vitamin A and human lung cancer. Int J Cancer 15:561–564.

Bollag W (1970) Vitamin A and vitamin A acid in the prophylaxis and therapy of epithelial tumors. Int J Vitam Res 40P:229–314.

Bollag W (1976) Prophylaxis of chemically induced benign and malignant epithelial tumors by vitamin A acid (retinoic acid). Eur J Cancer 8:689–693.

Brown E, Chan W, Smith JC Jr. (1976) Vitamin A metabolism during the repletion of zinc deficient rats. J Nutr 106:563–568.

Burrell RJW (1962) Esophageal cancer among Bantu in the Transkei. J Nat Cancer Inst 28:495–514.

Burrell RJW, Roach WA, Shadwell A (1966) Esophageal cancer in the Bantu of the Transkei associated with mineral deficiency in garden plants. J Natl Cancer Inst 36:201–214.

Calmon GH (1980) Retinoids for the prevention of epithelial cancers: Current status and future potential. Med Pediatr Oncol 8:177–185.

Chu EW, Malmgreen RA (1965) An inhibitory effect of vitamin A on the induction of tumors of forestomach and cervix in the Syrian hamster by carcinogenic polycyclic hydrocarbons. Cancer Res 25:884–894.

Cohen SM, Wittenberg JF, Bryan GT (1976) Effect of avitaminosis and hypervitaminosis A on urinary bladder carcinogenicity of N-[4-(5 nitro-2 furyl)-2-0 thiazolyl] formamide. Cancer Res 36:2334–2339.

Coordinating Group for Research on Etiology of Esophageal Cancer in North China (1975) The epidemiology and etiology of esophageal cancer in North China. A preliminary report. Chin Med J 1:167–183.

Crespi M, Munoz N, Grassi A, et al. (1979) Oesophageal lesions in Northern Iran: A premalignant condition. Lancet 2:217–220.

Cutler SJ, Young JL, Jr. (eds) (1975) Third National Cancer Survey: Incidence Data. National Cancer Institute Monograph 41, DHEW Publication No. (NIH) 75–787, U.S. Government Printing Office, Washington, D.C.

DeLuca LM (1977) The direct involvement of vitamin A in glycosyl transfer reactions of mammalian membranes. Vitam Horm 32:1–57.

DeLuca LM, Maestri N, Bonannani F, Nelson D (1972) Maintenance of epithelial differentiation. The mode of action of vitamin A. Cancer 30:1326–1331.

DeLuca LM, Sasak W, Adamo S, et al. (1980) Retinoid metabolism and mode of action. Environ Health Perspec 35:147–152.

Diamond I, Hurley LS (1969) Histopathology of zinc-deficient fetal rats. J Nutr 100:325–329.

Diamond I, Swenerton H, Hurley LS (1970) Testicular and esophageal lesions in zinc-deficient rats and their reversibility. J Nutr 101:77–84.

Doll R, Muir C, Waterhouse J (1970) Cancer incidence in five continents. Vol. 2. Union Internationale Contre Cancer.

Dowlatshahi D, Mobarhan S, Daneshbad A (1977) Clinical studies of carcinoma of the esophagus in the North Iran. Digestion 16:237.

Dowlatshahi K, Daneshbod A, Mobarhan S (1978) Early detection of cancer of esophagus along Caspian littoral. Lancet 1:125.

Dowlatshahi K, Miller RJ (in press) Opium as a promoter of oesophageal cancer in man.

Follis RH Jr. (1966) The pathology of zinc deficiency in zinc metabolism. Prasad AS, ed., Springfield, Ill.: CC Thomas, pp. 129–141.

Fong LYY, Sivak A, Newberne PM (1977) Zinc and copper concentration in tissues from esophageal cancer patients and animals. In: Hemphill DD, ed., Trace substances in environmental health-XI. A Symposium, Columbia: University of Missouri, 184–191.

Fong LYY, Siavak A, Newberne PM (1978) Zinc deficiency and methylbenzyl nitrosamine-induced esophageal cancer in rats. J Natl Cancer Inst 67:145–150.

Fujimaki Y (1926) Formation of carcinoma in albino rats fed on deficient diets. J Cancer Res 10:469–477.

Gabrial GH, Newberne PM (1979) Zinc deficiency, alcohol and esophageal cancer. In: Hemphill DD, ed., Trace substances in environmental health-XIII. A Symposium, Columbia: University of Missouri, pp 315–324.

Grubbs CJ, Moon RC, Sporn MB, Newton DL (1977) Inhibition of mammary cancer by retinyl methyl ether. Cancer Res 37:599–602.

Gudbjarnason S, Prasad A (1969) Cardiac metabolism in experimental alcoholism. In: Sardesai VM, ed., Biochemical clinical aspects of alcohol metabolism. Springfield, Ill: CC Thomas, p. 266.

Harris, CC, Sporn MB, Kaufman DG, et al. (1972) Histogenesis of squamous metaplasia in the hamster tracheal epithelium caused by vitamin A deficiency or benzo(a)pyrene ferric oxide. J Nat Cancer Inst 48:743–761.

Hewer T, Rose E, Ghadirian P, et al. (1978) Ingested mutagens from opium and tobacco pyrolysis products and cancer of the esophagus. Lancet 2:494–496.

Horie A, Kohchi S, Kuratsune M (1965) Carcinogenesis in the esophagus. II. Experimental production of esophageal cancer by administration of ethanolic solution of carcinogenes. Gann 56:429–441.

Joint Iran-International Agency for Research on Cancer (IARC) Study Group. (1977) Esophageal cancer studies in the Caspian littoral of Iran: Results of population studies—a prodrome. J Natl Cancer Inst 59:1127–1138.

Lasnitzki I, Goodman DS (1974) Inhibition of the effects of methylcholanthrene on mouse prostate organ culture by vitamin A and its analogs. Cancer Res 34:1564–1571.

Lotan R, Nicholson GL (1978) Inhibitory effect of retinoic acid or retinyl acetate on the growth of untransformed, transformed and tumor cells in vitro. J Natl Cancer Inst 59:1717–1722.

Mahboubi E, Kmet J, Cook PJ, et al. (1973) Oesophageal cancer studies in the Caspian littoral of Iran: The Caspian Cancer Registry. Br J Cancer 28:197–208.

Majumdar SK, Shaw GK,. O'Gorman PO, et al. (1982) Blood vitamin status (B1, B2, B6, folic acid and B12) in patients with alcoholic liver disease. J Vitam Nutr Res 52:266–277.

Malavielle C, Friesen M, Camus AM, et al. (1982) Mutagens produced by the pyrolysis of opium and its alkaloids as possible risk factors in cancer of the bladder and esophagus. Carcinogenesis 3:577–585.

Mandard AM, Chasle J, Marnay J, et al. (1981) Autopsy findings in 111 cases of esophageal cancer. Cancer 48:329–335.

Mandard AM, Marnay J, Helie H, et al. (1981) Absence d'effet de l'ethanol et des eaux de vie de cidre sur le tractus digestif supérieur et l'oesophage du rat Wistar. Bull Cancer 68:49–58. (English abstract).

McClain CJ, Van Thiel DH, Parker S, et al. (1979) Alterations in zinc, vitamin A, and retinol-binding protein in chronic alcoholics: A possible mechanism for night blindness and hypogonadism. Alcoholism: Clinical and Experimental Research 2:135–141.

Mobarhan S, Dowlatshahi K, Diba YY (1979) Hair zinc level from a normal population of northeast Iran with high incidence of esophageal carcinoma. Clin Res 28:598A.

Mobarhan S, Russel RM, Newberne P, Ahmed SB (1984) The effect of zinc deficiency and alcohol feeding on esophageal epithelium of rat. Nutr Rep Int (in press).

Moore T (1967) Effects of vitamin A deficiency in animals: Pharmacology and Toxicology of vitamin A. In: Sebrell WH, and Harris RS, ed., The Vitamins. Second edition, volume 1, New York: Academic Press, pp. 245–266, 280–294.

Nagel P, Mobarhan S, Layden T, Kunigk A (1982) Prevalence of protein calorie malnutrition (PCM) and micronutrient deficiency (MD) in alcoholics without liver disease. American College of Nutrition 23rd Annual Meeting: Abstract 84.

Narisawa T, Reddy BS, Wong CA, Weisburger J (1976) Effect of vitamin A deficiency on rat colon carcinogenesis of N-methyl-N'-nitro-N-nitrosoguanidine. Cancer Res 36:1379–1383.

Newberne PM, Rogers AE (1981) Vitamin A, retinoid and cancer. In: Newell GR, Ellison NM, eds., Nutrition and cancer: Etiology and treatment. New York: Raven Press, pp. 217–231.

Noetzel C, Mobarhan S, Nagel P, et al. (1983) Nutritional status and serum vitamin A levels in patients with esophageal cancer. Presented at Second International Conference on Disease of the Esophagus, Chicago, May 1983.

O'Neill CH, Hodges GM, Riddle PN, et al. (1980) A fine fibrous silica contaminant of flour in the high oesophageal cancer area of northeast Iran. Int J. Cancer 26:617–628.

Peto R, Doll R, Buckley JD, Sporn MB (1981) Can dietary betacarotene materially reduce human cancer rates? Nature 290:201–208.

Pottern LM, Morris LE, Blot WJ, et al. (1981) Esophageal cancer among black men in Washington, D.C.: I. Alcohol, tobacco and other risk factors. J Nat Cancer Inst 67:777–783.

Prasad AS, Oberleas D, Wolf P, Horwitz JP (1967) Studies on zinc deficiency: Changes in trace elements and enzyme activities in tissues on zinc deficient rats. J Clin Invest 46:549–557.

Ranadive KJ, Randadive SN, Shivapurkar NM, Gothoskar SV (1979) Betel quid chewing and oral cancer: Experimental studies on hamsters. Int J Cancer 24:835–843.

Rose EF (1981) A review of factors associated with cancer of the esophagus in Transkei. In: Cancer among black populations. New York: Alan R. Liss, pp. 67–75.

Rosenthan WS, Adham NF, Lopez R, Cooper-Mann JN (1973) Riboflavin deficiency in complicated chronic alcoholism. Am J Clin Nutr 26:856–860.

Russell RM (1980) Vitamin A and zinc metabolism in alcoholism. Am J Clin Nutr 33:2741–2749.

Sadeghi A, Behmard SH, Vesselinovitch SD (1979) Opium: A potential urinary bladder carcinogen in man. Cancer 43:2315–2321.

Sandstead HH (1973) Zinc nutrition in the United States: Perspectives in nutrition. Am J Clin Nutr 27:1251–1260.

Sandstead HH, Rinaldi RA (1968) Impairment of deoxyribonucleic acid synthesis by dietary zinc deficiency in the rat. J Cell Physiol 73:81–84.

Schweinsberg F, Schott-Kollat P (1976) Effect of vitamin A on formation, toxicity and carcinogenicity of nitroso-N-methylbenzylamine. Int Agency Cancer Res, 453–459.

Shingwekar AG, Mohanram M, Reddy V (1979) Effect of zinc supplementation on plasma levels of vitamin A and retinol-binding protein in malnourished children. Clin Chim Acta 93:97–100.

Smith JC Jr., McDaniel EG, Farr RR, Halstead JA (1973) Zinc: a trace element essential in Vitamin A metabolism. Science 181:954–955.

Solomons NW (1980) Zinc and the gastroenterologist: Implications for the practitioner. Pract Gastroenterol 15–20.

Sporn MB (1977) Retinoids and carcinogenesis. Nutr Rev 35:65–69.

Sporn MB, Chamon GH, Dunlop NM, et al. (1975) Activity of vitamin A analogs in cell cultures of mouse epidermis and organ cultures of hamster trachea. Nature 253:47–50.

Sporn MB, Dunlop NM, Newton DL, Smith JM (1976) Prevention of chemical carcinogenesis by vitamin A and its synthetic analogs (retinoids). Fed Proc 35:1332–1338.

Squire RA, Sporn MB,. Brown CC, et al. (1977) Histopathological evaluation of the inhibition of rat bladder carcinogenesis by 13-cis-retinoic acid. Cancer Res 37:2930–2936.

Sullivan JF, Lankford HG (1962) Urinary excretion of zinc in alcoholism and post-alcoholic cirrhosis: Am J Clin Nutr 10:153.

Sullivan JF, Lankford HG (1965) Zinc metabolism and chronic alcoholism. Am J Clin Nutr 17:57.

Thurnham D, Rathakette P, Hambidge KM, et al. (1982) Riboflavin, vitamin A and zinc status in Chinese subjects in a high risk area for oeosophageal cancer in China. Hum Nutr Clin Nutr 36C:337–349.

Tucker HF, Salmon WD (1955) Parakeratsis in zinc deficiency disease in the pig. Proc Soc Exp Biol Med 88:613–616.

Tuyns AJ, Masse LMF (1973) Mortality from cancer of the oesophagus in Brittany. Int J Epidemiol 2:241–245.

Tuyns AJ, Pequignot G, Jensen DM (1979) Role of diet, alcohol and tobacco in oesophageal cancer, as illustrated by two contrasting high-incidence areas in the North of Iran and the West of France. Front Gastrointest Res 4:101–110.

Van Rensburg SJ (1981) Epidemiologic and dietary evidence for a specific nutritional predisposition to esophageal cancer. J Natl Cancer Inst 67:243–251.

Wald N, Idle M, Boreham J, Bailey A (1980) Low serum-vitamin A and subsequent risk of cancer. Lancet 2:813–815.

Wolbach B, Howe PR (1925) Tissue changes following deprivation of fat-soluble A vitamin. J Exp Med 42:753–777.

Wolf G, Masushige S, Scheiber JB, et al. (1979) Recent evidence for the participation of vitamin A in glycoprotein synthesis. Fed Proc 38:2540–2543.

Wong Y-C, Buck RC (1971) An electron microscopic study of metaplasia of the rat tracheal epithelium in vitamin A deficiency. Lab Invest 24:55–66.

Wynder EL, Chan PC (1970) The possible role of riboflavin deficiency in epithelial neoplasia. II. Effect of skin tumor development. Cancer 26:1221–1224.

Wynder EL, Klein UE (1965) The possible role of riboflavin deficiency in epithelial neoplasia. I. Epithelial changes of mice in simple deficiency. Cancer 18:167–180.

Yang CS (1980) Research on esophageal cancer in China: A review. Cancer Res 40:2633–2644.

LYMPHOID PROLIFERATIONS OF THE GASTROINTESTINAL TRACT

LEONARD B KAHN, M.B. BCH., M. MED. PATH., M.R.C. PATH., AND RABIA MIR, M.D.

Lymphoproliferative disorders of the gastrointestinal tract may be broadly categorized into two groups: reactive lymphoid hyperplasia and malignant lymphoma. Although our knowledge of the causation of these disorders is fragmentary, recent advances in our understanding of the immune system has provided us with much new information concerning their pathophysiology. The application of newer techniques has enabled us to detect the various lymphocyte subpopulations and to determine the monoclonality or otherwise of lymphoproliferative lesions.

LYMPHOID HYPERPLASIA

Apart from the lymphoid tissue present in the oropharynx (Waldeyer's ring), the lymphoid tissue in the gastrointestinal tract is concentrated in the terminal small bowel in the form of Peyer's patches and is diffusely distributed throughout the small and large bowel in the form of solitary lymphoid follicles. In the pediatric age group, these lymphoid follicles in the colon frequently produce nodular filling defects measuring up to 2 mm in diameter (Laufer and Derek, 1978). Lymphoid tissue in the form of lymphocytes and predominantly IgA-producing plasma cells populate much of the lamina propria of the intestinal tract. As a consequence of a variety of antigenic stimuli, this gut-associated lymphoid tissue may undergo hyperplasia of either a localized or diffuse type. Although many of these reactions are morphologically readily recognizable, some may result in formation of lymphoma-like lesions (pseudolymphomas) and pose a diagnostic challenge to the surgical pathologist.

A variety of histologic features that have been used to distinguish these reac-

From the Long Island Jewish-Hillside Medical Center and the State University of New York at Stony Brook.

TABLE 1. Features Distinguishing Lymphoid Hyperplasia from Lymphoma

Feature	Lymphoid hyperplasia	Lymphoma
Reactive germinal centers	Present	Absent, but nodules may be present in follicular lymphomas
Cellular infiltrate	Polymorphic (mixed inflammatory cells); mature although scattered immunoblasts may be seen	Monomorphic and composed of mature or atypical (transformed) lymphoid cells
Fibrosis	May be present and result in nodular aggregates of lymphoid tissue	Usually not a feature
Peptic ulceration (stomach)	Frequently present	Absent
Cytoplasmic immunoglobulin	Polyclonal	Monoclonal
Depth of infiltrate	Not helpful	Not helpful

tive and neoplastic conditions are reproduced in Table 1. However, in this regard it must be stressed that few of these criteria are absolute predictors. Reactive germinal centers may be associated with a lymphoma and may represent either an immune response to the lymphoma or a precursor lymphoproliferative state (Figures 1 and 2). For similar reasons, a mixed inflammatory cell infiltrate and the demonstration of polyclonal cytoplasmic immunoglobulin (CIg) might accompany a lymphomatous process. A biopsy alone is thus frequently of limited value in differentiating lymphoma from pseudolymphoma. The presence of sheets of immature (transformed) lymphoid cells and the demonstration of production of monoclonal CIg by these cells in tissue sections using immunoperoxidase techniques are diagnostic of lymphoma. A negative immunoglobulin reaction is also frequently displayed by such cells and is helpful in the distinction from pseudolymphoma, in which a variety of Ig's may be present (Saraga et al., 1981).

Lymphoid hyperplasia may occur in a localized form in the stomach or the small or large intestine or it may occur in a more diffuse form in one or more of these organs (Ranchod et al., 1978). To date, more than 100 cases of localized gastric lymphoid hyperplasia have been reported (Mattingly et al., 1981), the majority associated with and probably representing an exaggerated response to chronic peptic ulceration (Hyjek and Kelenyi, 1982; Wright, 1973). The lymphoid hyperplasia may be so intense as to produce giant mucosal folds or such thickening at the margin of a peptic ulcer that the lesion simulates a malignant ulcer. The lymphoid hyperplasia may also take the form of multiple small mucosal nodules with or without umbilication. Most patients diagnosed as lymphoid hyperplasia have been subjected to some form of gastrectomy, but

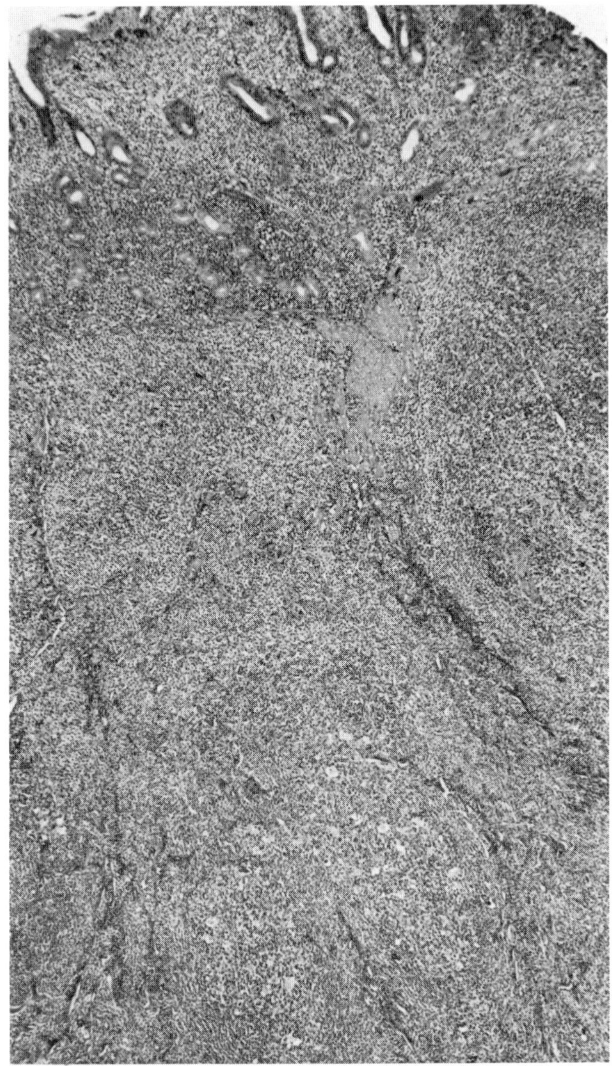

FIGURE 1. Diffuse gastric lymphoma and associated reactive lymphoid follicles (× 75)

Stroehlein and coworkers (1977) reported an uneventful 11-year follow-up of an untreated patient with gastric lymphoid hyperplasia that included periodic roentgenograms and endoscopy with biopsies.

Localized small intestinal lymphoid hyperplasia usually occurs in children and young adults in the terminal ileum and may present clinically as intussusception, recurrent abdominal pain, or hematochezia. Grossly it takes the form of a projecting mucosal nodule or a nodular indurated lesion. Localized rectal

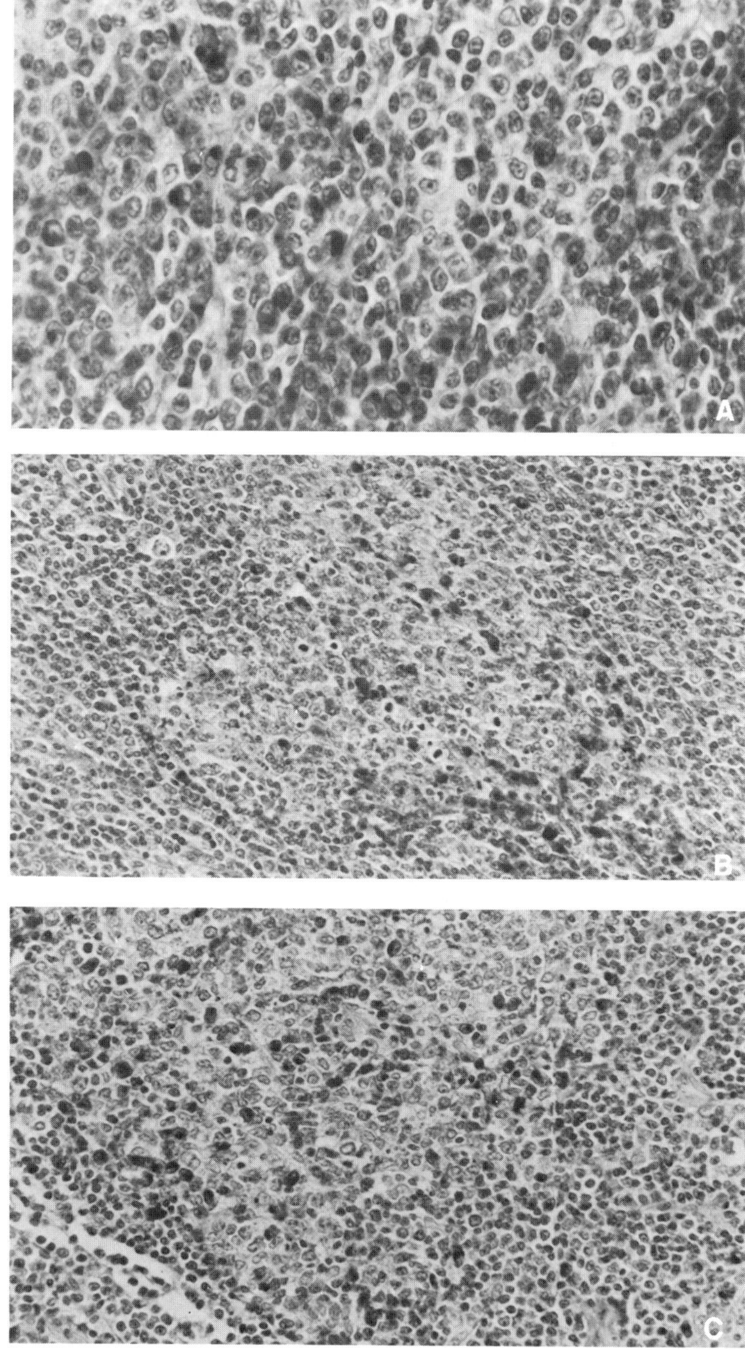

FIGURE 2. Same case as Figure 1. (**a**) Diffuse small lymphocytic lymphoma stain positively for κ light chain only ($\times$ 450). (**b**) Associated reactive follicles stain with anti-κ antiserum ($\times$ 225) and (**c**) anti-λ antiserum ($\times$ 225).

lymphoid hyperplasia occurs as a polypoid lesion usually in the second to fifth decades and presents as bleeding, prolapse, discomfort, diarrhea, constipation, or as an incidental finding.

Diffuse forms of lymphoid hyperplasia involving extensive areas of the small and/or large bowel may take the form of multiple mucosal nodules measuring up to 0.2 cm in diameter and have been referred to as enterocolitis lymphofollicularis. Such lesions have been shown to be present in 3% of all autopsies (Robinson et al., 1973), although as indicated previously, this finding is probably a normal one in the pediatric colon.

Diffuse intestinal nodular lymphoid hyperplasia may be associated with an immune deficiency state. Webster and coworkers (1977) were able to document the presence of nodular lymphoid hyperplasia of the intestines in 6 of 31 patients with acquired hypogammaglobulinemia. This usually takes the form of a late onset (second to fifth decade) variable immunodeficiency syndrome in which all three major Ig classes are variably diminished or absent. A selective deficiency of only IgA has been described in a few such cases but is extremely rare (Jacobson and deShazo, 1979). It is thought to result from failure of IgM-bearing lymphocytes to differentiate into IgA-producing plasma cells.

The nodules of hyperplastic lymphoid tissue usually involve only the small bowel but may, in addition, affect the large bowel (Nagura et al., 1979; Sauerbrei and Castelli, 1979; Mackenzie Crooks and Brown, 1980) and even the stomach (Munro and Simpson, 1974). Such patients are prone to develop sinopulmonary infections and diarrhea, often associated with giardiasis. The follicular lymphoid hyperplasia is usually associated with a diminished number of plasma cells in the lamina propria. Immunoperoxidase techniques have demonstrated that the follicles are populated by IgM-producing lymphocytes of polyclonal type (Nagura et al., 1979). These findings suggest that the nodules represent a proliferation of normal intestinal lymphoid cells in response to intestinal antigens with an accompanying unexplained arrest in differentiation to Ig-secreting plasma cells.

There is evidence that B-cell maturation is inhibited either by excessive T-lymphocyte suppression or lack of T-helper cell activity (Nagura et al., 1979). It has also been postulated that the lymphoid hyperplasia represents a compen-

FIGURE 3. Small bowel showing multiple smooth nodules of lymphoid hyperplasia and associated malignant lymphoma.

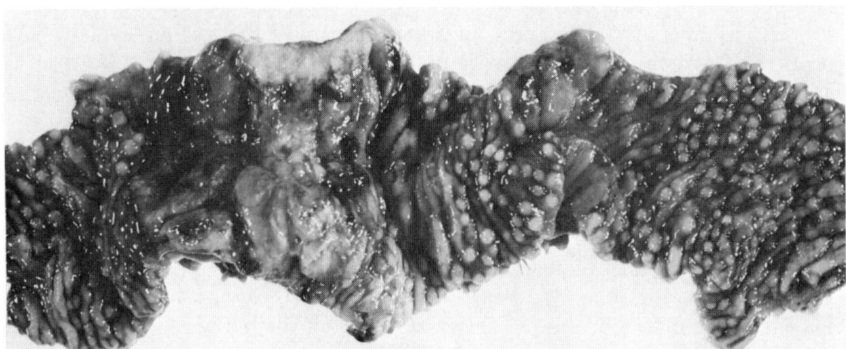

satory proliferation for defective Ig-secreting cells (Jacobson and deShazo, 1979). Patients with intestinal nodular lymphoid hyperplasia with or without an immunodeficiency syndrome have an increased tendency to develop gastrointestinal neoplasms, especially carcinoma, as was observed in 3 of 9 patients reported by Hermans and coworkers (1976). Intestinal lymphoma is a less frequent complication, but it has been reported as complicating four cases of nodular lymphoid hyperplasia (Figure 3) (Kahn and Novis, 1974; Lamers et al., 1980; Matuchansky et al., 1980; Gonzales-Vitale et al, 1982).

LYMPHOMA

Lymphomas are generally considered to be primary in the gastrointestinal tract when the signs and symptoms at the time of presentation are mainly confined to that system. Secondary involvement of the alimentary tract occurs during the course of extraabdominal lymphoma. Primary gastrointestinal lymphoma (PGL) constitutes about 5 to 9% of all non-Hodgkin's lymphoma (NHL), about 1 to 4% of all malignant gastrointestinal neoplasms (Saraga et al., 1981), about 3 to 5% of all malignant gastric neoplasms (Zornosa and Dodd, 1980), about 20% of all small-bowel tumors (Cox, 1979), and about 0.5% of all large-bowel tumors. In fact, the alimentary tract is the most frequent location of extranodal lymphoma.

Gastric lymphomas occur in the older age group and, in contrast to intestinal lymphomas, are rarely seen in children. Non-Hodgkin's lymphoma in children presents more frequently as primary gastrointestinal involvement (10 to 30%) and is the commonest gastrointestinal neoplasm in children. In children, the disease occurs most commonly in the terminal ileum and appendix and is associated with an incidence of marrow involvement and even leukemia approaching 25% (Nelson et al., 1977; Cox, 1979). American Burkitt's lymphoma primarily involves the gastrointestinal tract in children in a majority of cases. Of 30 cases reported by Arseneau et al. (1975), the gastrointestinal tract or an abdominal tumor of uncertain origin constituted the primary site of involvement in 19 patients.

Ten to 20% of patients with NHL are found to have gastrointestinal involvement at the time of initial examination with staging workup, and as many as 50% show such involvement at autopsy (Craig and Gregson, 1981; Zornosa and Dodd, 1980). Primary gastrointestinal lymphoma has been documented as a rare complication of both regional ileitis (Collins, 1977) and ulcerative colitis (Barki and Boult, 1981); as occurring in patients with congenital Wiskott-Aldrich syndrome (Faraci et al., 1975), and acquired immunodeficiency states such as those occurring in renal transplant patients (Jamieson et al., 1981; Kaslikova et al., 1981; Coggon et al., 1981); and as occurring in a familial setting (Maurer et al., 1976; Freedlander and Kissen, 1978). It may also complicate the enteropathy of dermatitis herpetiformis (Ramot et al., 1977) and of adult celiac disease. Primary gastrointestinal Hodgkin's disease is distinctly rare (Craig and Gregson, 1981). In our opinion, such a diagnosis should be made with great caution.

Primary gastrointestinal lymphoma is somewhat more common in the stomach than in the small bowel except in geographic areas with a high incidence of immunoproliferative small intestinal disease (IPSID), where small-bowel lesions predominate (Table 2) (Lewin et al., 1978; Weingrad et al., 1982; Henry

TABLE 2. Sites of Involvement by Primary Gastrointestinal Lymphoma

	Kahn et al. (S. Africa) 1972		Henry and Farrar-Brown (U.K.) 1977		Lewin et al. (U.S.) 1978		Weingrad et al. (U.S.) 1982		Totals	
Sites	No.	%	No.	%	No.	%	No.	%	No.	%
Stomach	19	33	51	41	48	43	76	73	194	48.9
Small bowel	34	60	53	42	50	45	15	14.5	154	38.8
Colon	4	7	21	17	13	12	13	12.5	49	12.3
Totals	57		125		111		104		397	

and Farrar-Brown, 1977; Kahn et al., 1972). The lymphoid tissue of Waldeyer's ring in the pharynx (Al-Saleem et al., 1970), the esophagus (Berman et al., 1979), and the appendix are rare sites of primary involvement. The clinical and macroscopic features of PGL do not differ significantly from other forms of gastrointestinal malignancy. The lesion may form a polypoid fungating mass or a malignant ulcer with heaped-up margins. It may more diffusely infiltrate the bowel wall, producing in the small bowel a diffuse thickening with aneurysmal dilatation of the involved segment or, in the stomach, a diffuse thickening with giant mucosal folds or a cobblestone appearance. Multicentric lesions are more common with PGL than with other forms of malignancy and may take the form of multiple lymphomatous polyps (Sheahan et al., 1971). Such polyps need to be distinguished from nodular lymphoid hyperplasia as discussed previously.

Considerable controversy exists with regard to histologic classification of the types of PGL seen in Westernized, developed countries. The problems are compounded by the many classifications for NHL that have appeared in recent years and that have been developed as a consequence of new information about the function of the immune system. The most widely accepted view is that these lymphomas represent the usual spectrum of those occurring in nodal locations. In our department, we are currently using both a modified Rappaport classification and the newly developed international lymphoma formulation (Table 3) (Rosenberg et al., 1982).

Diffuse large cell or "histiocytic" lymphomas of the Rappaport classification are by far the most frequent histologic type observed. Table 4 illustrates the histologic types of 117 cases of PGL seen at Stanford University and classified by the modified Rappaport classification (Lewin et al., 1978). Henry and Farrar-Brown (1977) expressed the view that tumors of plasma cell origin (extramedullary myelomas) constitute the largest group of PGL (39% in their series of 125 cases). Their evidence is derived from the light microscopic and ultrastructural resemblance of the tumor cells to plasma cells, but none of their patients had paraproteinemia nor evidence of myelomatosis. It seems likely that their cases of so-called extramedullary plasmacytoma represent immunoblastic transformation of malignant B-lymphocytes and lymphoplasmacytoid lymphomas.

TABLE 3. Non-Hodgkin's Lymphoma: International Formulation (Modified Rappaport Classification)

I. Low grade
   1. Small lymphocytic (well-differentiated lymphocytic)
      (a) With/without chronic lymphatic leukemia
      (b) With/without plasmacytoid features
   2. Follicular, small cleaved cell (nodular, poorly differentiated lymphocytic)[a]
   3. Follicular, mixed small cleaved and large cell (nodular, mixed lymphocytic-histiocytic)[a]

II. Intermediate grade
   1. Follicular, large cell (nodular, histiocytic)[a]
   2. Diffuse, small cleaved cell (diffuse, poorly differentiated lymphocytic)[a]
   3. Diffuse, mixed small and large cell (diffuse mixed lymphocytic-histiocytic)[a]
   4. Diffuse, large cell (diffuse, histiocytic)[a]

III. High grade
   1. Immunoblastic-plasmacytoid, clear cell, polymorphous types (histiocytic)
   2. Lymphoblastic convoluted and nonconvoluted cell types (lymphoblastic)
   3. Small noncleaved cell, Burkitt's

IV. Miscellaneous
   1. Mycosis fungoides
   2. Hairy cell leukemia
   3. Malignant histiocytosis
   4. Unclassified

[a]Exclusively or predominantly of follicle center cell origin.

A most interesting observation by Isaacson and colleagues (1979) in a study of 66 cases of PGL was that 33 of their cases were of true histiocytic origin. In addition to the observation of phagocytosis of red cells, platelets, and cell debris by tumor cells, these cells were shown, by immunoperoxidase techniques in 25 cases so studied, to contain all Ig classes and both light chain types, probably a consequence of phagocytic activity via Fc receptors or a result of antibodies directed against tumor antigens. They were also shown to contain muramidase and α_1-antitrypsin (AAT), enzymes produced by histiocytic cells (Figure 4). Elegant experiments using cell lysates from such tumors and study-

TABLE 4. Histologic Types: Stanford Series[a]

Type	No. (%)
Histiocytic, diffuse	70 (60%)
Lymphocytic	23 (20%)
Lymphoblastic (Burkitt and non-Burkitt)	10 (9%)
Hodgkin's	2 (2%)
Other	12 (9%)

[a]Ten cases are follicular; 8 cases had plasmacytoid features.

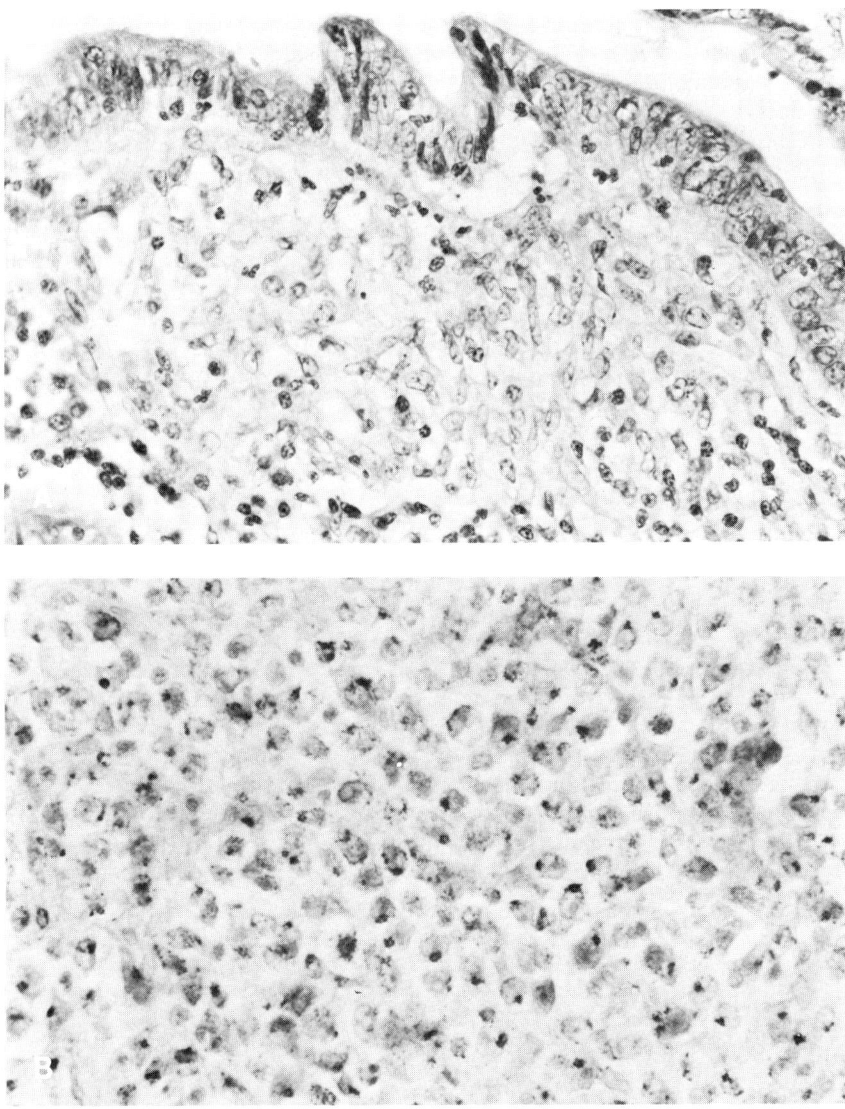

FIGURE 4. (**a**) Early mucosal infiltration of mildly atypical histiocytes in malignant histiocytosis of intestine. (**b**) Focal paranuclear immunoperoxidase reaction for AAT. *Source:* Wright (1980).

ing immunodiffusion patterns confirmed that the positive staining for AAT was due to AAT identical to serum AAT and that this material was synthesized by these cells rather than taken up from the environment (Isaacson et al., 1981).

The serum lysozyme level has also been shown to be elevated in these patients, but not in cases of uncomplicated celiac disease (Hodges et al., 1979).

In 22 of their 33 cases of true histiocytic lymphoma, the distribution of organ involvement (bowel, mesenteric nodes, bone marrow, spleen, and liver) and the predominantly sinusoidal pattern of histologic involvement suggested a diagnosis of histiocytic medullary reticulosis ("malignant histiocytosis of the intestine"). Some, but not all, of these patients had a clinical course compatible with celiac disease, suggesting to Isaacson and coworkers (1980) that this type of lymphoma may complicate that disease. The mucosa remote from the lymphoma exhibited villous atrophy and plasma cell infiltration. The presence of an atrophic spleen in many cases and HLA typing conforming to types found in celiac disease is further corroborative evidence for the existence of underlying celiac disease. However, these patients uniformly fail to show a response to a gluten-free diet, but this may relate to the late stage of the disease when a lymphoma has already become clinically manifest. In more recent studies, Isaacson and coworkers were able to demonstrate "early" microscopic involvement of mucosa or mucosal crypts by malignant histiocytes causing small foci of ulceration (Figure 4) (Isaacson, 1980). In some patients, ulcerative jejunitis was found in the absence of small bowel lymphoma. The authors suggested that malignant histiocytes might even be present in such lesions, but that the histiocytes were too sparse to be recognized and were also obscured by the many inflammatory cells present. They considered this lesion to represent the earliest phase of malignant histiocytosis of the intestine (Isaacson and Wright, 1978, 1980).

Apart from the immunologic studies of Isaacson and coworkers (1980), only a few other studies of PGL using immunologic techniques have been published (Table 5). In contrast to the findings of Isaacson and coworkers (1980), the positively staining lymphomas were found to be of B-cell type. In the largest series studied to date, Saraga and coworkers (1981) demonstrated monoclonal antibody in 26 of 70 cases. Seven cases showed a bitypic staining pattern, while the remainder failed to demonstrate any positive staining. In contrast to nodal NHL where 75% of B-cells are κ-producing, 90% of the Ig-positive PGLs were of λ-light chain type and 21 of the 33 were positive for light chain only. Seo and coworkers (1982) found monoclonal Ig in 9 of 18 gastric lymphomas studied (8κ; 1λ); 5 cases were negative for Ig and 4 contained muramidase, suggesting a true histiocytic derivation. Yamanaka and coworkers (1980) demonstrated monoclonal IgM (3κ; 1λ) in 4 of 5 cases of PGL. The presence of malignant T-lymphocytes in the gastrointestinal tract has been reported in a single case of Sezary's syndrome (Cohen et al., 1978).

We have performed immunoperoxidase study on 76 cases of PGL using a panel of antisera for λ, κ, J-chain, AAT, lysozyme, and human serum albumin. In all cases, paraffin-embedded tissue was used and a more sensitive avidin-biotin-peroxidase complex method was used (Hsu et al., 1981). The diagnosis of B-cell lymphoma was established on the basis of either monotypic staining for the light chains and/or positive staining for J chain. The presence of intracytoplasmic albumin was interpreted as indicative of passive absorption and correlated with bitypic staining for light chains. Cases diagnosed as being of monocyte/macrophage origin showed positive reaction for lysozyme and/or AAT and/or α_1 anti-chymotrypsin. Twenty-two cases (29%) were of B-cell derivation, and 20 cases (26%) showed κ, λ with or without albumin indicating pas-

TABLE 5. Immunologic Findings in Gastrointestinal Lymphoma: A Review of the Literature

Reference	Number of cases studied	Sites	Technique	Results[a]
Isaacson et al., 1979	34	Stomach, small intestine, ileocecal	Paraffin embedded tissue, immunoperoxidase (PAP) prior trypsin digestion	14λK, Lyso.[b] and AAT 11λK, Lyso.[c] 9(−)
Yamanaka et al., 1980	5	Stomach	Direct and indirect immunofluorescence on frozen tissue sections	5(+)anti-B cell serum: (3μK, 1μλ)
Saraga et al., 1981	70	Stomach, small and large intestine	Paraffin embedded tissue, immunoperoxidase (PAP)	37(−) 33(+)Clg: (13λ, 6lλK,[d] 3Yλ, 3μλ, 2αλ, 1Jλ, 1Jμλ, 1αK, 1αYλ, 1YλK, 1α)
Seo et al., 1982	18	Stomach	Paraffin embedded tissue, immunoperoxidase (PAP)	5(−) 5μK 2YK 1Yλ 1αK 4 Lyso.

[a]Y = gamma heavy chain, α = alpha heavy chain, μ = mu heavy chain, K = kappa light chain, λ = lambda light chain, J = marker for B-lymphocytes.
[b]Performed in only 9 cases. [c]Performed in only 7 cases. [d]Negative for lysozyme.

sive absorption. Twenty-seven of the cases (36%) failed to stain with any of the antisera used. Only 7 cases stained with one or more of the histiocytic enzyme markers. However, a large number of cases showed the presence of considerable admixture of nonneoplastic, reactive histiocytic type cells. The existence of true histiocytic lymphomas of the gastrointestinal tract has been questioned. We agree with Isaacson and colleagues that such tumors do indeed exist but, in our experience, they constitute a very small group.

Several factors must be borne in mind in interpreting the results of immunoperoxidase stains in PGL. It is important that adequate controls using antisera on known histologic preparations be run in parallel. The interpretation of monoclonality is dependant on the presence of homogeneous fields of tumor cells, a proportion of which stain exclusively for only one light chain type (Figure 5). The number of such positively staining malignant cells may vary from less than 50% to nearly 100%. In some instances, reactive polyclonal lymphoid and plasma cells, including lymphoid follicles, are present within or, more commonly, at the periphery of the tumor and usually account for less than 10% of all positively staining cells. A negative staining reaction in malignant cells may be a consequence of loss of antigen resulting from tissue storage or processing, small concentrations of the antigen, gene deletion, or poor expression for the antigen. Lymphomas composed of small mature-looking lymphocytes

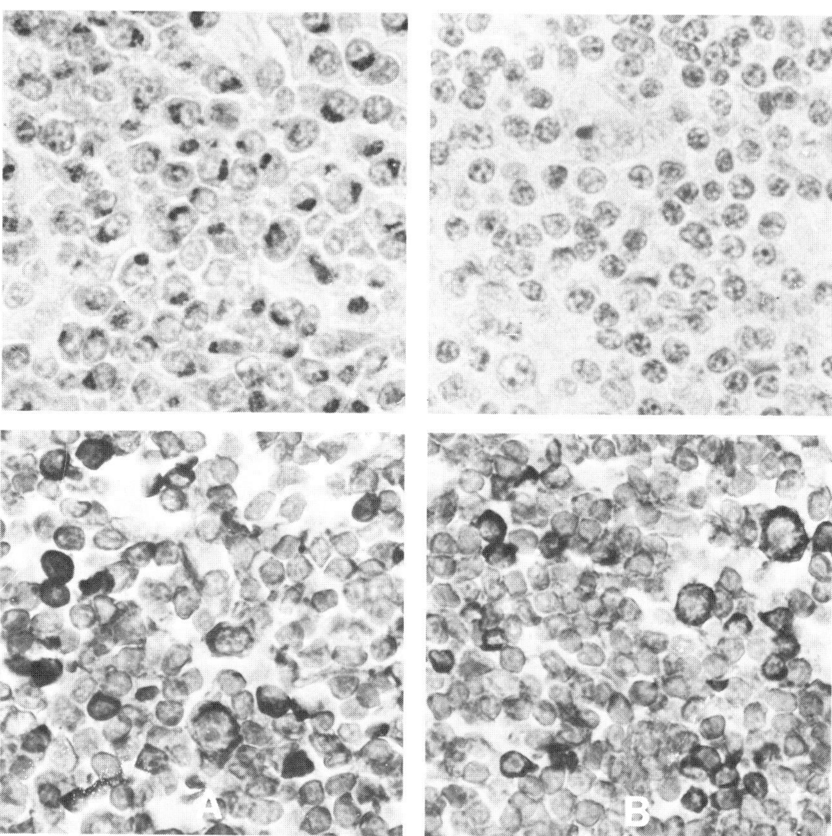

FIGURE 5. Small lymphocytic gastric lymphoma with plasmacytoid features are shown in the upper panels. All cells stain for κ light chain in (**a**) paranuclear location (× 550), in contrast to (**b**) negative staining for λ light chain (× 550). Gastric pseudolymphoma in the lower panels stain for both light chain types (× 550).

(well-differentiated lymphocytic of Rappaport) usually contain no cytoplasmic Ig. A positive immunologic reaction for monoclonal Ig or immunoglobulin is also very helpful in differentiating PGL from undifferentiated gastric carcinoma, especially in small peroral biopsies. Other helpful distinguishing features include demonstration of intracytoplasmic mucin and desmosomes in carcinoma cells (Figures 6 and 7).

Malabsorption may be the chief manifestation of two varieties of PGL. First, lymphoma may complicate long-standing celiac disease and has been reported in 6 to 10% of such patients (Brandt et al., 1978). It should be suspected when new symptoms (pain, weight loss, fever, diarrhea) appear in a well-controlled patient with celiac disease lasting more than 10 years. Such patients may also have significantly elevated serum lysozyme levels (Hodges et al., 1979). As discussed previously, Isaacson and coworkers (1980) believe that lymphomas

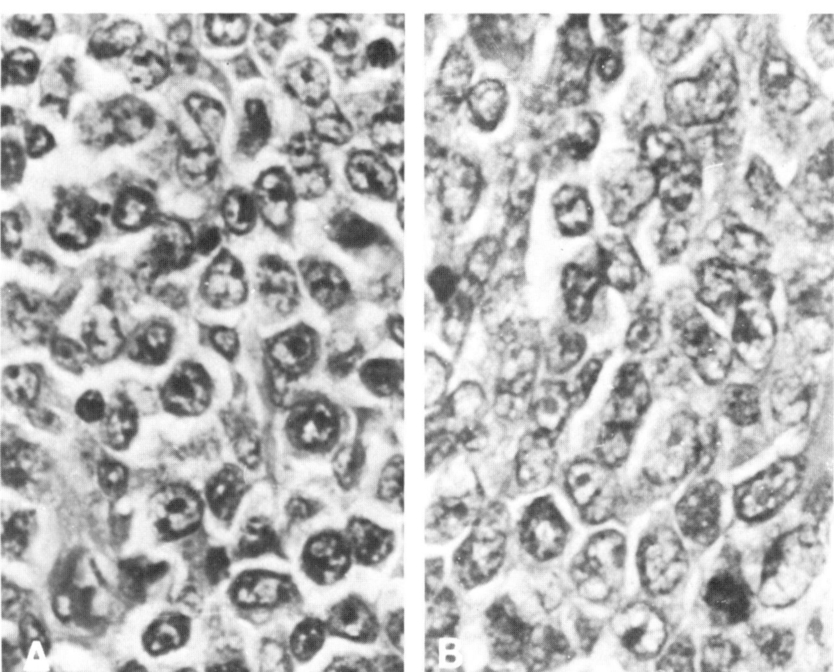

FIGURE 6. (**a**) Close morphologic resemblance of immunoblastic lymphoma (× 1000) to (**b**) undifferentiated gastric carcinoma (× 900).

developing in this selected group of patients are of true histiocytic origin. It has been postulated that a T-cell deficiency known to occur in adult celiac disease may have some bearing on the development of the lymphoma (Brandt et al., 1978).

Malabsorption is also the prime manifestation of so-called immunoproliferative small intestinal disease (IPSID). Immunoproliferative small intestinal disease was first documented in Peru in 1963 and has subsequently been described within the past two decades among population groups living in areas of depressed socioeconomic conditions (south and eastern Mediterranean countries, North Africa, and South Africa) (Al-Saleem and Zardawi, 1979; Lewin et al., 1976; Nassar et al., 1978; Haghighi et al., 1978; Novis et al, 1973). It has a distinctive ethnic (Arabs, Sephardic Jews of Israel, Mulattos of Cape Province of South Africa) and age (20 to 40 years) distribution. Clinically, malabsorption is the outstanding feature; the patients also exhibit impaired growth, abdominal pain, and finger clubbing. An immunopathy is present in a variable proportion (up to 69%) of cases (Al-Saleem and Zardawi, 1979) and involves a portion of the Fc fragment of IgA without light chains. Such cases are referred to as alpha-heavy chain disease. The abnormal protein can be demonstrated in serum, urine, intestinal fluid, and cell cytoplasm (Rambaud et al., 1980).

Pathologically, two patterns of disease are seen within the bowel represent-

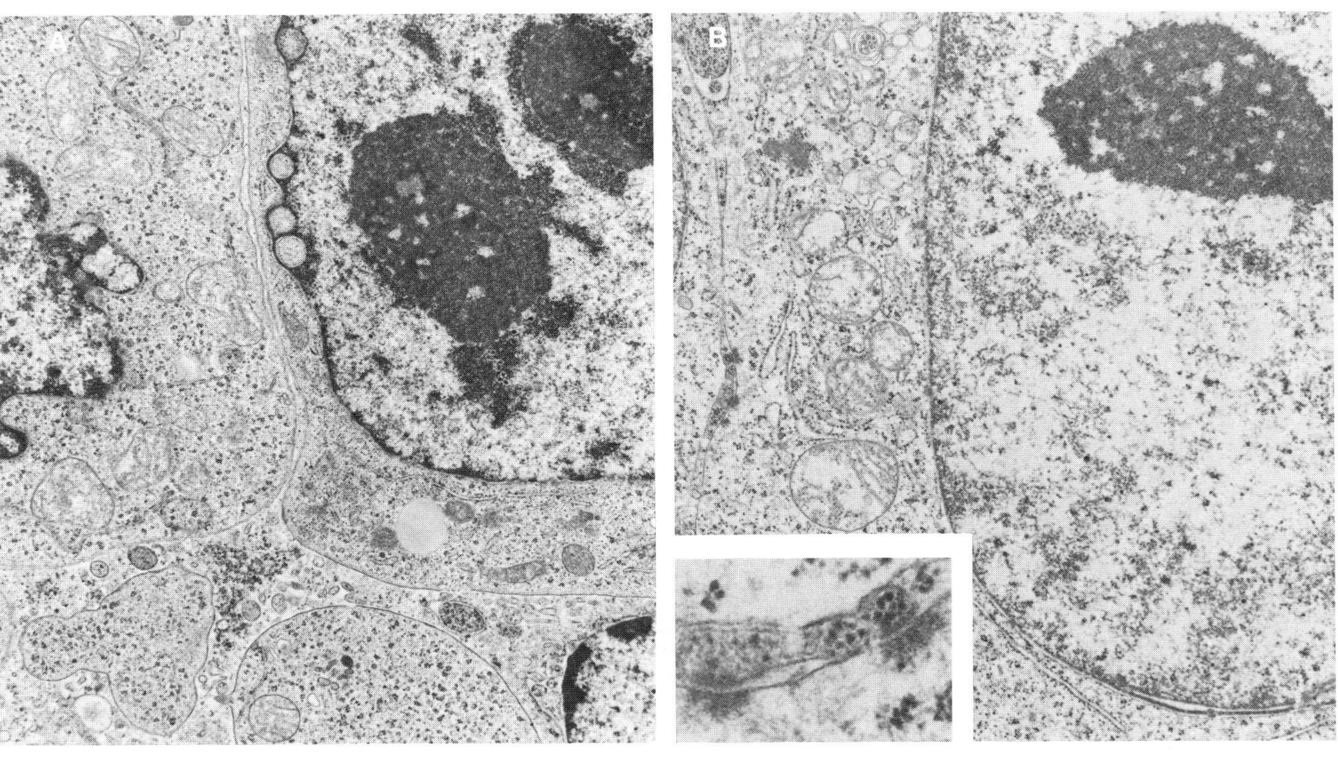

FIGURE 7. Electron micrographs from same cases as Figure 6. (**a**) Immunoblast with numerous polyribosomes and stacked RER (× 12,000) and (**b**) carcinoma cells with desmosomes (× 12,000).

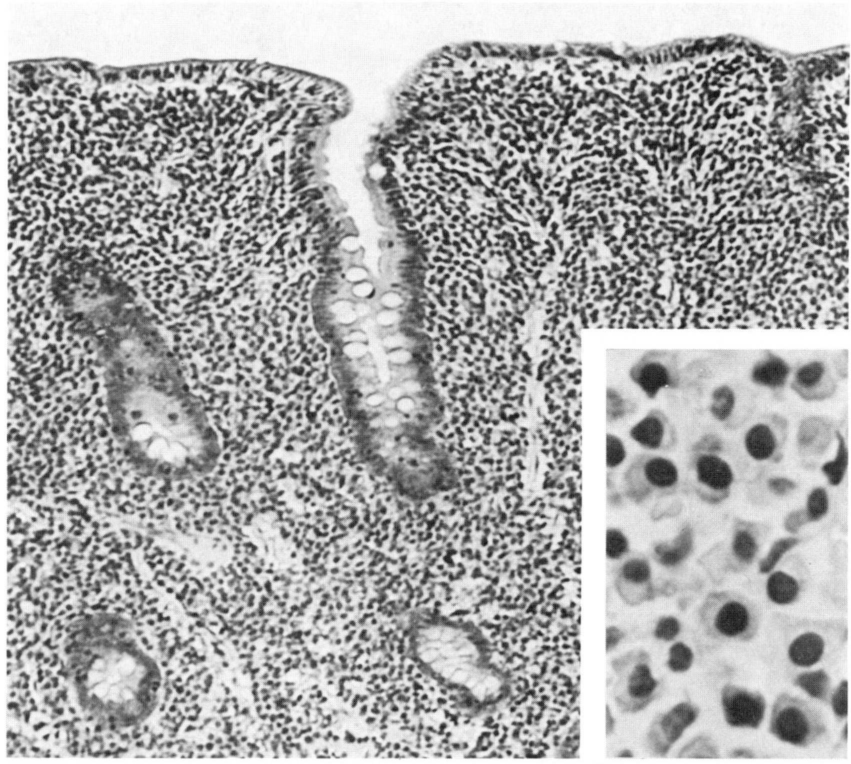

FIGURE 8. Villous atrophy and dense lymphoplasmacytic infiltrate in small bowel in IPSID (× 125; inset × 800). *Source:* Kahn and Novis (1974).

ing two phases of the disease. Initially, a dense mucosal infiltration of mature-looking plasma cells with or without lymphocytes involves the entire length of the small bowel and causes partial effacement of the villi (Figure 8). These cells have been shown, by immunologic techniques, to be synthesizers of the defective protein (Selzer et al., 1979; Brouet et al., 1977; Isaacson, 1979; Pangalis and Rappaport, 1977). It is uncertain whether these cells are inflammatory, premalignant, or malignant, but it appears that, at this state, the disease may be reversible, as evidenced by reports of complete long-term response to broad spectrum antibiotics. The clonality of these cells cannot be determined because of the absence of light chains. A variety of designations have been appended to this stage of the process, namely,

Pure lymphoplasmacytic proliferation with alpha-heavy chains (Al-Saleem and Zardawi, 1979).

Alpha-heavy chain disease and massive plasma cell infiltration without lymphoma (Lewin et al. 1976).

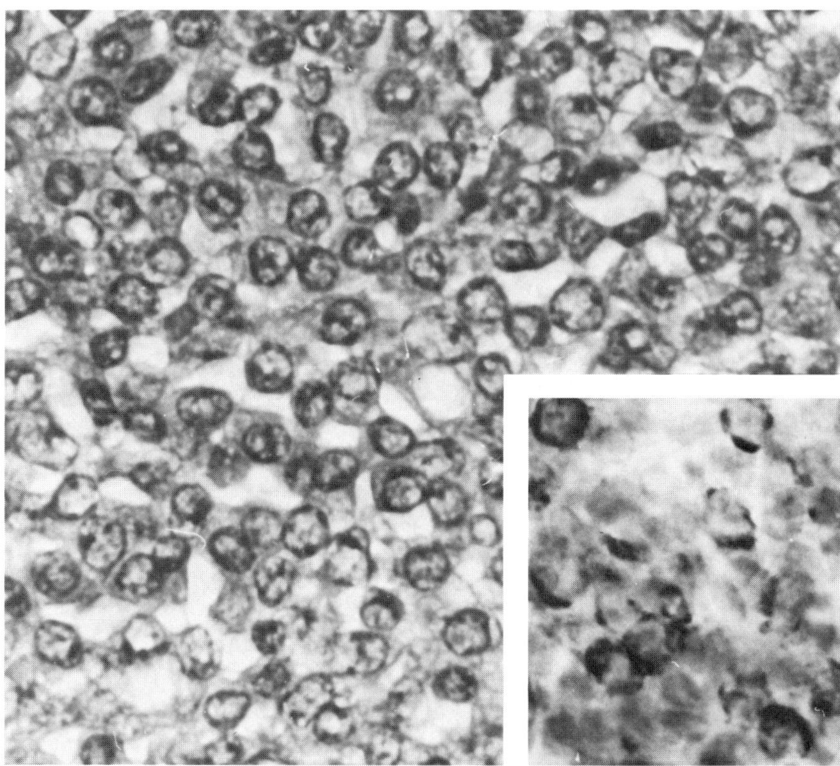

FIGURE 9. Mesenteric lymph node with lymphoma from another case of IPSID. The inset shows positive immunoperoxidase staining for alpha-heavy chain (× 1000).

Intestinal phase of alpha-heavy chain disease (Tabbane et al., 1976).

Immunoproliferative disease of the small intestine, Stage O (Nassar et al., 1978).

Alpha-heavy chain disease, Stage A (Galian et al., 1977).

Immunocytic enteropathy (Al-Saleem and Zardawi, 1979).

A malignant lymphoma of immunoblastic type subsequently involves the upper small intestine and/or mesenteric nodes and usually remains confined to the abdomen. In 6 of the 10 cases studied immunologcially, the lymphoma cells were shown to be synthesizing the abnormal protein (Figure 9) (Selzer et al., 1979; Brouet et al., 1977; Isaacson, 1979; Pangalis and Rappaport, 1977; Ramot et al., 1977). This phase of the disease has also been referred to by a variety of names such as,

Lymphoplasmacytic lymphoma with diffuse lymphoplasmacytic proliferation (Al-Saleem and Zardawi, 1979).

Neoplastic phase of alpha-heavy chain disease (Tabbane et al., 1976).

Primary intestinal lymphoma, "Mediterranean type" (Lewin et al., 1976).

Immunoproliferative disease of the small intestine, Stages I–IV (Nassar et al., 1978).

Alpha-heavy chain disease, Stages B–D (Galian et al., 1977).

Primary lymphoma of the upper small intestine (Nasr et al., 1970).

This form of intestinal lymphoma is thought to result from intestinal antigenic stimulation, possibly infectious, starting during infancy in populations living under adverse socioeconomic situations. Borochowitz et al. (1979) have shown that infants severely stressed by enteritis during the first 6 months of life develop thymic atrophy with persistent cell-mediated immune deficiency, which could contribute to the development of lymphoma. However, other factors must be involved because the disease has not been described in many third world countries.

Unusual variants of alpha-chain disease include a respiratory form, as well as a case from Durham, North Carolina, in a patient with multiple lymphomatous polyps but an absence of malabsorption and plasma cell infiltration of the bowel (Cohen et al., 1978). Apart from alpha-chain disease, other dysproteinemias may be associated with immunoproliferative gastrointestinal disease, for example,

1. IgA myeloma protein, κ-type, in a 30-year-old Spanish female with malabsorption, massive plasma cell infiltration of the small bowel, and immunoblastic lymphoma of bowel and mesentery (Chantar et al., 1974).
2. IgA myeloma protein, κ-type, in a 20-year-old Algerian female with gastric myeloma (Preud'homme et al., 1980).
3. IgA myeloma protein, κ-type, and Bence Jones proteinuria with dense mucosal plasma cell infiltration without villous atrophy in the small bowel (Tangun et al., 1975).
4. Biclonal IgM, λ-type and Y_1-heavy chain with gastric lymphoma (Virella et al., 1977).
5. Y-heavy chain with plasmacytoid gastric lymphoma (Papac et al., 1978).
6. Y_1-heavy chain in a 12-year-old Turkish child with malabsorption and a diffuse lymphoplasmacytic infiltration of the lamina propria of the small bowel and mesenteric nodes (Bender et al., 1978).
7. IgG_3, κ-type protein with nodular lymphoid hypoplasia of stomach, small bowel, and mesenteric nodes (Kopec et al., 1974).

A number of factors have been considered as having significance with reference to prognosis in PGL. Of these, location in the stomach is associated with a better prognosis (12 to 60% five-year survival rate, mean $\pm$ 35%) (Mattingly et al., 1981; Saraga et al. 1981; Contreary et al., 1980) than location in the small bowel (12 to 48% five-year survival rate, mean $\pm$ 30%) (Saraga et al., 1981; Contreary et al., 1980). In most series, infiltration of the lymphoma through the entire thickness of the wall has an adverse effect on prognosis (Saraga et al., 1981; Lim et all, 1977; Nelson et al., 1977; Fu and Perzin, 1972). In some series, large size (greater than 10 cm) (Saraga et al., 1981; Fu and Perzin, 1972) and node involvement (Lim et al., 1977; Nelson et al., 1977; Contreary et al., 1980) have been associated with shorter survival times. Survival has also been shown to be improved in patients whose tumor cells are immunoglobulin producing (Saraga et al., 1981). Surprisingly, the histologic type of the lymphoma has proved to be the least helpful prognostic parameter (Saraga et al., 1981; Lim et al., 1977; Nelson et al., 1977). However, lymphomas of small cell type (diffuse, well-differentiated lymphoma with or without plasmacytoid features) and nodular lymphomas have a better prognosis (Lim et al., 1977; Weingrad et al., 1982).

The most widely accepted therapeutic approach to PGL has been resection of all bowel-bearing tumors, where technically feasible, followed by radiotherapy and/or chemotherapy, depending on the clinical stage of the disease (Nelson et al., 1977). Resection of the tumor is important because of a significant incidence of perforation following radiotherapy and/or chemotherapy. Gastrointestinal bleeding or perforation, probably as a consequence of therapy, was noted in 25% of 48 cases of PGL of histiocytic type (Rosenfelt and Rosenberg, 1980).

In immunoproliferative forms of intestinal lymphoma, a staging laparotomy is recommended to exclude lymphoma in patients with diffuse lymphoplasmacytic infiltrates seen in peroral biopsies. A trial of broad spectrum antibiotics is indicated when no such lymphoma is evident. Most recurrences and deaths from PGL occur within 16 months of therapy (Nelson et al., 1977).

We wish to express our sincere appreciation to the following individuals for their tireless efforts on our behalf in completing this work: Susan G. Richer, H.T.L. (A.S.C.P.), histology technician in immunopathology, who handled all the immunohistochemistry preparations in our studies; William Oxberry, electron microscopy technologist, who assisted in the preparation of the photomicrographs; and Joan M. Sullivan, R.M.A., C.M.A., secretary to the chairman, who sorted through our notes and prepared the manuscript in the proper format.

REFERENCES

Al-Saleem T, Harwick R, Robbins R, Blady JV (1970) Malignant lymphoma of the pharynx. Cancer 26:1383-1387.

Al-Saleem T, Zardawi IM (1979) Primary lymphomas of the small intestine in Iraq: A pathologic study of 145 cases. Histopathology 3:89–106.

Arseneau JC, Canellos GP, Banks PM, et al. (1975) American Burkitt's lymphoma: A clinicopathologic study of 30 cases. Clinical factors relating to prolonged survival. Am J Med 58:314–321.

Barki Y, Boult I (1981) Two uncommon malignancies complicating chronic ulcerative colitis. J Can Assoc Radiol 32:136–137.

Bender SW, Danon F, Preud'homme JL, et al. (1978) Gamma heavy chain disease simulating alpha chain disease: A case report. Gut 19:1148–1152.

Berman M, Falchuk KR, Trey C, Gramm HF (1979) Primary histiocytic lymphoma of the esophagus. Dig Dis Sci 24:883–886.

Borochowitz D, Dutz W, Kohout E, Vessal K (1979) Gastrointestinal mucosa and primary gastrointestinal lymphoma. Isr J Med Sci 15:397–404.

Brandt L, Hagander B, Norden A, Stenstam M (1978) Lymphoma of the small intestine in adult celiac disease. Acta Med Scand 304:467–470.

Brouet JC, Mason DY, Danon F, et al. (1977) Alpha-chain disease: Evidence for common clonal origin of intestinal immunoblastic lymphoma and plasmacytic proliferation. Lancet 1:861.

Chantar C, Escartin P, Plaza AG, et al. (1974) Diffuse plasma cell infiltration of the small intestine with malabsorption associated to IgA monoclonal gammapathy. Cancer 34:1620–1630.

Coggon DNM, Rose DH, Ansell ID (1981) A large bowel lymphoma complicating renal transplantation. Br J Radiol 54:418–420.

Cohen HJ, Gonzalvo A, Krook J, et al. (1978) New presentation of alpha heavy chain disease: North American polypoid gastrointestinal lymphoma. Cancer 41:1161–1169.

Collins WJ (1977) Malignant lymphoma complicating regional enteritis: Case report and review of the literature. Am J Gastroenterol 68:177–181.

Contreary R, Nance FC, Becker WF (1980) Primary lymphoma of the gastrointestinal tract. Am Surg 191:593–598.

Cox JD (1979) Prognostic factors in malignant lymphoreticular tumors of the small bowel and ileocecal region: A review of 50 case histories. Int J Radiol Oncol Biol Phys 5:185–190.

Craig O, Gregson R (1981) Primary lymphoma of the gastrointestinal tract. Clin Radiol 32:63–71.

Faraci RP, Hoffstrand HJ, Witebsky FG, et al. (1975) Malignant lymphoma of the jejunum in a patient with Wiskott-Aldrich syndrome. Surgical treatment. Arch Surg 110:218–220.

Freedlander E., Kissen LJ (1978) Gut lymphoma presenting simultaneously in two siblings. Br Med J 1:80–81.

Fu Y-S, Perzin KH (1972) Lymphosarcoma of the small intestine. A clinicopathologic study. Cancer 29:645–659.

Galian A, Lecestre MJ, Scotto J, et al. (1977) Pathological study of alpha chain disease with special emphasis on evolution. Cancer 39:2081–2101.

Gonzales-Vitale JC, Gomez LG, Goldblum RM, et al. (1982) Immunoblastic lymphoma of small intestine complicating late-onset immunodeficiency. Cancer 49:445–449.

Haghighi P, Kharazim A, Gerami C, et al. (1978) Primary upper small intestinal lymphoma and alpha-chain disease. Am J Surg Pathol 2:147–157.

Henry K, Farrar-Brown G (1977) Primary lymphomas of the gastrointestinal tract. 1. Plasma cell tumors. Histopathology 1:53–76.

Hermans PE, Dias-Buxo JA, Stabo JD (1976) Idiopathic late-onset immunoglobulin deficiency. Clinical observation in 50 patients. Am J Med 61:221–237.

Hodges JR, Isaacson P, Eade OE, Wright R (1979) Serum lysozyme levels in malignant histiocytosis of the intestine. Gut 20:854–857.

Hsu SM, Raine L, Ganger H (1981) The use of avidin-biotin-peroxidase complex (ABC) in immunoperoxidase techniques: A comparison between ABC and unlabeled antibody (PAP) procedures. J Histochem Cytochem 19:577.

Hyjek E, Kelenyi G (1982) Pseudolymphomas of the stomach: A lesion characterized by progressively transformed germinal centres. Histopathology 6:61–68.

Isaacson P (1979) Middle East lymphoma and alpha-chain disease. An immunohistochemical study. Am J Surg Pathol 3:431–441.

Isaacson P (1980) Malignant histiocytosis of the intestine: The early histologic lesion. Gut 21:381–386.

Isaacson P, Wright DH (1978) Malignant histiocytosis of the intestine. Its relationship to malabsorption and ulcerative jejunitis. Hum Pathol 9:661–677.

Isaacson P, Wright DH, Judd Ma, Mepham BL (1979) Primary gastrointestinal lymphoma. A classification of 66 cases. Cancer 43:1805–1819.

Isaacson P, et al. (1980) Malabsorption and intestinal lymphomas. In: Wright D, ed., Recent advances in gastrointestinal pathology. Philadelphia: WB Saunders, pp. 193–212.

Isaacson P, Jones DB, Millward-Sadler GH, et al. (1981) Alpha-1 antitrypsin in human macrophages. J Clin Pathol 34:982–990.

Jacobson KW, deShazo RD (1979) Selective immunoglobulin A deficiency associated with nodular lymphoid hyperplasia. J Allergy Clin Immunol 64:516–521.

Jamieson NV, Thiru S, Calne RY, Evans DB (1981) Gastric lymphomas arising in two patients with renal allografts. Transplant 31:224–225.

Kahn LB, Novis B (1974) Nodular lymphoid hyperplasia of the small bowel associated with primary small bowel reticulum cell lymphoma. Cancer 33:837–844.

Kahn LB, Selzer G, Kaschula ROC (1972) Primary gastrointestinal lymphoma. A clinicopathologic study of 57 cases. Am J Digest Dis 17:219–232.

Kaslikova J, Kocandrle V, Zastava V, et al. (1981) Multiple immunoblastic sarcoma of the small intestine following renal transplantation. Transplant 31:481–482.

Kopec M, Swierczynska Z, Pazdur J, et al. (1974) Diffuse lymphoma of the intestines with a monoclonal gammapathy of IgG_3 Kappa type. Am J Med 56:381–385.

Lamers CBHW, Wagener DJT, Assman KJM, van Tongeren JHM (1980) Jejunal lymphoma in a patient with primary adult-onset hypogammaglobulinemia and nodular lymphoid hyperplasia of the small intestine. Dig Dis Sci 25:553–557.

Laufer I, Derek, D (1978) Lymphoid follicular pattern: A normal feature of the pediatric colon. AJR 130:51–55.

Lewin KJ, Kahn LB, Novis BH (1976) Primary intestinal lymphoma of "Western" and "Mediterranean" type alpha chain disease and massive plasma cell infiltration. A comparative study of 37 cases. Cancer 38:2511–2528.

Lewin KJ, Ranchod M, Dorfman RF (1978) Lymphomas of the gastrointestinal tract. A study of 117 cases presenting with gastrointestinal disease. Cancer 42:693–707.

Lim FE, Hartman AS, Tan EGC, et al. (1977) Factors in the prognosis of gastric lymphomas. Cancer 39:1715–1720.

Mackenzie Crooks DJ, Brown WR (1980) The distribution of intestinal nodular lymphoid hyperplasia in immunoglobulin deficiency. Clin Radiol 31:701–706.

Mattingly SS, Cibull ML, Ram MD, et al. (1981) Pseudolymphoma of the stomach. A diagnostic and therapeutic dilemma. Arch Surg 116:25–29.

Matuchansky C, Morichau-Beauchant M, Touchard G, et al. (1980) Nodular lymphoid hyperplasia of the small bowel associated with primary jejunal malignant lymphoma. Gastroenterology 78:1587–1592.

Maurer HS, Gotoff SP, Allen L, Bolan J (1976) Malignant lymphoma of the small intestine in multiple family members. Association with an immunologic deficiency. Cancer 37:2224–2231.

Munro A, Simpson JG (1974) Nodular lymphoid hyperplasia of the stomach and small intestine with hypogammaglobulinemia. Br J Surg 61:953–954.

Nagura H, Kohler PF, Brown WR (1979) Immunocytochemical characterization of the lymphocytes in nodular lymphoid hyperplasia of the bowel. Lab Invest 40:66–73.

Nasr K, Haghighi P, Bakhandek K, Bagshenas M (1970) Primary lymphoma of the upper small intestine. Gut 11:673–678.

Nassar VH, Salem PA, Shahid MI, et al. (1978) "Mediterranean abdominal lymphoma" or immunoproliferative small intestinal disease. Part II: Pathological aspects. Cancer 41:1340–1354.

Nelson DF, Cassady JR, Traggis D, et al. (1977) The role of radiation therapy in localized resectable intestinal non-Hodgkin's lymphoma in children. Cancer 39:89–97.

Novis BH, Kahn LB, Banks S (1973) Alpha chain disease in Subsaharan Africa. Am J Digest Dis 18:679–688.

Pangalis GA, Rappaport H (1977) Common clonal origin of lymphoplasmacytic proliferation and immunoblastic lymphomas in intestinal alpha chain disease. Lancet 2:880.

Papac RJ, Rosenstein RW, Richards F, Yesner RL (1978) Gamma heavy chain disease seen initially as gastric neoplasm. Arch Int Med 138:1151–1153.

Preud'homme J-L, Galian A, Danon F, et al. (1980) Extramedullary plasmacytoma with gastric and lymph node involvement. An immunologic study. Cancer 46:1753–1758.

Rambaud J-C, Modigliani R, Nguyen Phuoc BK, et al. (1980) Non-secretory alpha-chain disease in intestinal lymphoma. N Engl J Med 303:53.

Ramot B, Levanon M, Hahn Y, et al. (1977) The mutual clonal origin of the lymphoplasmacytic and lymphoma cell in alpha heavy chain disease. Clin Exp Immunol 27:440.

Ranchod M, Lewin KJ, Dorfman RF (1978) Lymphoid hyperplasia of the gastrointestinal tract. A study of 26 cases and review of the literature. Am J Surg Pathol 2:383–400.

Robinson MJ, Padron S, Rywlin AM (1973) Enterocolitis lymphofollicularis. Morphologic, pathologic and serum immunoglobulin patterns. Arch Pathol 96:311–315.

Rosenberg S (Chairman of Writing Committee) (1982) National Cancer Institute sponsored study of classifications of non-Hodgkin's lymphomas. Summary and description of a working formulation for clinical usage. Cancer 49:2112–2135.

Rosenfelt F, Rosenberg SA (1980) Diffuse histiocytic lymphoma presenting with gastrointestinal tract lesions. The Stanford experience. Cancer 45:2188–2193.

Saraga P, Hurlimann J, Ozello L (1981) Lymphomas and pseudolymphomas of the alimentary tract. An immunolgoic study with clinicopathologic correlations. Hum Pathol 12:713–723.

Sauerbrei E, Castelli M (1979) Hypogammaglobulinemia and nodular lymphoid hyperplasia of the gut. J Can Assoc Radiol 30:62–63.

Selzer G, Sherman G, Callihan TR, Schwartz Y (1979) Primary small intestinal lymphoma and alpha-heavy chain disease. A study of 43 cases from a pathology department in Israel. Isr J Med Sci 15:111–123.

Seo IS, Binkley WB, Warner TFCS, Warfel KA (1982) A combined morphologic and immunolgoic approach to the diagnosis of gastrointestinal lymphomas. I. Malignant lymphomas of the stomach (A clinicopathologic study of 22 cases.) Cancer 49:493–501.

Sheahan DG, Martin F, Baginsky S, et al. (1971) Multiple lymphomatous polyposis of the gastrointestinal tract. Cancer 28:408–425.

Stroehlein JR, Weiland LH, Hoffman HN, Judd ES (1977) Untreated gastric pseudolymphoma. Dig Dis 22:465–470.

Tangun Y, Saracbasi Z, Inceman S, et al. (1975) IgA myeloma globulin and Bence-Jones proteinuria in diffuse plasmacytoma of the small intestine. Ann Intern Med 83:673.

Tabbane S, Tabbane F, Cammoun M, Mourali N (1976) Mediterranean lymphoma with alpha heavy chain monoclonal gammopathy. Cancer 38:1989–1996.

Virella G, Monteiro O, Lopes-Virella MF, et al. (1977) Asynchronous development of two monoclonal proteins (IgM λ and y_1 chains) in a patient with abdominal lymphoma. Cancer 39:2247–2253.

Webster ADB, Kenwright S, Ballard J, et al. (1977) Nodular lymphoid hyperplasia of the bowel in primary hypogammaglobulinaemia: Study of in vivo and in vitro lymphocyte function. Gut 18:364–372.

Weingrad DN, Decosse JJ, Sherlock P, et al. (1982) Primary gastrointestinal lymphoma: A 30-year review. Cancer 49:1258–1265.

Wright D, ed. (1980) Recent advances in gastrointestinal pathology. Philadelphia: WB Saunders.

Wright JE (1973) Pseudolymphoma of the stomach. Hum Pathol 4:305–318.

Yamanaka N, Ishii Y, Koshiba H, et al. (1980) A study of surface markers in gastrointestinal lymphoma. Gastroenterology 79:673–677.

Zornosa J, Dodd CD (1980) Lymphoma of the gastrointestinal tract. Semin Roentgenol 15:272–287.

CHEMOTHERAPY OF ADVANCED GASTROINTESTINAL MALIGNANCIES

FREDERICK P SMITH, M.D., F.A.C.P.,
STEVEN LANGE, M.D., ROBERT SILGALS, M.D.,
AND PHILIP S SCHEIN, M.D., F.A.C.P.

Gastrointestinal malignancy is the leading cause of cancer mortality in the United States. More than 190,000 new patients are anticipated for 1983 (Silverberg, 1982). Whereas surgery remains the only modality with curative potential, the majority of patients present with advanced tumors not amenable to surgical cure. Even when resection is possible, the patient remains at high risk for recurrence. Consequently, survival statistics have not changed greatly in the last 30 years. However, some important advances in the management of gastrointestinal malignancies have been realized in the last decade. Techniques of radiation therapy have been improved. Active chemotherapy protocols are being developed. Combined modality programs are finding a place in the management of certain subsets of patients. In this chapter we will briefly review chemotherapy of advanced gastrointestinal malignancies and describe potential areas for future studies.

ESOPHAGEAL CANCER

Approximately 9000 new cases of esophageal cancer are diagnosed each year (Silverberg, 1982). In general, the primary therapy for esophageal tumors entails surgical resection and/or radiation therapy. The results in terms of control of disease and of patient survival have been disappointing. Chemotherapy has often been reserved for patients who fail primary local therapy and for patients with disseminated disease. These patients are often markedly debilitated and, subsequently, less than ideal candidates for aggressive therapy. As a result, the efficacy of chemotherapy in esophageal cancer has only limited evaluation and the available reports show a wide fluctuation in response rates.

From the Vincent T. Lombardi Cancer Research Center, Georgetown University, Washington, D.C.

Only recently have investigators attempted to add chemotherapy to the primary management of these patients in combined modality programs.

Single Agent Therapy

Response rates for single antineoplastic agents have, in general, not exceeded 20%. Remission durations have been short, ranging from 6 to 8 weeks. Bleomycin appears to have some activity (Rosenbaum and Carter, 1970). Initial European studies with this drug reported an encouraging 54% response rate. However, subsequent trials have failed to confirm these results, with experience in the United States showing response rates ranging from 0 to 17% (Bonadonna et al., 1972; Wasserman et al., 1975). 5-Fluorouracil has been demonstrated to have marginal activity, with responses occuring in 14 to 17% of patients (Desai et al., 1979; Livingston and Carter, 1970; Wasserman et al., 1975). The nitrosourea CCNU also has only borderline efficacy, with objective tumor regressions noted in 3 of 19 patients (Moertel, 1976). Cis-diamine-dichloroplatinum has recognized activity in epidermoid carcinomas of the head and neck and, subsequently, has been studied in esophageal cancer. Results vary from 4 responses in 10 patients (Ravry and Moore, 1980) to only one response in 17 patients (Davis et al., 1980).

Doxorubicin has also been studied, again with inconsistent findings. Kolaric and coworkers (1977) reported one complete and five partial responses in 18 patients given doxorubicin at a dose of 40 mg/mm administered on 2 consecutive days every 3 weeks. In contrast, the Eastern Cooperative Oncology Group (ECOG) (Ezdinli et al., 1980) obtained only one response in 20 patients treated with doxorubicin at a dose of 60 mg/mm every 3 weeks.

Other drugs that have showed initial encouraging activity for esophageal cancer include methyl-GAG and vindesine (Falkson, 1971; Kelsen et al., 1979; Knight et al., 1979; Schnider et al., 1974). These reports represent preliminary information and will require further study.

Combination Chemotherapy

The majority of trials investigating combination chemotherapy in esophageal cancer have used bleomycin and cis-platinum either alone or with other drugs. Kelsen and coworkers (1978) obtained responses in 12 of 65 patients (18%) treated with bleomycin and cis-platinum. Median survival of patients was 4 months from initiation of therapy. Hentek and colleagues (1979) reported responses in 5 of 8 patients with the addition of methotrexate to the bleomycin and cis-platinum. In a study of the combination of mitomycin-C, bleomycin, and cis-platinum, Lad recorded 7 responses in 13 patients. However, the median survival of all patients was only 7 weeks (Lad, 1980). More recently, Kelsen and coworkers (1982) reported encouraging results with the combination of vindesine, cis-platinum, and bleomycin. Of 53 patients evaluable for response, 29 partial remissions were recorded, including 6 of 14 patients with metastatic disease and 16 of 28 patients with locoregional disease. Median remission duration in patients with metastatic disease was 8 months. Although these latter results are quite encouraging, it should be noted that no prospective randomized trials comparing various combination chemotherapy regimens have been reported.

Combined Modality Therapy

With the prediction of esophageal cancer for local progression and with the attendant complications of failure of local control, combined modality therapy should represent an important treatment advance. Preliminary data suggest that this mode of therapy may result in an overall improvement in the treatment of this disease. Kolaric and coworkers (1976) combined bleomycin with radiation therapy in 24 consecutive patients with inoperable esophageal carcinoma. An objective response rate of 62% was noted compared with 26% in a previous group treated with radiation alone. The same investigators similarly documented improvement of response rates when doxorubicin (33% response rate alone) was combined with radiation (62% response rate) in a randomized study (Kolaric, 1977). Response durations averaged 3.2 months in the doxorubicin-treated group and 8.6 months in the patients treated with combined therapy. Finally these authors studied 31 patients in a prospective randomized trial that compared combination chemotherapy of bleomycin and doxorubicin with a similar combination with radiation (Kolaric et al., 1980). Only 3 of 16 patients (19%) in the former group responded compared with 3 complete responses and 6 partial responses (60% total response rate) in the combined modality group. Only one study to date has not produced a significant difference in response rates when comparing chemotherapy with combined modality therapy (Earle et al., 1980).

The improved response rates seen with combined modality treatment have raised the question of whether initial chemotherapy and radiation would improve the results of subsequent surgery. Leichman and colleagues devised a program of initial radiation therapy and chemotherapy with cis-platinum and 5-FU followed by surgery. Seven of 11 patients treated in this manner were tumor free at the time of operation (Leichman et al., 1981). Although the results are preliminary, the data suggest that the ability to resect the primary tumor may be enhanced by prior combination therapy. In addition, Kelsen and coworkers (1982) reported their results with preoperative chemotherapy. Twenty-three of 28 patients treated with cis-platinum, vindesine, and bleomycin preoperatively had resectable tumors. Fifteen patients underwent resections with curative intent. All patients received postoperative radiation. Although these results are preliminary and survival data are not yet available, the results are encouraging when compared with historical series. Given the known response rates of advanced esophageal cancer to chemotherapy and radiation and the early results of these two trials, such combined modality approaches to this tumor seem most reasonable and in need of further study.

GASTRIC CANCER

Gastric cancer represents the sixth leading cause of cancer mortality in the American male (Silverberg, 1982). A dramatic decrease in the incidence of the disease has occured since 1930, when gastric malignancy was the leading cause of cancer death in the United States. In the last decade, we have learned that carcinoma of the stomach is the most responsive gastrointestinal adenocarcinoma tract to chemotherapy. Several drugs are active. The benefit of combination chemotherapy in advanced disease has been demonstrated by several investigators. Trials designed to evaluate the efficacy of adjuvant therapy in patients at high risk for relapse after surgery are well under way.

Single Agent Therapy

5-FU, the most extensively evaluated single agent, has an objective response rate of approximately 20% (Comis and Carter, 1974). Mitomycin-C has also been demonstrated to have definite activity. Response rates of 15 to 30% have been reported in a collective series of more than 200 evaluable patients (Comis and Carter, 1974). However, response durations are relatively short (12 to 24 weeks). Initial concern about the potential for late and prolonged bone marrow suppression with mitomycin-C has largely been alleviated by altering the frequency of drug administration. Improved hematologic tolerance with maintenance of therapeutic efficacy has been demonstrated with the drug given every 6 to 8 weeks instead of more frequently.

Doxorubicin appears to be the most active single agent in gastric cancer. Response rates ranging from 22 to 36% have been reported in three independent trials (Gastrointestinal Tumor Study Group, 1979; Moertel, 1976; Moertel and Lavin, 1979). Unfortunately, the median duration of response is relatively short at approximately 4 months. The nitrosoureas, in particular BCNU and methyl CCNU, seem at best to have marginal activity with response rates of less than 20% (Kovach et al., 1974; Moertel et al., 1976). Hydroxyurea, DTIC, mechlorethamine, and chlorambucil also have only marginal efficacy (Goldsmith et al., 1972; Hurley et al., 1961; Moore et al., 1968). Recently, the folate antagonist triazinate has been demonstrated to have activity; the Gastrointestinal Tumor Study Group (GITSG) has reported responses in 4 of 19 patients with advanced measurable gastric cancer (Bruckner, 1982).

Combination Therapy

Several trials of combination chemotherapy have been reported and are summarized in Table 1. Combinations of 5-FU and a nitrosourea have been extensively evaluated. In a randomized phase III trial, 5-FU plus BCNU was compared with each drug used alone (Kovach et al., 1974). The combination produced a 41% objective response rate compared with 29% for 5-FU and 17% for BCNU. The median survival for patients treated with the combination regimen was 7 months and was not significantly longer than with single agent therapy. However, the combination achieved a statistically significant survival benefit at 18 months, with 27% of patients alive who received 5-FU plus BCNU. Subsequently, the ECOG reported its experience in 146 previously untreated patients comparing 5-FU plus methyl-CCNU with methyl-CCNU alone (Moertel et al., 1976). The combination regimen again produced a significantly superior response rate; namely, 40% versus 8%. Unfortunately, three more recent

TABLE 1. Combination Chemotherapy Regimens in Gastric Cancer

Drug regimen	Number of responses/ number of patients	Response rate (%)	Reference
5-FU + BCNU	14/34	41	Kovach et al., 1974
5-FU + methyl-CCNU	12/30	40	Moertel et al., 1976
	12/49	24	Moertel and Lavin, 1979
	6/29	21	O'Connell et al., 1980
	1/18	6	Baber et al., 1976
5-FU + mitomycin-C + cytosine arabinoside	15/27	55	Kazua et al., 1972
	6/16	38	DeJager et al., 1974
	3/18	17	Gastrointestinal Tumour Study Group, 1979
5-FU + adriamycin + mitomycin-C	6/11	55	Bitran et al., 1979
	26/62	42	MacDonald et al., 1980
	8/20	40	Panettiere and Heilbrun, 1979
5-FU + mitomycin-C	17/53	32	Moertel and Lavin, 1979
5-FU + adriamycin + methyl-CCNU	7/15	47	Moertel and Lavin, 1979
	8/22	36	Lacave et al., 1979
5-FU + adriamycin + cis-platinum	10/35	29	Woolley et al., 1981

trials have raised questions concerning the efficacy of 5-FU in combination with a nitrosourea. Response rates of less than 25% with no apparent survival benefit over single agent therapy have been recorded in studies of the GITSG (Gastrointestinal Tumor Study Group, 1979; O'Connell et al., 1980) and the Southeast Oncology Group (Baker et al., 1963).

The Japanese initiated combination chemotherapy trials using mitomycin-C shortly after demonstrating its single agent activity. In 1972 a 55% response rate in 27 patients treated with 5-FU, mitomycin-C, and cytosine arabinoside was reported. However, the median duration of response was less than 4 months and a survival advantage was not apparent (Kazua et al., 1972). Subsequent trials have produced more modest remission rates. DeJager and coworkers (1974) reported responses in 6 of 16 patients (38%) treated with an identical program. The GITSG (1979) using a modified dosing schedule, reported 3 responses in 18 patients.

The combination of 5-FU, doxorubicin (Adriamycin) and mitomycin-C (FAM) developed at the Vincent T. Lombardi Cancer Center at Georgetown University has been shown to be an active regimen in the treatment of gastric cancer. In a phase II trial in 62 previously untreated patients with measurable metastatic disease, an objective response rate of 42% was achieved. Responding patients showed a significant survival advantage over nonresponders; 12.5 months versus only 3.5 months. In general, the regimen was well tolerated, with moderate myelosuppression being the major toxicity (MacDonald et al., 1980).

The activity of FAM in gastric cancer has subsequently been confirmed. Bitran and colleagues (1979) reported a 55% response rate in 11 patients. A Southwest Oncology Group study compared FAM with sequential administration of the same three agents. A 40% response rate was seen in 20 patients treated with FAM in the conventional schedule. Only 24% of the patients treated with the sequential schedule responded, indicating the importance of drug scheduling when using this regimen (Panettiere and Heilbrun, 1979). Similarly, Bunn and colleagues (1978) reported only an 11% response rate in 18 patients treated with a sequential four-drug combination of 5-FU and methyl CCNU followed 4 weeks later by doxorubicin and mitomycin-C. Karlin and coworkers (1980) evaluated the combination of FAM plus methyl CCNU. This FAMMe regimen produced an objective response rate of 42%, and the authors concluded that the addition of methyl CCNU did not improve on the results of FAM alone.

Other combinations have also been investigated. In a randomized prospective trial, the GITSG reported a 47% objective response rate with a combination of 5-FU, doxorubicin, and methyl CCNU (FAMe) versus a 17% rate with 5-FU, methyl CCNU, and cytosine arabinoside and a 24% response rate with Adriamycin alone. Patients treated with the FAMe combination showed a statistically significant improvement in survival comparison with the other groups (Moertel and Lavin, 1979). Finally Lacave and Brugarolas in Spain have published confirmatory evidence of the superiority of doxorubicin-containing regimens. In a randomized prospective trial, an objective response was obtained in 36% of patients with FAMe compared with a 9% response rate with 5-FU and methyl-CCNU (Lacave et al., 1979). These data strongly suggest that the inclusion of doxorubicin in combination chemotherapy regimens for gastric cancer is essential if the best response rates are to be obtained.

Recently, triazinate (Bakers antifol), an inhibitor of dihydrofolate reductase, was shown to have activity in gastric cancer (Bruckner et al., 1978). With this information, we have added triazinate to the standard FAM schedule in an attempt to improve response rates in patients with metastatic disease. The triazinate is given 1 hour before the 5-FU to take advantage of the potential interaction between antifols and pyrimidines. To date, 12 patients have been treated and three responses have been observed (unpublished data).

Combined Modality Therapy

In a compilation of data from several studies, Comis evaluated the role of surgery in nearly 9000 cases of gastric cancer. Of 4587 patients considered to have resectable tumors preoperatively, 33% had evidence of residual disease after surgery (1982). Similarly, in a retrospective review of Mayo Clinic cases, Moertel (1969) classified 64 of 284 cases of gastric cancer as regional in terms of extent of disease. In addition, other patients with gastric cancer will not be surgical candidates because of local spread or involvement of adjacent organs despite the absence of distant metastases. In these subsets of patients, the entire extent of tumor can often be encompassed in a single radiation port with only minimal potential toxicity to adjacent organs such as liver and kidney. These patients can be classified as having locally unresectable or locally advanced gastric cancer provided that the radiation port is no larger than 20 cm^2 (Schein et al., 1982).

Several studies have suggested that these patients may benefit from a combined modality approach using both radiation and chemotherapy. In 1969, Moertel and colleagues reported the results of a randomized trial comparing radiation therapy with and without sensitization with 5-FU in patients with locally advanced gastric cancer. Radiation therapy alone showed no benefit in terms of patient survival when compared with an historical control group that received supportive care only. Radiation plus 5-FU given during the first 3 days of therapy produced only a small increase in median survival. However, 12% of patients in the combination modality arm were alive at 5 years. No patients who received radiation alone survived longer than 18 months (Moertel et al., 1969).

Subsequently, the GITSG designed a trial to further clarify the roles of chemotherapy and radiation therapy in the subset of patients with locally advanced disease. Patients were prospectively randomized to receive either chemotherapy alone (5-FU plus methyl-CCNU) or a combination of radiation therapy with 5-FU sensitization followed by 5-FU plus methyl CCNU. An initial review of the study indicated that the chemotherapy arm was superior to the combined modality arm with 1 year survival at 68% versus 44%, respectively. In addition, patients treated with the combined modality program experienced significantly more toxicity (Schein and Childs, 1978). However, a more recent analysis after longer follow-up has demonstrated a late survival benefit for the radiation plus chemotherapy group. A plateau in survival at approximately 20% has developed after 2 to 3 years in the combined modality group. In contrast, the chemotherapy alone group has showed a continued probability of late relapse and death (GITSB, 1982). Hematologic and nutritional complications were higher in the combined modality group and may have contributed to the poorer survival during the first year of therapy. A closer monitoring of blood counts and more aggressive nutritional support might improve prognosis. In addition, the delay in initiation of chemotherapy in the patients treated with radiation first may have allowed for early progression of occult metastatic disease.

Nonetheless, the improved long-term survival in the group of patients receiving combined modality therapy suggests an important role for this approach in patients with locally advanced tumors. At the Vincent T. Lombardi Cancer Research Center, we have incorporated FAM with radiation in locally advanced upper-gastrointestinal malignancies. One cycle of FAM is followed by split-course irradiation with 5-FU sensitization to a total of 4500 rad. After a brief interval, FAM is resumed to complete six additional cycles. Twenty-one patients with locally advanced gastric cancer have been treated. On preliminary analysis, the median survival is in excess of 13 months in this group (Schein, 1983). This encouraging result needs further confirmation in prospectively randomized comparative studies.

PANCREATIC CANCER

Adenocarcinoma of the pancreas has shown a steadily increasing incidence in the United States over the past 4 decades (Silverberg, 1982). Surgery remains the only therapeutic modality with curative potential, but less than 15% of cases will be candidates for resection because of the extent of the tumor (Gudjonsson et al., 1979). Even with "curative" surgery, the 5-year survival is less than 5% (Carter and Comis, 1975; Gudjonsson et al., 1979). Only in the past decade have systematic evaluations of other treatment modalities been performed.

Single Agent Therapy

5-FU has been the most extensively evaluated single agent. Although response rates varying from 5 to 67% have been reported, a 15 to 25% response rate is generally accepted as valid (Carter and Comis, 1975; Hurley and Ellison, 1960). The duration of response has been short (2 to 4 months), and no evidence exists that 5-FU prolongs survival. Mitomycin-C has been reported to have activity comparable to 5-FU (MacDonald et al., 1977). A review of the literature showed a 27% response rate in 44 patients collected from several small trials (Carter and Comis, 1975). The nitrosoureas are relatively inactive in pancreatic carcinoma. BCNU produced no responses in 31 patients (Moertel, 1973). Moertel and coworkers (1976) recorded 2 responses in 15 patients treated with methyl-CCNU, while ECOG reported only a 9% response rate in 34 patients (Douglass et al., 1976). In contrast, streptozotocin, a naturally occurring methyl-nitrosourea, does seem to have moderate activity (Broder and Carter, 1971; DuPriest et al., 1975; Stolinsky, 1972). A collective response rate of 36% (8/22) has been reported in a review of the literature (Carter and Comis, 1975).

The GITSG has recently completed a series of phase II trials in an attempt to identify additional drugs with single agent activity in pancreatic carcinoma (Schein et al., 1978). Doxorubicin produced 2 partial responses in 15 previously untreated patients and no responses in 10 patients who had previously received chemotherapy. Methotrexate and actinomycin D were found to have minimal activity. The GITSG evaluated ICRF-159, B-deoxytheoguanosine, and galactitol and found no evidence of significant activity (Kaplan, 1978). Alkylating agents have been evaluated in only a small number of patients without evidence of substantial activity (Horton, 1980; Hurley et al., 1961; Solom et al., 1963; Wintrobe and Huguley, 1948).

Combination Chemotherapy

Despite the identification of only a small number of active single agents, there has been continued interest in combination chemotherapy for pancreatic carcinoma (see Table 2). Kovach and colleagues (1974) randomized 82 patients between treatement with 5-FU, BCNU, and a combination of the two. An objective response was recorded in 30% of patients treated with the combination regimen, 16% treated with 5-FU alone, and 0% treated with BCNU. However, no survival differences could be shown among the three groups. Lokich and Skarin (1972) noted similar results with four responses in 15 patients receiving 5-FU and BCNU.

TABLE 2. Combination Chemotherapy in Pancreatic Cancer

Drug regimen	Number of responses/ number of patients	Response rate (%)	Reference
5-FU + BCNU	10/30	33	Moertel and Lavin, 1979
	4/15	27	Lokich and Skarin, 1972
5-FU + MeCCNU		17	Buroker et al., 1978
	3/15	19	O'Connell et al., 1980
		10	Horton, 1980
5-FU + mitomycin-C		30	Burober et al., 1978
5-FU + streptozotocin		21	Aberhalden, 1977
Streptozotocin +	10/23	43	Wiggans et al., 1978
mitomycin-C + 5-FU	7/22	32	Aberhalden, 1977
5-FU + adriamycin	10/27	37	Smith, 1980
+ mitomycin-C	6/15	40	Bitran et al., 1979

The combination of 5-FU and methyl-CCNU has produced response rates of 15 to 20% in several trials (Buroker et al., 1978; O'Connell et al., 1980). Buroker and coworkers (1978) reported a 30% rate of tumor regression with 5-FU plus mitomycin-C.

In 1974, we initiated a phase II trial of combination chemotherapy with streptozotocin, mitomycin-C, and 5-FU (SMF) (Wiggans et al., 1978). Twenty-three consecutive cases with advanced measurable disease were entered into this trial. Ten of 23 (43%) achieved an objective response, with one patient demonstrating a complete remission with regression of biopsy proven hepatic metastases. The responders demonstrated a median survival of 10 months as compared with 3 months for the nonresponders. The median survival for all cases was 6 months. Four of 23 patients (17%) lived one year or longer. In a randomized study, Aberhalden and coworkers have obtained similar results with objective responses in 7 of 22 patients (32%) treated with a modified SMF regimen. Three complete responses were reported. A combination of 5-FU and streptozotocin showed a 21% response rate (Aberhalden et al., 1977). Subsequently, we initiated a pilot study of 5-FU, doxorubicin (Adriamycin), and mitomycin-C (FAM) (Smith et al, 1980). Ten of 27 patients (37%) with advanced measurable disease had an objective response. The median survival of responding patients was 12 months, compared with 3.5 months for nonresponders. The median survival of all patients was 6 months. This experience has been confirmed by Bitran and coworkers (1979), who reported responses in 6 of 15 patients.

Bruckner and colleagues (1978, 1980) have published preliminary reports on the use of hexamethylmelanine, mitomycin-C and 5-fluorouracil (Hex-MF) in 15 patients with pancreatic cancer. Six (40%) had objective tumor regression, and the median survival for the entire group is reported to be in excess of 42 weeks, longer than that observed in past series.

A controlled, prospective randomized study of chemotherapy in unresectable pancreatic cancer has been reported by Mallinson and coworkers (1980). Forty patients were randomized either to be followed with supportive care or to be treated with a combination of cyclyphosphamide, 5-fluorouracil, vincristine, and methotrexate followed by maintenance with 5-fluorouracil and mitomycin-C. The 21 treated patients had a median survival of 44 weeks, compared with 9 weeks for the control group, a highly significant difference ($P = .0006$). Although no objective tumor measurements were undertaken, symptomatic improvement appeared to be achieved more frequently in the treated group. In analyzing their study, the authors demonstrate a reasonable balance of age, sex, disease localization, and duration of symptoms prior to diagnosis. They do not analyze for location of the primary tumor nor for performance status—two potentially important prognostic factors.

In this trial, the patient numbers were small; the possible contribution of 125 patient-visits in the treated group compared with 38 in the control was not taken into account; the lack of assessment of tumor regression rate and its impact on the very good survival (44 weeks) leaves open to question the activity of the drug regimen; and, as previously mentioned, an analysis of additional potentially important prognostic factors should have been performed. This should therefore be viewed as an important first step in attempting to confirm the efficacy of chemotherapy for inoperable pancreatic cancer.

Combined Modality Therapy

As is the case with gastric cancer, a significant number of patients with pancreatic cancer present with locally advanced disease not amenable to surgical cure but without evidence of distant metastases. In a review of 5075 cases of primary pancreatic malignancies, Baylor and Berg (1973) found that 29% of adenocarcinomas either were confined to the pancreas or involved regional nodes or adjacent organs. Similarly, Moertel (1969) reported that 67 of 145 patients with pancreatic cancer had regional disease only. Initial results with radiation therapy alone in patients without distant metastases have been disappointing, with little or no benefit in comparison with supportive care only. A potential benefit for combined modality therapy was first supported by a Mayo Clinic study (Moertel et al, 1979). Split-course radiation therapy to a total of 3500 to 4000 rad with 5-FU sensitization was compared with radiation therapy alone. No improvement in survival was observed in the radiation alone arm when compared with historical controls. However, the combined modality group showed an improvement in mean survival (10.4 months versus 6.3 months without 5-FU) but not median survival.

Subsequently, the GITSG (1979) evaluated the role of higher dose split-course radiation therapy. Patients were prospectively randomized to receive either 6000 rad, 6000 rad with 5-FU sensitization followed by weekly 5-FU, or 4000 rad with 5-FU. Median and 1-year survival in the combined modality arms was statistically superior to the radiation alone arm. In addition in the combined modality groups, median survival was somewhat longer in patients receiving 6000 rad plus 5-FU (39 versus 31 weeks). However, this difference is not statistically significant. ($P = .09$), and the survival curves overlapped at 60 weeks of follow up.

To further address the problem of local control, we studied fast neutron therapy for locally advanced pancreatic cancer. Fast neutrons have a theoretical advantage over conventional photon irradiation in that the oxygen enhancement ratio is small, namely, oxygen is not required for maximal effectiveness. Consequently, neutrons may be more effective for deep-seated anoxic tumors in the pancreas (Catterall, 1974). Seventeen patients were treated with 1716 rad of 15 MEV fast neutrons with and without 5-FU sensitization. In a retrospective comparison with the GITSG study, no survival advantage could be demonstrated while toxicity in terms of hemorrhagic gastritis was considerable (MacDonald et al., 1978). Newer techniques including I-125 implantation at time of surgery (Shipley, 1980) and intraoperative radiation (Wood et al., 1982) are currently being investigated. Results including response rates and patient survival are not yet available.

With the demonstration of activity of FAM chemotherapy in metastatic pancreatic cancer, this combination was tested in 17 patients with locally advanced disease (Smith, 1981). The results of chemotherapy alone appeared comparable to those of the combined modality treatment of the GITSG (1979). The median survival of all patients was 8 months. Distant metastases were seen in only one third of patients evaluated; local progression accounted for 75% of treatment failures. As a result, we have now treated 21 patients with FAM-radiation-FAM as described for locally advanced gastric cancer. Although the analysis is preliminary, a median survival in excess of 13 months has been observed and treatment tolerance appears acceptable (Schein, 1983).

COLORECTAL CANCER

Colorectal cancer is the second leading cause of cancer death in the United States. In excess of 123,000 new cases are now diagnosed each year. Almost 50% of patients will develop disseminated disease within 5 years of diagnosis. Despite extensive investigations of chemotherapy, little progress has been made over the last 30 years, and nearly all patients who develop recurrent or metastatic colon cancer will die of their disease.

Single Agent Therapy

More than 40 chemotherapeutic agents have been evaluated in the treatment of colon cancer. However, only three classes of drugs have been shown to have definite, albeit limited, activity: the fluorinated pyrimidines, the nitrosoureas, and mitomycin-C (Heal and Schein, 1977).

Since its introduction in 1957, 5-FU has been extensively evaluated. Currently it provides the basis for standard chemotherapy in this disease (Moertel et al., 1969). In a review of the world literature, Wasserman and colleagues (1975) were able to show an overall response rate of only 21% in more than 2000 patients treated with 5-FU. Multiple investigations have examined various dosages and routes and schedules of administration to determine the most efficacious manner of using this drug. The routine of administration appears to be important. Originally, given the frequency of liver metastases in colon cancer, it was theorized that oral 5-FU might be more effective because of delivery by the portal circulation. In randomized studies, however, investigators have documented higher response rates with intravenous therapy as compared with oral administration (Ansfield et al., 1977; Bateman et al., 1975; Hahn et al., 1975). Erratic gastrointestinal absorption may well account for these differences.

In addition, high loading doses (for example 15 mg/kg/day for 5 consecutive days) and continuous infusions have been compared with the more standard weekly intravenous injections. In general, small increases in response rates have been found with the more aggressive regimens. However, patient survival does not appear to be improved and toxicity is usually more severe (Ansfield et al., 1977; Jacob et al., 1971; Leone, 1974; Moertel et al., 1969; Seifert et al., 1975). Overall, there appears to be little reason to favor the more aggressive schedules.

Trials are underway to investigate novel approaches to the administration of 5-FU. Machover and colleagues have studied the combination of 5-FU with high-dose folinic acid. Their rationale is based on biochemical and cell culture studies that demonstrate that high levels of intracellular folates may increase the cytotoxic effects of pyrimidines on thymidylate synthetase. A preliminary report is encouraging, with objective responses occuring in 56% of previously untreated patients and 21% of previously treated patients (Machover et al., 1982).

Other investigations have evaluated the sequential administration of methotrexate followed by 5-FU because of cell culture and animal tumor models that suggest a cytotoxic synergism with this sequence. Two explanations for the synergism have been proposed. Pretreatment with methotrexate has been shown to increase intracellular levels of 5-FU and its nucleotide derivitives. 5-FU is then incorporated into RNA. The enhanced cytotoxicity of the methotrexate-5-FU sequence is explained by the increased incorporation of 5-FU into RNA rather than by the binding of 5-FU to thymidylate synthetase (Benz and Cadman, 1981; Cadman et al., 1979). Alternatively, other investigators propose that treatment with methotrexate increases intracellular levels of dihydrofolates by blocking the action of dihydrofolate reductase. The high levels of DHF result in a tighter binding of 5-FU to thymidylate synthetase. The increased cytotoxicity is a result of this binding (Fernandez and Bertino, 1980). Clinical data regarding the sequential administration of methotrexate and 5-FU are preliminary and contradictory. Weinerman and colleagues (1982) reported a 42% response rate in a group of 29 patients, some of whom had received previous chemotherapy. However, we have observed only one response in 16 previously untreated patients given methotrexate and 5-FU in the same sequence (Cantrell et al., 1982).

The nitrosoureas have been demonstrated to have some activity in colon cancer. The experience is greatest with methyl-CCNU, and a response rate of approximately 15% has been reported (Moertel, 1975). In one controlled trial, MeCCNU was found to be comparable to 5-FU (Moertel, 1973). Methyl-nitrosoureas such as streptozotocin and chlorozotocin also have been demonstrated to have marginal activity (response rates less than 20%) (Horton et al., 1975; Hoth et al., 1978; Moertel, 1971).

Numerous other agents have been investigated in colon cancer. Only mitomycin-C has been shown to be even marginally effective, with reported response rates of 12 to 16% (Moertel, 1975; Wasserman, 1975). Agents with minimal or no activity include cyclophosphamide, methotrexate, L-PAM, adriamycin, hydroxyurea, vincristine, and several experimental agents (Bedikian et al., 1980, 1981; Carrol et al., 1980; Mitchell et al., 1981; Nair et al., 1980; Padilla, 1978; Wasserman, 1975).

Combination Chemotherapy

Combination chemotherapy of metastatic colorectal carcinoma thus far has not been proved superior to single agent 5-FU. Initial studies of the combination of 5-FU and methyl CCNU either alone (Posey and Morgan, 1977), with vincristine (MOF) (Falkson and Falkson, 1976; Moertel et al., 1975), or with vincristine and streptozotocin (MOF-strep) (Kemeny, 1978) reported response rates of 35% or better. Unfortunately, these results have not stood the test of time. The ECOG recently published the results of their trials with combination chemotherapy; 5-FU plus MeCCNU; 5-FU plus methyl-CCNU plus DTIC; and 5-FU plus MeCCNU plus vincristine plus DTIC were all tested. Response rates in the four regimens ranged from 9 to 18%. No statistical differences were found in either response rates or patient survival (Engstrom et al., 1982). The GITSG has reported their results with the MOF-strep regimen in previously untreated patients with good performance status. A response rate of only 9% was recorded (Smith et al., 1982). Other investigators have similarly reported disappointing results with combination chemotherapy (Lokich et al., 1977; Weitz, 1983). At this time, it appears that little progress has been made in the chemotherapy of colorectal carcinoma since the introduction of 5-FU. New effective agents will have to be identified before response rates and patient survival improve. All new agents introduced into clinical trials should be tested in this disease in the hope of finding more effective therapy.

CONCLUSION

Modest but significant advances have been made in the chemotherapeutic and combined modality treatment of advanced gastric and pancreatic cancer over the past decade. These treatment programs are now being evaluated in adjuvant trials with encouraging preliminary results.

In metastatic gastric and pancreatic cancer, future studies should be directed to refining and improving combination chemotherapy regimens. This goal will necessitate phase II studies of new antineoplastic agents, an often tedious but necessary exercise. In designing future studies, consideration should be given to the exploration of pharmacologic interactions, such as that of 5-fluorouracil with leucovorin. For locally advanced upper gastrointestinal malignancies, combined modality studies with combination chemotherapy plus radiation therapy are to be encouraged.

In contrast to the upper gastrointestinal tumors, little impact has been made on the chemotherapy of large bowel cancer. Consequently, the major thrust in advanced cancer must entail phase II studies of new agents (or novel methods of delivery) to find active drugs for this disease (see Chapter 10 of this book by Ensminger and Gyves).

REFERENCES

Aberhalden, RT, Bukowski, RM, Groope, CW, et al. (1977) Streptozotocin (STZ) and 5-FU with and without mitomycin-C (Mito) in the treatment of pancreatic adenocarcinoma. Proc Am Soc Clin Oncol 18:301.

Ansfield R, Klotz J, Nealon T, et al. (1977) A phase III study comparing the clinical utility of four regimens of 5-FU. Cancer 39:34-40.

Baker LH, Talley RW, Matter R, et al. (1976) Phase III comparison of the treatment of advanced gastrointestinal cancer with bolus weekly 5-FU vs methyl-CCNU plus bolus weekly 5-FU. Cancer 38:1-7.

Bateman J, Irwin L, Pugh N, et al. (1975) Comparison of intravenous and oral administration of 5-FU for colorectal cancer. Proc Am Soc Clin Oncol 16:24.

Baylor SM, Berg JW (1973) Cross classification and survival characteristics of 5000 cases of cancer of the pancreas. J Surg Oncol 5:335-358.

Bedikian AY, Valdivieso M, Maroun F, et al. (1980) Evaluation of vindesine and MER in colorectal cancer. Cancer 46:463-467.

Bedikian AY, Stroehlein FR, Karlin DA, et al. (1981) Clinical evaluation of Aziridinyl benzoquinone (AZQ, NSC 182986) in patients with advanced colorectal cancer. Proc Am Soc Clin Oncol. 22:452.

Benz C, Cadman E (1981) Modulation of 5-FU metabolism and cytotoxicity by antimetabolite pretreatment of human colorectal adenocarcinoma. Cancer Res 41:994-999.

Bitran JD, Desser RK, Kozloff MF, et al. (1979) Treatment of metastatic pancreatic and gastric adenocarcinomas with 5-FU, Adriamycin, and mitomycin C (FAM). Cancer Treat Rep 63:2049-2051.

Bonadonna G, DeLena M, Monfaridine S, et al. (1972) Clinical trials with bleomycin in solid tumours. Eur J Cancer Clin Oncol 8:205-215.

Broder LE, Carter SK (1971) Streptozotocin: Clinical brochure. Therapy Evaluation Program, National Cancer Institute, Bethesda, Maryland.

Bruckner HW, Ambinder E, Storch JA et al. (1978) Useful new combination of hexamethylmelamine, 5-fluorouracil infusion and mitomycin-C or MeCCNU. Clin Res 26:431A.

Bruckner HW, Storch J, Chamberlin K, et al. (1980) Combination chemotherapy for pancreatic cancer. Proc Am Soc Clin Oncol 21:420.

Bruckner HW, Lokich J, Stablein D (1982) Studies of Baker's antifol, methotrexate and razoxane in advanced gastric cancer: GITSG report. Cancer Treatm Rep 66:1713-1717.

Bunn PA, Nugent J, Ihde DC, et al. (1978) 5-FU, methyl CCNU (MeCCNU), Adriamycin and mitomycin-C in advanced gastric cancer. Proc Am Soc Clin Oncol. 19:358.

Buroker T, Kin PN, Heilbrun L, et al. (1978) 5-FU infusion with mitomycin-C (MMC) vs 5-FU infusion with methyl-CCNU (ME) in the treatment of advanced upper gastrointestinal cancer. Proc Am Soc Clin Oncol. 19:310.

Cadman E, Heimer R, Davis L (1979). Enhanced 5-FU nucleotide formation after methotrexate administration: Explanation for drug synergism. Science 205:1135-1137.

Cantrell JE, Burchet R, et al. (1982) Phase II study of sequential methotrexate, 5-FU therapy in advanced measurable colorectal cancer. Cancer Treatm Rep 66:1563-1565.

Carrol DC, Gralla RJ, Kemeny NE (1980) Phase II evaluations of N-(phosphonacetyl-L-aspartic acid (PALA) in patients with advanced colorectal carcinoma. Cancer Treatm Rep 64:349-351.

Carter SK, Comis RL (1975) Adenocarcinoma of the pancreas: Current therapeutic approaches, prognostic variables and criteria of response. In: Staquet, MF ed., Cancer therapy: Prognostic factors and criteria of response. New York: Raven Press, p. 237-253.

Catterall M (1974) A report of three years' fast neutron therapy from the Medical Research Council's cyclotron at Hammersmith Hospital, London. Cancer 34:91-95.

Comis RL (1982) The therapy of stomach cancer, In: Carter SK, Glatsein E, Livingston RB, eds. Principles of cancer treatment. New York: McGraw-Hill, pp. 420–426.

Comis RL, Carter SK (1974) Integration of chemotherapy into combined modality treatment of solid tumours. III Gastric cancer. Cancer Treatm Rev 1:221–238.

Davis S, Shanmugathasa M, Kessler W (1980) Cis-dichlorodiamineplatinum (11) in the treatment of esophageal carcinoma. Cancer Treatm Rep 64:709–711.

DeJager G, Magill GB, Goldberg RB, Krakoff IH (1974) Mitomycin-C 5-FU, and cytosine arabinoside (MFC) in gastrointestinal cancer. Proc Am Soc Clin Oncol 15:178.

Desai D, Gelber R, Ezdinli E, Falkson G (1979) Chemotherapy of advanced esophageal carcinoma. Proc Am Soc Clin Oncol 20:381.

DeVita VT, Hellman S, Rosenberg S (1982) Cancer principles and practice of oncology. Philadelphia: Lippincott, pp. 523–527.

Douglass HO Jr, Lavin PT, Moertel CG (1976): Nitrosureas: Useful agents for treatment of advanced gastrointestinal cancer. Cancer Treatm Rep 60:769–780.

DuPriest RW, Huntington M, Massey WH, et al. (1975) Streptozotocin therapy in cancer patients. Cancer 35:358–367.

Earle J, Gelber RD, Moertel CG, Hahn RG (1980) A controlled evaluation of combined radiation and bleomycin therapy for squamous cell cancer of the esophagus. Int J Radiat Oncol Biol Phys 6:821–826.

Engstrom PF, MacIntyre J, Douglass HO, et al. (1982) Combination chemotherapy of advanced colorectal cancer utilizing 5-FU, semustine dacarbazine, vincristine and hydroxyurea. Cancer 49:1555–1560.

Ezdinli EZ, Gelber R, Desai D, et al. (1980) Chemotherapy of advanced esophageal carcinoma: Eastern Cooperative Oncology Group experience. Cancer 46:2149–2153.

Falkson G, (1971) Methyl-GAG (NSG-32946) in the treatment of esophagus cancer. Cancer Chemother Rep 55:209–212.

Falkson G, Falkson HC (1976) fluorouracil, methyl-CCNU and vincristine in cancer of the colon. Cancer 38:1468–1470.

Fernandez DJ and Bertino JR (1980) 5-fluorouracil and methotrexate synergy: Enhancement of 5-fluorodeoxyuridylate binding to thymidylate synthetase by Dihydropteroypoly glutamates. Proc Natl Acad Sci USA 77:5663–5667.

Gastrointestimal Tumor Study Group (1979) Comparative therapeutic trial of radiation with and without chemotherapy in pancreatic carcinoma. Int J Radiat Oncol Biol Phys 5:1643–1647.

Gastrointestinal Tumor Study Group (1979): Phase II-III chemotherapy studies in advanced gastric cancer. Cancer Treatm Rep 63:1871–1876.

Gastrointestinal Tumor Study Group (1982) A comparison of combination chemotherapy and combined modality therapy for locally advanced gastric carcinoma. Cancer 49:1771–1777.

Goldsmith MA, Friedman MA, Carter SK (1972): Clinical brochure: 5-(3-3-dimethyl-1-triazeno) carboxamide (DTIC, DIC). National Cancer Institute, Bethesda, Maryland.

Gudjonsson B, Livstone EM, Spiro HM (1979) Cancer of the pancreas: Diagnostic accuracy and survival statistics. Cancer 42:2494–2506.

Hahn RJ, Moertel CG, Shutt AJ, Bruckner HW (1975) A double blind comparison of intensive 5-FU by oral vs intravenous route in the treatment of colorectal carcinoma. Cancer 35:1031–1035.

Heal JM, Schein PS (1977) Management of gastrointestinal cancer. Med Clin North Am 61:991–999.

Hentek V, Vogl EE, Kaplan BH, Greenwald E (1979) Combination chemotherapy of advanced esophageal cancer (ECa) with methotrexate (M), Bleomycin (B) and diamminedichloroplatinum (D). Proc Am Soc Clin Oncol 20:400.

Horton J, (1980) Trials of single agent and combination chemotherapy in advanced cancer of the pancreas. Proc Am Soc Clin Oncol 21:420.

Horton J, Mittelman A, Taylor SG, et al. (1975) Phase II trials with procarbazine (NSC-77213), streptozotocin (NSC-85998), 6-thioquanine (NSC-752) and CCNU (NSC-79037) in patients with metastatic cancer of the large bowel. Cancer Chemother Rep 59:333-340.

Hoth D, Butler T, Winokur S, et al. (1978) Phase II study of chlorozotocin. Proc Am Soc Clin Oncol 19:381.

Hurley JD, Ellison EH (1960) Chemotherapy of solid cancer arising from the gastrointestinal tract. Ann Surg 152:568-582.

Hurley JD, Ellison EH, Casey LL (1961) Treatment of advanced cancer of the gastrointestinal tract with antitumor agents. Gastroenterology 41:557-562.

Jacobs EM, Reeves WJ, Wood DA, et al. (1971) Treatment of cancer with weekly intravenous 5-FU. Cancer 27:1302-1305.

Kaplan RS (1978) Phase II trial of ICRF-159, B-2-deoxythioguanosine (B-2-TGdR), and galactitol (Gal) in advanced measurable pancreatic carcinoma. Proc Am Soc Clin Oncol 19:335.

Karlin DA, Pradeep SM, Heifetz LG et al. (1980) Phase I-II study of 5-fluorouracil, adriamycin, mitomycin-C, and methyl CCNU (FAMMe) chemotherapy for advanced upper gastrointestinal cancer. Proc Am Soc Clin Oncol 21:169.

Kazua O, Kurita S, Nishimura M, et al. (1972) Combination therapy with mitomycin-C (NSC 26980), 5-FU (NSC 19893) and cytosine arabinoside (NSC 63878) for advanced cancer in man. Cancer Chemother Rep 56:373-385.

Kelsen DP, Cvitkovic E, Bains M, et al. (1978) Cis-dichlorodiammineplatinum (11) and bleomycin in the treatment of esophageal carcinoma. Cancer Treatm Rep 62:1041-1046.

Kelsen DP, Bains M, Golbey R, Woodcock T (1979) Vindesine in the treatment of esophageal carcinoma. Proc Am Soc Clin Oncol 20:338.

Kelsen DP, Bains M, Hilaris B, et al. (1982) Combination chemotherapy of esophageal carcinoma using cisplatin, vindesine, and bleomycin. Cancer 49:1174-1177.

Kemeny N, Yagoda A, Goldberg R (1978) Methyl-CCNU (MeCCNU), 5 Fluorouracil (5-FU), Vincristine and Streptozotocin (MOF-STREP) for metastatic colorectal carcinoma. Proc Am Soc Clin Oncol 19:354.

Knight WA, Livingston RB, Fabian C, Costanzi J (1979) Methylglyoxal bis-guanyl-hydrozone (methyl GAG MGBG) in advanced human malignancy. Proc Am Soc Clin Oncol 20:319.

Kolaric K, Maricic Z, Dujmovic I, Roth A (1976) Therapy of advanced esophageal cancer with bleomycin, irradiation and combination of bleomycin with radiation. Tumori 62:255-262.

Kolaric K, Maricic Z, Roth A, Dujmovic I (1977) Adriamycin alone and in combination with radiotherapy in the treatment of inoperable esophageal cancer. Tumori 63:485-491.

Kolaric K, Marici Z, Roth A, Dujmovic I (1980) Combination of bleomycin and adriamycin with and without radiation in the treatment of inoperable esophageal cancer. Cancer 45:2265-2273.

Kovach JS, Moertel CG, Schutt AJ (1974) A controlled study of combined 1,3 bis (2-chloroethyl)-1-nitrosourea and 5-FU therapy for advanced gastric and pancreatic cancer. Cancer 33:563-567.

Lacave AJ, Brugarolas A, Buesa JM, et al. (1979) Methyl CCNU (Me), 5-fluorouracil (F), adriamycin (A) (MeFA) versus Me F in advanced gastric cancer. Proc Am Soc Clin Oncol 20:310.

Lad TE (1980) Platinum, mitomycin-C and bleomycin chemotherapy of esophageal carcinoma. Proc Am Soc Clin Oncol 21:419.

Leichman L, Steiger Z, Seydel HG, Haas CD (1981) Potentially curative combined modality therapy for inoperable carcinoma of the esophagus. Proc Am Soc Clin Oncol 22:458.

Leone LA (1974) The chemotherapy of colorectal cancer. Cancer 34:972-976.

Livingston RB, Carter SK, (1970) Single agents in cancer chemotherapy New York: Plenum Publishers.

Lokich JJ, Skarin AT (1972) Combination chemotherapy with 5-fluorouracil (5-FU) and 1,3-bis(2chloroethyl)-1-nitrosourea (BCNU) for disseminated gastrointestinal cancer. Cancer Chemother Rep 56:653–657.

Lokich JJ, Skarin AT, Mayer RJ, Frei E (1977) Lack of effectiveness of combined 5-FU and methyl CCNU therapy in advanced colorectal cancer. Cancer 40:2792–2796.

MacDonald JS, Widerlite L, Schein PS (1977) Biology, diagnosis and chemotherapeutic management of pancreatic malignancy. Adv Pharmacol Chemother 14:107–142.

MacDonald JS, Smith F, Ornitz R, et al. (1978) Phase I-II trial of fast neutron radiation with and without 5-fluorouracil for locally advanced pancreatic (LAP) and gastric carcinoma. Proc Am Soc Clin Oncol 19:377.

MacDonald JS, Schein PS, Woolley PV, et al. (1980) 5-FU, doxorubicin, and mitomycin-C (FAM) combination chemotherapy for advanced gastric cancer. Ann Intern Med 93:533–536.

Machover D, Schwartzenberg L, Goldschmidt E, et al. (1982) Treatment of advanced colorectal and gastric adenocarcinoma with 5-FU combined with high dose folinic acid: A pilot study. Cancer Treatm Rep 66:1803–1807.

Mallinson CN, Rade MO, Cocking B, et al. (1980): Chemotherapy in pancreatic cancer; results of a controlled prospective randomized multicenter trial. Br Med J 281:1589–1591.

Mitchell E, Killen J, Willis L, et al. (1981) Phase II studies of 1-(2-chloroethyl)-3-(2,6 dioxo-1-piperidyl) 1-nitrosourea (PCNU, NSC 95446) in colorectal carcinoma, melanoma and hypernephroma. Proc Am Soc Clin Oncol 22:455.

Moertel CJ (1969) Natural history of gastrointestinal cancer. In: Moertel CJ, Reitemeir RJ, eds., Advanced Gastrointestinal cancer/clinical management and chemotherapy. New York: Hoeber Medical Division, Harper & Row, p. 3.

Moertel CG (1973) Therapy of advanced gastrointestinal cancer with the nitrosoureas. Cancer Chemother Rep 4:27–34.

Moertel CG (1975) Clinical management of advanced gastrointestinal cancer. Cancer 36:675–682.

Moertel (1976) Chemotherapy of gastrointestinal cancer. Clin Gastroenterol 5:777–793.

Moertel CG, Lavin PT (1979) Phase II-III chemotherapy studies in advanced gastric cancer. Cancer Treatm Rep 63:1863–1869.

Moertel CG, Childs DS, Reitemeier R, et al. (1969) Combined 5-FU and supervoltage radiation therapy of locally advanced unresectable gastrointestinal cancer. Lancet 2:865–867.

Moertel CG, Mittelman JA, Bakermeier RF, et al. (1976) Sequential and combination chemotherapy of advanced gastric cancer. Cancer 38:678–682.

Moertel CG, Reitemeier RF, Hahn RG (1969) Therapy with the fluourinated pyrimidines. In: Moertel CG, Reitemeier RJ, eds., Advanced gastrointestinal cancer. New York: Hoeber Medical Division, Harper & Row, p. 86.

Moertel CG, Reitemeier RF, Schutt AJ, et al. (1971) Phase II Study of Streptozotocin (NSC 85998) in the treatment of advanced gastrointestinal cancer. Chemother Rep 55:303–307.

Moertel CG, Schutt AJ, Hahn RG, Reitemeier RJ (1975) Therapy of advanced colorectal cancer with a combination of 5-FU methyl-1,3 cis (2-chloroethyl)-1-nitrosourea and vincristine. J Nat Cancer Inst 54:69–71.

Moertel CG, Schutt AJ, Reitemeier RF, Hahn RG (1976) Therapy for gastrointestinal cancer with the nitrosoureas alone and in drug combination. Cancer Treatm Rep 60:729–732.

Moore G, Bross I, Ausman R, et al. (1968) Effects of chlorambucil (NSC3088) in 374 patients with advanced cancer. Cancer Chemother Rep 52:661–666.

Nair, KG, Moayeri H, Mittelman A (1980) A phase II study of fluorodopan in the treatment of advanced colorectal cancer. Cancer Treatm Rep 64:697–699.

O'Connell M, O'Fallen P, Lavin P, et al. (1980) A comparative assessment of combination chemotherapy in advanced gastric carcinoma. Proc Am Soc Clin Oncol 21:420.

Padilla F, Corren J, Buroker T, Vaitkevicius VK (1978) Phase II Study of Baker's antifol in advanced colorectal cancer. Cancer Treatm Rep 62:553–555.

Panettiere FJ, Heilbrun L (1979) Experience with two treatment schedules in the combination chemotherapy of advanced gastric carcinoma. In: Carter SK and Crooke CT, eds., Mitomycin-C: Current status and new developments. New York: Academic Press, pp. 145–157.

Posey LE, Morgan LR (1977) Methyl-CCNU and 5-FU in carcinoma of the large bowel. Cancer Treatm Rep 61:1453–1458.

Ravry MJ, Moore M (1980) A Phase II pilot study of Cis-platinum (11) (DDP) in advanced squamous cell esophageal carcinoma (SCE). Proc Amer Soc Clin Oncol 21:353.

Rosenbaum C, Carter SK (1970) Clinical brochure; bleomycin (NSC 125066, "bleo" BLM). National Cancer Institute, Bethesda, Maryland.

Schein PS, Childs D (1978) A controlled randomized evaluation of combined modality therapy (5000 rad, 5-FU and MeCCNU), vs 5-FU and MeCCNU alone for locally unresectable gastric cancer. Proc Am Soc Clin Oncol 19:329.

Schein PS, Lavin PT, Moertel CG, et al. (1978) Randomized phase II clinical trial of adriamycin, methotrexate and actinomycin-D in advanced measurable pancreatic carcinoma. Cancer 42:19–22

Schein PS, Smith FP, Woolley PV, Ahlgren JD (1982) Current management of advanced and locally unresectable gastric carcinoma. Cancer 50:2590–2596.

Schein, PS, Smith FP, Dritschillo A, et al. (1983) Phase I-II trial of combined modality FAM (5-fluorouracil, adriamycin and mitomycin-C) plus split course radiation (FAM-RT-FAM) for locally advanced gastric (LAG) and pancreatic (LAP) cancer: A mid-Atlantic oncology program. Proc Am Soc Clin Oncol 2;126.

Schnider BI, Colski J, Jones R, Carbone P (1974) Effectiveness of methyl GAG (NSC-32946) administered intramuscularly. Cancer Chemother Rep 58:689–695.

Seifert P, Baker LH, Reed ML (1975) Comparison of continuously infused 5-FU with bolus injection in treatment of patients with colorectal adenocarcinoma. Cancer 36:123–128.

Shipley WV, Nardi GL, Cohen AM, et al. (1980) Iodine-125 implant and external beam irradiation in patients with localized pancreatic carcinoma: A comparative study to surgical resection. Cancer 45:709–714.

Silverberg E (1982) Cancer statistics 1982. CA 32:15–31.

Smith FP, Ellenberg SS, Mayer RJ, et al. (1982) Phase II study of MOF-STREP (Methyl-CCNU, vincristine, 5-fluorouracil, streptozotocin) in advanced measurable colorectal carcinoma. A GITSG trial. Proc AACR 23:149.

Smith FP, Hoth DF, Levin B, et al. (1980) 5-FU, adriamycin and mitomycin-C (FAM) chemotherapy for advanced adenocarcinoma of the pancreas. Cancer 46:2014–2018.

Smith FP, Wooley PV, Korsmeyer S, et al. (1981) Combination chemotherapy with 5-fluorouracil, adriamycin and mitomycin-C (FAM) for locally advanced pancreatic cancer equivalence to external beam therapy and implications for future trials. Proc Am Soc Clin Oncol 17:455.

Solom J, Alexander MJ, Steinfield JL (1963): Cyclophosphamide: A clinical study. JAMA 183:165–170.

Strolinsky DC, Sadoff L, Braunwald J, Bateman JR (1972) Streptozotocin in the treatment of cancer. Cancer 30:61–67.

Wasserman TH, Comis R, Goldsmith M, et al. (1975) Tabular analysis of the clinical chemotherapy of solid tumors. Cancer Chemother Rep 6:399.

Weinerman B, Schachter B, Schipper H, et al. (1982) Sequential methotrexate and 5-FU in the treatment of colorectal cancer. Cancer Treatm Rep 66:1553–1555.

Weltz MD, Perry DJ, Blom J, Butler WM (1983) Methyl CCNU 5-fluorouracil, vincristine, and streptozotocin (MOF-STREP) in metastatic colorectal carcinoma. Clin Oncol 1:135.

Wiggans RG, Woolley PV, MacDonald JS, et al. (1978) Phase II trial of streptozotocin, mitomycin C and 5-FU (SMF) in the treatment of advanced pancreatic cancer. Cancer 41:387–391.

Wintrobe M, Huguley C (1948) Nitrogen mustard for Hodgkin's disease, lymphosarcoma, the leukemias and other disorders. Cancer 1:159–160.

Wood WC, Shipley WU, Gunderson LL, et al. (1982) Intraoperatic irradiation for unresectable pancreatic carcinoma. Cancer 49:1272–1275.

Woolley PV, Smith F, Estevez R, et al. (1981) A phase II trial of 5-FU, adriamycin and Cis-platinum (FAP) in advanced gastric cancer. Proc Am Soc Clin Oncol 21:455.

PANCREATIC CANCER IN THE HAMSTER MODEL

PARVIZ M POUR, M.D., AND TERENCE A LAWSON, PH.D.

Although there are adequate animal models for many of the most common and uncommon types of human cancer, the induction of pancreatic exocrine carcinomas similar to those in humans has proved difficult. The situation has been especially dismal because the incidence of this disease is increasing throughout the world, but its etiology is not well understood, prognosis is poor, and therapeutic attempts are largely unsuccessful. The development in our institute of a model for pancreatic tumors that closely resembles in morphologic and biologic properties the equivalent human neoplasms (Pour, 1980; Pour and Levitt, 1979; Pour and Wilson, 1980; Pour et al., 1975b) has brought much encouragement and hope for understanding the basic problems surrounding the disease. Selective tumor induction by a single dose of carcinogen has made our animal model a unique tool for studying various aspects of pancreatic cancer.

CHARACTERIZATION OF THE MODEL

There are definitive characteristics and particularities of experimental pancreatic ductal (ductular) cancer, compared with other types of induced neoplasms. The species-specificity in tumor induction is, for example, one of the more interesting and striking features of pancreatic cancer. Among the many species thus far tested, only the Syrian (golden) hamster is susceptible to pancreatic ductal (ductular) carcinogenesis (Pour and Wilson, 1980). This conceptually interesting issue has led us to investigate certain anatomic-histologic and physiologic characteristics of this species to understand the reasons for the species specificity. Anatomically, the hamster pancreas differs in certain aspects from that of other mammals (Ogrowsky et al., 1980; Takahashi et al., 1977). The

From the Eppley Institute for Research in Cancer and the Department of Pathology and Laboratory Medicine, University of Nebraska Medical Center, Omaha.

most striking anatomic feature of the organ is its λ-shape and three lobes (duodenal, gastric, and splenic), consisting of a small head and splenic and gastric lobes in retro- and anterogastric positions, respectively. There is a common duct formed by the pancreatic duct and the common bile duct. Anatomic differences seem irrelevant to the etiology and mechanism of the disease in humans and in hamsters. However, the particular relationship between the common bile and pancreatic ducts in hamsters make bile reflux impossible and may be evidence against the suggested bile reflux theory in the etiology of pancreatic cancer. Measurement of physiologic aspects surrounding the pattern of pancreatic secretion under unstimulated and secretagogue-stimulated conditions (Helgeson et al., 1980a, 1980b) indicated no marked difference between hamsters and other species; however, the reported data should be regarded as inconclusive, and more subtle studies are required for clarification.

Histologic features of the hamster pancreas do not differ from those in humans or in species unresponsive to development of pancreatic ductal (ductular) neoplasms (Pour, 1978; Pour and Wilson, 1980). Therefore, neither physiologic, anatomic, or histologic patterns appear decisive for disease development; the basic mechanisms may lie at the cellular and subcellular levels, especially those concerned with the metabolic machinery. This view is supported by the finding that specific molecular structures of the carcinogens are necessary for their pancreatic carcinogenic effect and there seem to be species differences in metabolism of these carcinogens (see below). Moreover, among the laboratory species examined, only Syrian hamsters have spontaneous pancreatic ductal (ductular) neoplasms (Pour et al., 1976, 1979a; Takahashi and Pour, 1978). This factor could account for the influence of genetic factors in development of pancreatic ductal (ductular) cancer, as previously suggested by an epidemiologic and in vitro studies (Blot et al., 1978; Danes and Lynch, 1982). Variations in the quality and quantity of some drug-metabolizing enzymes between pancreatic acinar and ductal/ductular cells in rats and hamsters (Kawabata et al., 1984) may also reflect genetic influence.

PANCREATIC CARCINOGENS AND THEIR METABOLISM

The nitrosamines that induce pancreatic ductular (ductal) neoplasms in Syrian hamsters are shown in Figure 9. Characteristic of all these carcinogens is the presence of 2-hydroxy- or 2-oxo- groups. The 2-oxo- derivatives are the more potent, but among them, *N*-nitrosobis(2-oxopropyl)-amine (BOP) is a more selective pancreatic carcinogen (Pour et al., 1978).

The metabolism of carcinogens by pancreatic cells has been demonstrated through a series of experiments. Scarpelli and coworkers (1980), as well as our own in vitro studies, showed that pancreatic tissue is capable of metabolizing carcinogens, such as *N*-nitroso-2,6-dimethyl morpholine (NDMM) and BOP, to their ultimate carcinogen, probably by a mixed function oxidase. Reznik-Schüller and coworkers (1980) demonstrated incorporation of labeled NDMM into acinar cells. However, since autoradiographic studies were performed long after injection of the radiolabeled carcinogen, one may assume that the observed labeling of the acinar cells, actively engaged in protein synthesis, may well represent the degradation (noncarcinogenic) product of the original compound. The latter possibility would mediate against Reznick's conclusion that acinar cells are the primary target of the carcinogen. Nevertheless, pancreatic ductal/ductular cells have been shown to contain specific carcinogen metabolizing enzymes (Kawabata et al., 1984), and studies in isolated pancreatic cells have revealed that ductal/ductular cells are able to metabolize BOP directly (Pour and Lawson, 1983d).

Our metabolic in vivo studies (Gingell et al., 1976, 1979; Gingell and Pour, 1978) demonstrated that BOP is metabolized to *N*-nitroso(2-hydroxypropyl) (2-oxopropyl)amine (HPOP) and *N*-nitrosobis(2-hydroxypropyl)amine (BHP). Since additional studies revealed methylation of pancreatic DNA after BOP (Lawson et al., 1981), further metabolism of HPOP or BHP to a methylating agent was obvious. 7-Methylguanine, but not O-6-methylguanine, was found in hydrolysates of pancreatic DNA (Lawson, unpublished results).

Studies on DNA damage in target tissue (pancreas), nontarget tissue (salivary gland), and intermediate tissue (liver) after BOP treatment showed extensive DNA damage in all three organs. However, whereas the damage was largely repaired in the salivary gland by 4 weeks, some DNA damage persisted in the liver and pancreas. When high BOP doses were used, considerable DNA damage was still evident in the pancreas, but not in the liver, at 6 weeks (Lawson et al., 1982). These data correlate with BOP carcinogenicity in hamsters (Pour et al., 1977a) and indicate that its tumorigenicity is probably related to DNA-methylation, which opens questions as to the nature of the methylating intermediate of the carcinogen. According to Krüger (1973), *N*-nitrosomethyl(2-oxopropyl)amine (MOP) would be the most likely proximate carcinogen. Although our original study failed to demonstrate MOP in blood and urine of BOP-treated hamsters (Pour et al., 1980a), later experiments using tissue homogenates revealed the presence of MOP in liver and pancreas soon after BOP administration (Lawson et al., 1981; Pour et al., 1981a). Since higher MOP concentrations were found in the pancreas than in the liver and because MOP was found to be an extremely potent pancreatic carcinogen (Pour et al., 1980a), it seemed conceivable that MOP was a more proximate carcinogenic metabolite of BOP, and HPOP was an intermediate metabolite. Studies to elucidate the metabolic routes to MOP from BOP are underway in our institute.

The formation of MOP as a proximate pancreatic carcinogen from BOP and other related carcinogens is an attractive process and might also explain the existing species differences in neoplastic response. Comparative studies by us (Lawson, unpublished; Pour et al., 1979c) on hamsters (responsive to BOP) and rats (nonresponsive) showed that BOP and, to a greater extent, MOP concentrate in the hamster pancreas. No concentrating effects were seen in rats for either compound. BOP metabolism in rats, rather, was directed to formation of BHP and HPOP, which are less specific and less carcinogenic to the hamster pancreas than BOP (Pour et al., 1975a). The apparent preferential synthesis of the less carcinogenic metabolites of BOP by rats correlates with BOP's overall weaker carcinogenicity in rats compared with hamsters (Pour et al., 1979c).

HISTOGENESIS OF PANCREATIC CANCER

There are three opinions concerning the histogenesis of exocrine pancreatic cancer. Some investigators point to the formation of exocrine ductal (ductular) tumors from dedifferentiated acinar cells (Bockman et al., 1978; Flaks et al.,

1980); our experience in experimental and human material (Pour, 1981; Pour and Salmasi, 1979; Pour and Wilson, 1980; Pour et al., 1982d) definitely implicates the ductal (ductular) cells of the pancreas as the tumor progenitor cells and the third group (Scarpelli and Rao, 1978; Scarpelli et al., 1983) considers both of the above-mentioned possibilities. Our view is consistent with the embryologic development of the pancreas; that is, the ductular (tubular) cells are the brickstone of both endocrine and exocrine pancreatic tissues. We are also in line with general concepts on tumor histogenesis in various other tissues, which have implicated "stem cells" as the most capable unit for proliferation and neoplasia. The mixed cellularity of neoplasms composed of cells in various stages of differentiation and of different cytologic patterns, as can be seen also in pancreatic cancer, is most consistent with this notion.

From the embryologic and phylogenetic viewpoints (Like and Orci, 1972; Pictet and Rutter, 1972), the dedifferentiation theory is difficult to understand, since it is based on the concept that during the neoplastic process the acinar

FIGURE 1. Proliferation and distention of periinsular *(left)* and intrainsular ductules. (H & E, × 195)

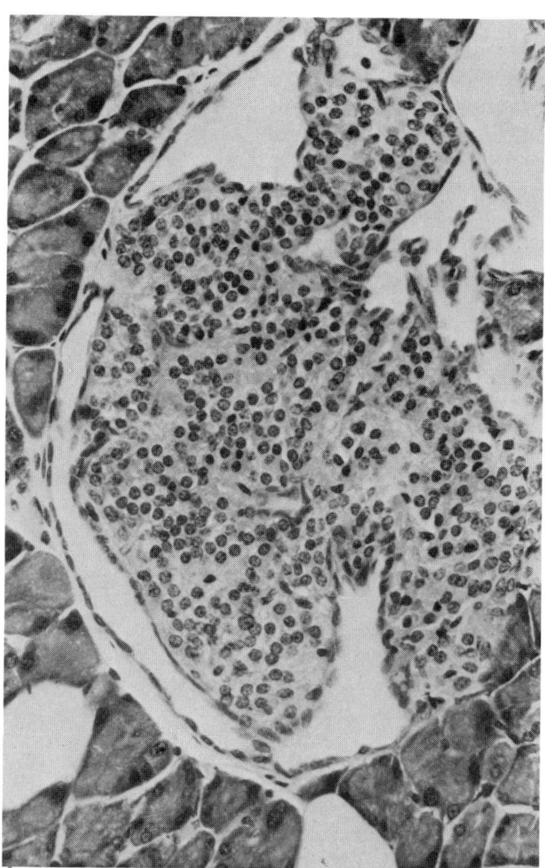

cells, which are functionally highly specialized cells, progressively change their phenotypic and genotypic characteristics to become undifferentiated ductular (tubular) cells. The latter then proliferate and differentiate toward a variety of cells, including islet cells, as will be outlined later. We know of no similar examples of experimental or human neoplasms in which development requires dedifferentiation of highly differentiated and specialized cells. We believe, with many others, that neoplasia in any organ, including the pancreas, is due to the abnormal, exaggerated growth of (stem) cells that repeat the embryonic process (Pierce and Cox, 1977).

Our studies (Pour 1978, 1980, 1981; Pour and Wilson, 1980; Pour et al., 1979b) show that peri- and intrainsular ductules, known also to occur in other species (for references see Bensley, 1911; Boquist et al., 1974; Edström and Boquist, 1973; Pour and Wilson, 1980), centroacinar cells, and cells scattered along the ducts, but especially in the ductules, represent the germinative (stem cell) unit of the pancreas (Walters, 1965). This view is further based on findings during

FIGURE 2. Distention and ramification of peri- and intrainsular ductules in a well-demarcated, partly encapsulated, and remarkably enlarged islet. (H & E, × 30)

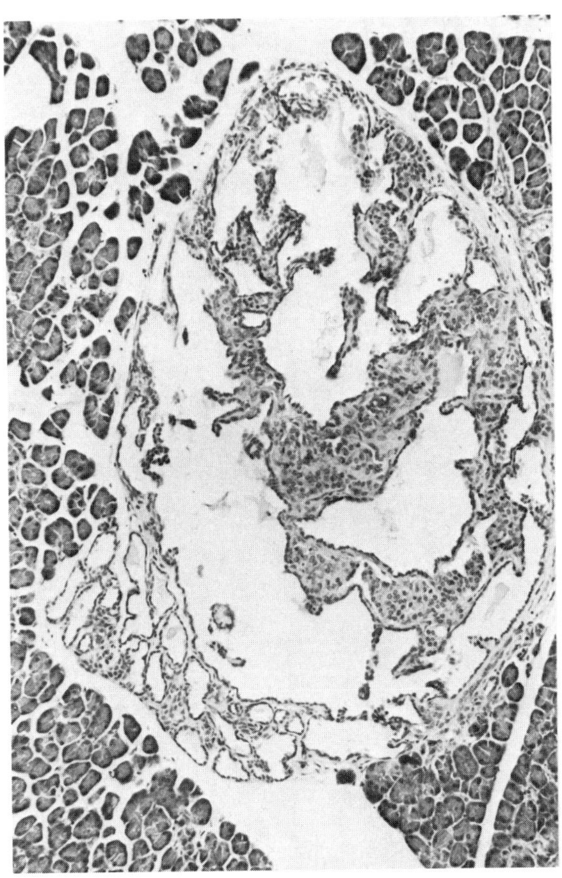

the neoplastic process, beginning with (a) proliferation of peri- and intrainsular ductular cells, leading to formation of branched and extended ductules culminating in formation of ductular adenoma (Figures 1 and 2); (b) hypertrophy and hyperplasia of centroacinar cells, resulting in occlusion of excretory channels of acini with subsequent acinar cell necrosis and their later replacement by ductular cells (Figures 3–5) and formation of pseudoductules (precursors of either adenomas or carcinomas); (c) proliferation of stem cells within the ductal epithelium, culminating in multifocal intraductal epithelial growth and resulting in development of polyps or carcinomas.

In all instances, the proliferating cells often tend to differentiate toward insular cells and retain their ability to do so even at advanced stages of carcinogenesis (Figures 6 and 7), as has also been demonstrated in human material (Schlosnagle and Campbell, 1981). In many instances, a variety of islet cells—including insulin-, glucagon-, or somatostatin-containing cells—can be identified within ductular adenomas or carcinomas. There is accumulating evidence

FIGURE 3. Ductular adenoma, which has developed within an islet. The remnant of islet cells is seen in the upper right corner. (H & E, × 195)

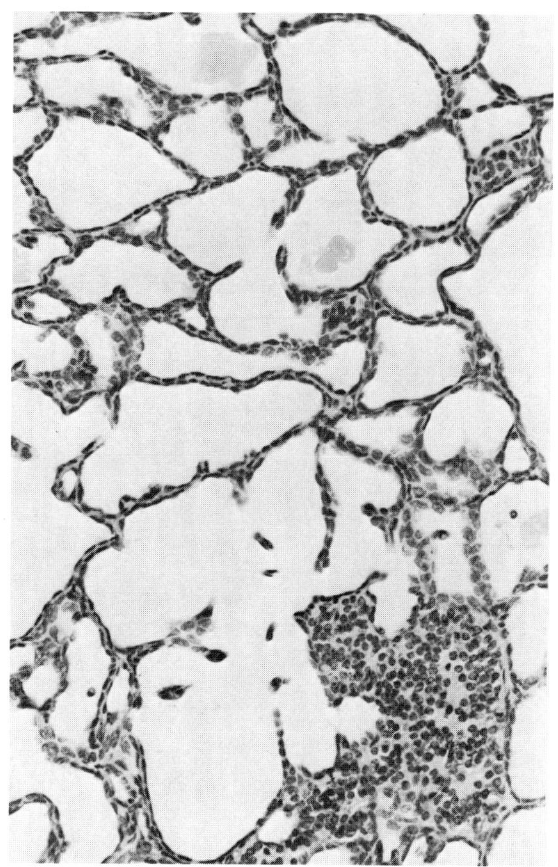

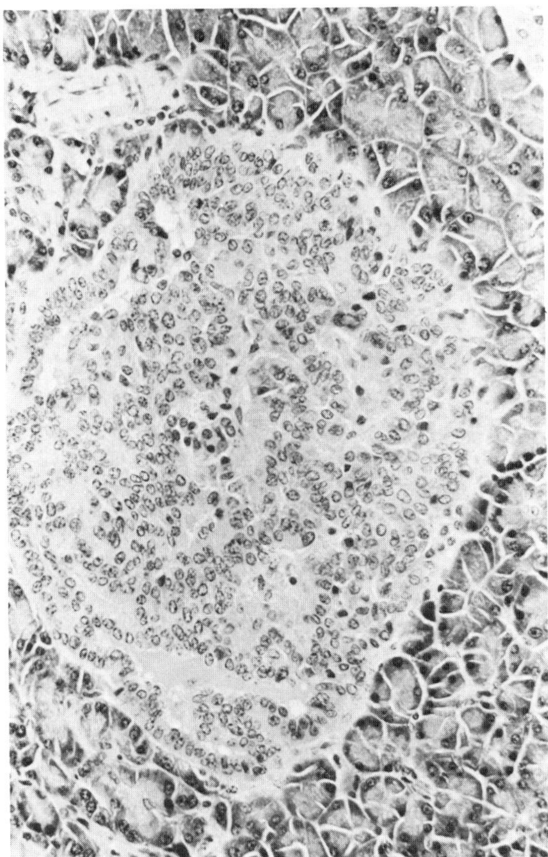

FIGURE 4. Hyperplastic, slightly distended and mucus-containing periinsular ductule extending within the islet *(top)* (H & E, × 195)

for the presence of the same and other types of endocrine cells in human exocrine pancreatic cancer (Eusebi et al., 1981; Kodama and Mori, 1983; Reid et al., 1982; Schlosnagle and Campbell, 1981). Identification of these endocrine cells in tumor metastases (Eusebi et al., 1981) also confirms our view that islet cells are an integral part of cancer. Nevertheless, the wide variety of metaplastic changes, including pyloric and goblet cell metaplasia of pancreatic ductular and ductal epithelium and formation of islet cells arising from them, reflects the enormous potential of tumor progenitor cells to differentiate and underlines our concept of the stem cells as the principal pancreatic cells for proliferation and neoplasia.

Studies such as those conducted by Flaks et al. (1980) cannot be considered conclusive for the dedifferentiation of acinar cells into ductular cells, mainly because in such experiments weekly administration of carcinogen is associated with concomitant noncarcinogenic (degeneration, regeneration) and carcinogenic processes, which can make interpretation difficult. Nevertheless, recent

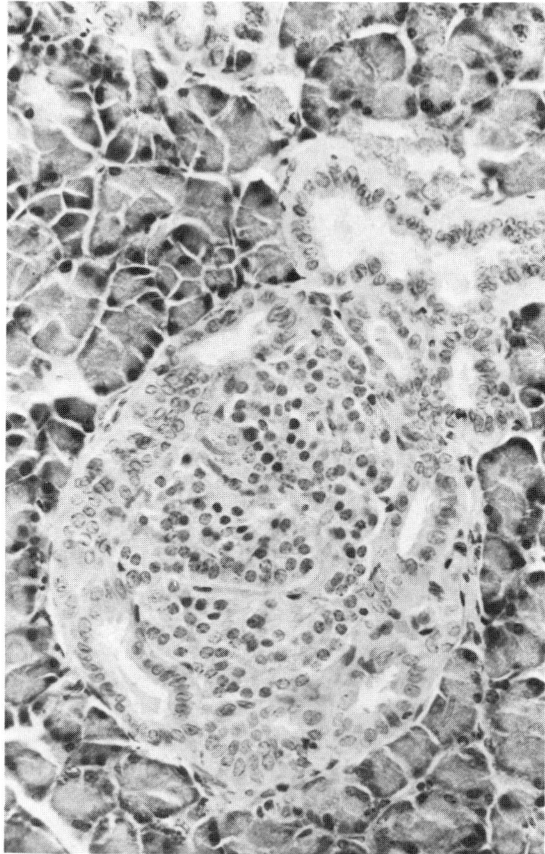

FIGURE 5. Hyperplastic periinsular ductules with focal pleomorphism of cells. (H & E, × 195)

ultrastructural studies by us and by others (Moore et al., 1983) could not confirm acinar cell dedifferentiation during pancreatic carcinogenesis.

There is other circumstantial evidence for the ductular cells as primary tumor progenitor cells:

1. Pulse labeling of pancreatic tissue by [^{3}H]thymidine after treatment with BOP showed significant labeling of ductular cells, beginning from 8 to 10 postcarcinogenic weeks. There was little or no labeling of acinar cells (Pour and Wilson, 1980; Pour et al., 1981a).
2. Remarkable ductulitis and insulitis were seen in the pancreas of hamsters bearing homologous, transplanted pancreatic carcinoma induced by BOP (Runge et al., 1978). Since many tumors retain some antigen normally present on the cell type from which they originate (Schwentker, 1934), it was thought that the host reaction to these (ductular) antigens present in large concentrations in transplanted carcinoma had elicited an immunologic reaction with formation of antibody, which could have resulted in a

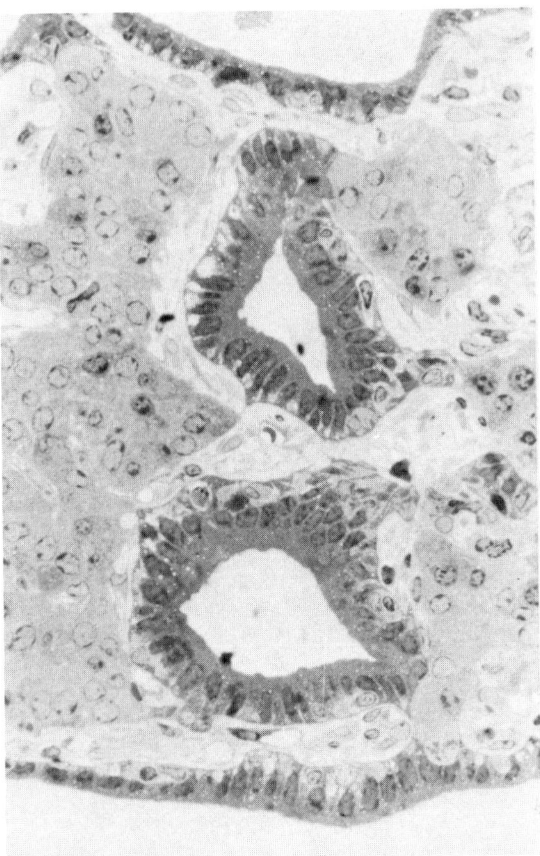

FIGURE 6. Budding of islet cells (light cells) from the base of malignant ductular epithelium (dark cells). (Giemsa, Epon, × 195)

cross-reaction with normal host pancreatic ductular constituents. The immunoperoxidase reaction using hamster IgG confirmed our view (Pour et al., 1981a).

3. In some areas of many induced hyperplastic and neoplastic lesions, a number of glycogen-containing cells, which in some instances presented the major bulk of tumors, were found (Figure 8). As far as is known, the centroacinar cells are the only embryonic pancreatic cells capable of synthesizing and storing glycogen (Like and Orci, 1972).
4. Human pancreatic adenocarcinomas, including a poorly differentiated cancer, expressed surface determinants detectable by monoclonal antibody to duct cell surface marker (Parsa et al., 1982).

If stem cells are considered tumor progenitor cells scattered through the pancreatic ductal, but specifically through ductular epithelium, our proposed classification (Pour, 1980; Pour and Wilson, 1980) of induced pancreatic cancer

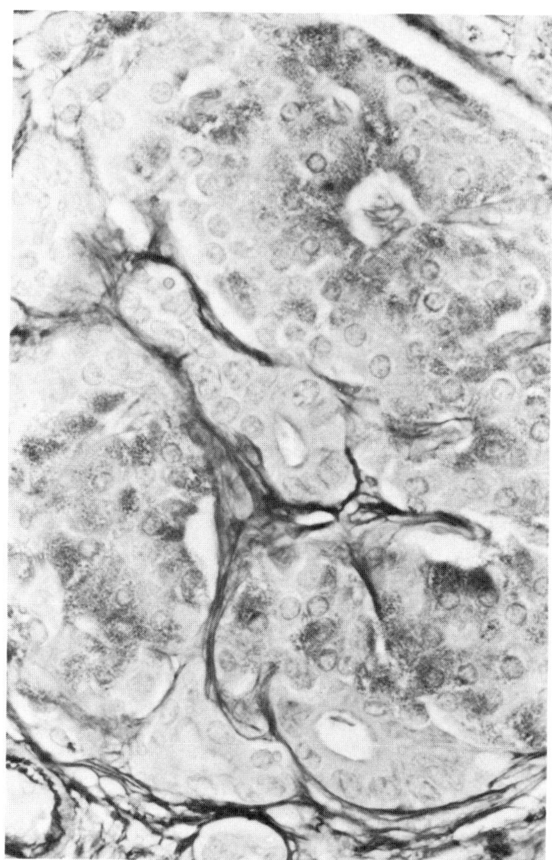

FIGURE 7. A mixed ductular-insular tumor. B cells have dark granulation. (Gomori's Aldehyde Fuchsin, × 195)

as originating from ducts or ductules becomes an issue of academic interest and does not seem to bear any prognostic or etiologic significance.

MECHANISMS OF PANCREATIC CARCINOGENESIS

The view that HPOP could be the proximate pancreatic carcinogen (Pour et al., 1979d) was supported by the observation that the compound occurs in equilibrium of an open and a cyclic hemiacetal form (Figures 9 and 10), the latter resembling the pyranose form of hexose sugars, on the one hand, and the glucose moiety of streptozotocin (SZ), on the other (Pour et al., 1979d). Since the specific affinity of SZ for pancreatic islet cells is possibly mediated through the sugar moiety of the compound as a carrier of the carcinogenic moiety (Wilander and Tjälve, 1975), we assumed the cyclic glucose-like structure of HPOP may facilitate its uptake into the pancreatic cells, although this carcinogen was

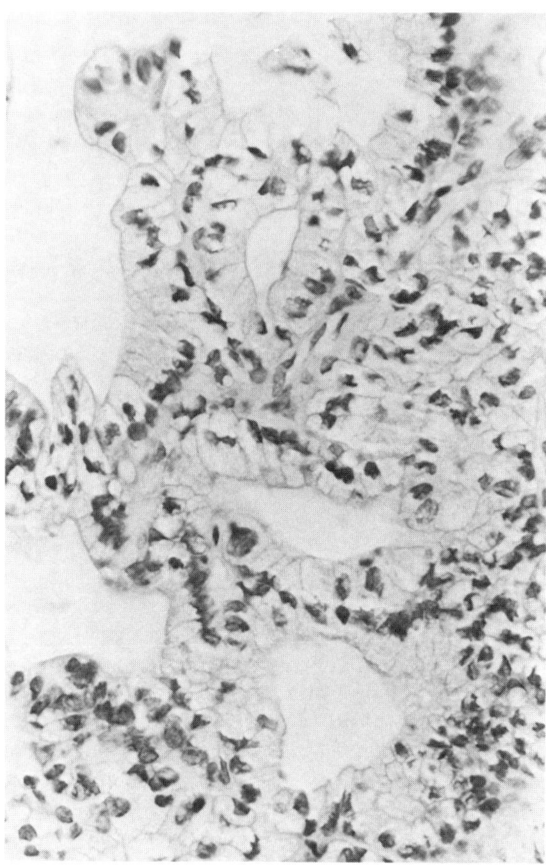

FIGURE 8. Clear cell carcinoma of the pancreas. Special staining revealed presence of glycogen in tumor cells. (H & E, × 195)

shown to be less specific for the pancreas than was BOP (Pour et al., 1979d). Supporting the importance of cyclic structure for pancreatotropic effect was the pancreatic carcinogenic effects of N-nitrosobis(2-oxobutyl)amine and N-nitroso(2-oxobutyl) (2-oxopropyl)amine, both of which occurred in cyclic form (Figure 11), even after a single injection (Pour and Raha, 1981).

The apparent difference in the target tissue of SZ (primarily islet cells) and of HPOP (primarily ductular cells) seemed nonfundamental, based on our studies indicating a mutual response of both endocrine and exocrine pancreatic tissues to HPOP, morphologically expressed by the development of mixed ductular-insular, as well as insular, neoplasms. Theoretically speaking, the noncyclic form of HPOP or of its metabolites (MOP) may affect the ductular cells, and the cyclic form, the islet cells.

To explore this possibility, we tested the effect of N-nitroso-2-methoxy-2,6-dimethylmorpholine (NDMN), an analogue of HPOP, with the difference that

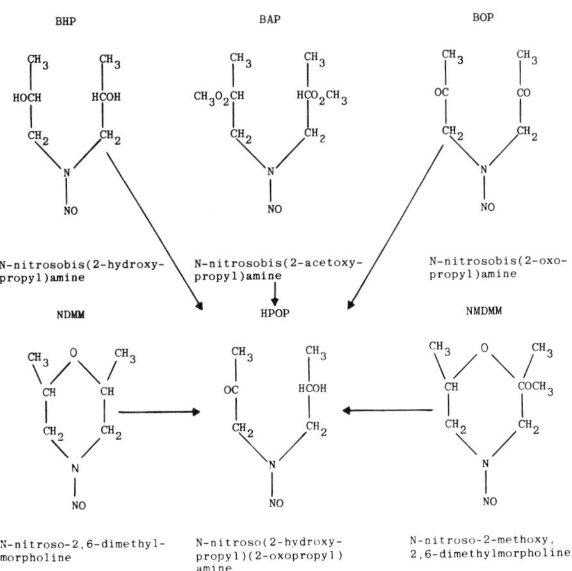

Figure 9. Chemical structure of pancreatic carcinogens.

its molecule in contrast to that of HPOP was found in vitro to impose a totally cyclic structure. If our hypothesis was correct, this compound should primarily affect islet cells, as does SZ. The results of our study with this compound (Pour et al., 1981b) confirmed one of our views, but disagreed with another. Contrary to the in vitro results, NDMN was found to be metabolized in vivo to the same degree to HPOP and BHP (Gingell et al., 1980). Supporting our view was the finding that the 2-methoxy derivative did, in fact, show a striking affinity for the islet cells. As with SZ, a single high dose of the 2-methoxy compound led to selective destruction of islet cells within 3 days and killed the animals in a diabetic coma. Islet cells in the surviving hamsters showed signs of regeneration, in a manner similar to the situation after SZ application, and after 60 to 72 hours almost all islets appeared normal. Approximately 40 weeks later, and again in analogy with SZ, some hamsters developed islet cell neoplasms. However, in contrast to the effect of SZ, almost all surviving hamsters developed ductal/ductular and mixed ductular-insular cell tumors. Interestingly, however, weekly application of the 2-methoxy compound in subdiabetogenic doses induced only ductal/ductular or mixed ductular-insular neoplasms, but not pure islet cell tumors (Pour et al., 1981b).

Our explanation for this phenomenon is as follows: We have shown (Pour and Donnelly, 1978) that the carcinogenic effect for the pancreas from all these carcinogens is most probably mediated through blood rather than bile-reflux mechanisms. Furthermore, the blood supply of the exocrine pancreas is mediated by the efferent branches of the insular arteries, and, accordingly, substances circulating in the blood travel to the islet first and to exocrine tissue later. This is also true for substances such as insulin, which has been suggested

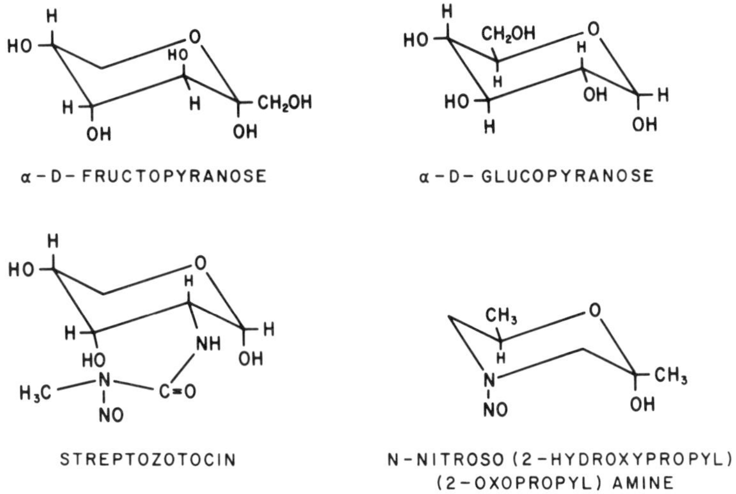

α-D-FRUCTOPYRANOSE

α-D-GLUCOPYRANOSE

STREPTOZOTOCIN

N-NITROSO (2-HYDROXYPROPYL) (2-OXOPROPYL) AMINE

Figure 10. Cyclic structure of HPOP and its comparison with pyronase form of sugars and with sugar moiety of streptozotocin.

to be responsible for increased protein synthesis in the acinar cells immediately surrounding the islets, causing a "halo" or "zoning" effect (for references see Pour et al., 1981b).

As described earlier, the first morphologic alteration of the pancreas after carcinogen treatment is necrosis of the acinar cells immediately surrounding islets and proliferation of periinsular and intrainsular ductules. Hence, apparently, the periinsular region is specifically affected by the carcinogen, possibly because the carcinogen via blood circulation reaches the islet cells, where it is taken up preferentially due to its sugarlike molecule (of NDMN or its metabolite HPOP). The high concentration of carcinogen may lead to selective

Figure 11. Cyclic forms of HBOP and HBOB.

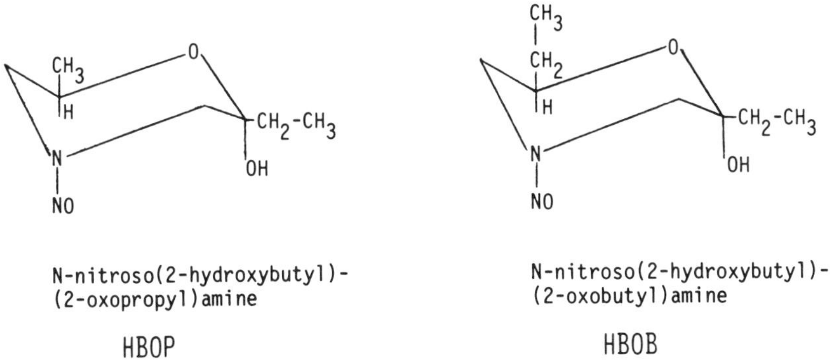

N-nitroso(2-hydroxybutyl)-(2-oxopropyl)amine

HBOP

N-nitroso(2-hydroxybutyl)-(2-oxobutyl)amine

HBOB

destruction of the B-cells, as did NDMN, whereas the low, noncytotoxic concentration could be metabolized to MOP, the more proximate pancreatic carcinogen. Based on the concentration gradient of MOP in the postinsular capillaries, the periinsular region becomes a preferential site of the carcinogenic effect.

If our hypothesis were true, islet cell damage would alter BOP metabolism. Therefore, we decided to test the effect on BOP carcinogenesis of alloxan (Pour et al., 1982c), which, when given to hamsters at a dose of 60 mg/kg, causes islet cell degeneration within 2 hours. In surviving hamsters, these cells regenerate completely 2 weeks after the alloxan administration (House et al., 1956; Nace et al., 1956). Therefore, we gave a single BOP injection to the first group (group 1) at the peak of islet cell degeneration (at 2 hours) and to the second group (group 2) at a time (2 weeks) when islet cell regeneration was considered complete. Surviving hamsters were killed 46 weeks after BOP injection in each group to guarantee the same postcarcinogen exposure time overall. The results fully agreed with our expectations in that 32% of group 1 hamsters developed pancreatic tumors compared with 92% in group 2 and 90% in group 3. The difference in tumor incidence between groups 1 and 3 was statistically significant ($P < .005$). Since alloxan does not affect all the islet cells (Edström and Boquist, 1973; Trandaburu and Ionescu, 1971), and according to some reports a few surviving B-cells show even a higher activity (Edström and Boquist, 1973), the induction of a few tumors in group 1 can be explained.

The question as to whether or not a higher alloxan dose would have destroyed a larger number of islets and hence further reduced the tumor incidence in our experiment was answered by Bell and Strayer (1982). These authors investigated the possible role of diabetes as a predisposing factor in pancreatic carcinogenesis and found that SZ prevented pancreatic cancer induction, when given at 50 mg/kg on three consecutive days, followed by weekly subcutaneous BOP injections of 5 mg/kg each. Only one hamster had focal hyperplasia of the ductules in the SZ-pretreated group (compared with 100% in controls), whereas all others had normal-appearing exocrine pancreas, but markedly small, atrophic islets.

These results nevertheless indicate the significance of islets in pancreatic exocrine tumor formation. The presence of various carcinogen-metabolizing enzymes in concentrations much higher than those found in acinar, ductal, and ductular cells (J. Baron, personal communication) further support this view. Islet cells apparently are not only involved in carcinogen metabolism but also participate in tumor formation and undergo functional deterioration. This view may best explain the known association between pancreatic cancer and altered glucose metabolism. Future work may clarify this important point.

MODIFICATION OF PANCREATIC CARCINOGENESIS

In agreement with epidemiologic data, a diet high in unsaturated fat fed for life after a single carcinogen injection increased the pancreatic tumor yield in our model in a statistically significant fashion (Birt et al., 1981). However, a high fat diet fed before carcinogen administration did not change the tumor yield. This finding indicates that diet influences the growth (promotional) phase, but it has no effect on the initiation phase, of pancreatic carcinogenesis. On the other hand, a protein-free diet fed during both initiation and promotional stages of carcinogenesis inhibited tumor development (Pour et al., 1982a). The latter experiment, along with epidemiologic data, suggests that a dietary imbalance rather than an excess or deficiency of individual dietary ingredients is decisive in modifying pancreatic carcinogenesis.

Among other modifiers of pancreatic carcinogenesis, partial pancreatectomy (PP) appears of interest. Whereas a single injection of BOP 1 week after PP significantly increased the number, size, and multiplicity of pancreatic tumors, a significant tumor reduction was found in hamsters that received carcinogen immediately after PP (Pour et al., 1983b). Since tumor incidence was also similarly low in sham-operated hamsters treated with carcinogen immediately after the operation, interaction of the carcinogen with the narcotic used (pentobarbital) or the immediate consequences of the surgery (hypothermia, shock) were thought responsible for tumor inhibition. This mechanism is obviously different from the effect of chronic ethanol consumption, which has also been shown to inhibit pancreatic carcinogenesis (Tweedie et al., 1981).

BIOLOGIC MARKERS OF EXPERIMENTAL PANCREATIC CANCER

Most induced pancreatic adenocarcinomas produce considerable amounts of mucin, which was found to be immunogenic in rabbits and of blood group A-like specificity (Runge and Pour, 1980). Our limited studies showed that the same antigenic property has also been shared in some cases of human pancreatic cancer (Pour et al., 1981a). These and similar antigens of a glycoprotein type (Berry and Amerigo, 1980; Dunzendorfer et al., 1981; Feizi et al., 1979; Iwaki et al., 1982; Kuhns and Schoentag, 1981; Metzgar et al., 1982; Salmon, 1979) may provide useful parameters for early detection and possibly also therapy of cancer.

COMPARATIVE STUDIES

Based on our comparative morphologic studies, hyperplastic, preneoplastic, and neoplastic lesions in humans and hamsters show striking similarities, including the occurrence of mixed ductular-insular neoplasms (Pour, 1981; Pour and Wilson, 1980; Pour et al., 1979b; Pour et al., 1982d). As in hamsters, human ductular cells are apparently the primary progenitor cells of tumors, including squamous cell cancer (Pour et al., 1982d). The latter is rarely found in hamsters, but the overall data nevertheless demonstrate a similar histogenesis of pancreatic cancer in the two species. Furthermore, biologic similarities exist between pancreatic cancer in the hamster and in humans, including the remarkable potential of tumors to invade, metastasize, cause vascular thrombosis, and produce mucin with blood group A-like antigenic properties. There are yet other remarkable similarities, including a striking multiplicity of lesions and the influence of diet on tumor growth.

These findings open up questions as to possible mutual etiologic factors in human disease. The increasing evidence of the presence of various nitroso compounds in the environment, and especially the possibility of in vivo formation of these carcinogens (Tannenbaum, 1981), support this view. Of significant interest was the finding in our institute (Issenberg et al., 1983) of BHP in commercial samples of triisopropanolamine at concentrations of 21 to 270 ng/g and in diisopropanolamine at concentrations of 20 to 1300 ng/g. Isopropanolamines are used in many products, including cosmetics, corrosion inhibitors, detergents, gas conditioning, textiles, electroplating, metal cleaning and rust removal, leather fat liquoring and tanning, and photographic emulsions, fuel and lubricant additives, and sensitizers. Exposure to some of these materials has been thought to be associated with an increased risk of pancreatic cancer (Bross et al., 1978; Hanis et al., 1982; Monson and Fine, 1978). Investigation of all the areas in which isopropanolamines are used in large quantities is necessary to determine whether BHP is formed in quantities sufficient to present a hazard to the general public using the product. Pancreatic cancer induction in our model by application of BHP to the skin (Pour et al., 1977b, 1980c) underlines the significance of such studies.

SUGGESTED DIRECTION OF FUTURE WORK

The search in the environment for carcinogens similar in structure to those that experimentally induce pancreatic cancer, along with studies on the elucidation of a relationship between the molecular structure and the pancreatotropic effect of the carcinogens, should be emphasized. At the same time, from a practical viewpoint the model should be used to evolve cancer prevention methods. Control of human exposure to environmental carcinogens in our civilized world may be impossible. Ultimately, an understanding of promotion in neoplastic development may be more important for human cancer prevention than extensive analyses of causative environmental carcinogens. Diet deserves particular attention in this approach. Because of the important role of the pancreas in digestion, the organ's physiologic functions and diseases may be determined by factors influenced by diets. These include dietary composition, as well as other exogenous or endogenous factors. Considering the obvious dialogue between the endocrine and exocrine pancreas (Pour, 1981), the elucidation of factors that could influence normal function and growth of the (exocrine-endocrine) pancreas appears a comprehensive, but rewarding, task. The search for tumor-specific antigens should be continued and their use in early detection and therapy as specific drug delivery systems tested. Elucidation of tumor histogenesis in humans and in the model requires further studies. Attempts to develop new pancreatic cancer models and to screen several species for occurence of "spontaneous" pancreatic cancer may shed some light on the problem.

REFERENCES

Bell RH, Strayer DL (1982) Pretreatment with streptozotocin prevents development of N-nitrosobis(2-oxopropyl)amine (BOP)-induced pancreatic cancer in the Syrian hamster. Pancreas Club, Inc. Annual Meeting 1982. University of Chicago Medical Center, Chicago.

Bensley RR, (1911) Studies on the pancreas of the guinea pig. Am J Anat 12:297–388.

Berry CL, Amerigo J (1980) Blood group antigens in vascular tumors. Evaluation of the immunoperoxidase technique. Virchows Arch A Pathol Anat Histol 388:167–174.

Birt DF, Salmasi S, Pour P (1981) Enhancement of experimental pancreatic cancer in Syrian golden hamsters by dietary fat. J Natl Cancer Inst 67:1327–1332.

Blot WJ, Fraumeni JF, Stone BJ (1978) Geographic correlates of pancreas cancer in the United States. Cancer 42:373–380.

Bockman DE, Black O Jr, Mills LR, Webster PD (1978) Origin of tubular complexes developing during induction of pancreatic adenocarcinoma by 7,12-dimethylbenz(a)anthracene. Am J Pathol 90:645–658.

Boquist L, Hellman B, Lernmark A, Talzedval I-B (1974) Influence of the mutation (diabetes) on insulin release and islet morphology in mice of different genetic backgrounds. J Cell Biol 62:77–89.

Bross IDJ, Viadana E, Houten L (1978) Occupational cancer in men exposed to dust and other environmental hazard. Arch Environ Health 32:300–307.

Danes BS, Lynch HT (1982) A familial aggregation of pancreatic cancer: An *in vitro* study. JAMA 247:2798–2802.

Dunzendorfer U, Schumann W, Drahovsky D, Ohlenschlager G (1981) Glycopeptides (FSH, LH, TSH, prolactin) and glycoproteins in patients with genitourinary cancer. Oncology 38:110–115.

Edström C, Boquist L (1973) Alloxan diabetes in duct ligated rats. Acta Pathol Microbiol Scand 81A:1–10.

Eusebi V, Capella C, Bondi A, Sessa F, Vezzadini P, Mancini AM (1981) Endocrine-paracrine cells in pancreatic exocrine carcinomas. Histopathology 5:599–613.

Feizi T, Picard J, Kapadia A, Slavin G (1979) Changes in the expression of the major blood group antigens ABH and their precursor antigens H in human gastric cancer tissues. Protides Biol Fluid Proc Colloq 27:221–224.

Flaks B, Moore MA and Flaks A (1980) Ultrastructural analysis of pancreatic carcinogenesis. III. Multifocal cystic lesions induced by N-nitrosobis(2-hydroxypropyl)amine in the hamster exocrine pancreas. Carcinogenesis 1:693–706.

Gingell R, Pour P (1978) Metabolism of the pancreatic carcinogen N-nitrosobis(2-oxopropyl)amine after oral and intraperitoneal administration to Syrian hamsters: Brief communication. J Natl Cancer Inst 60:911–913.

Gingell R, Wallcave L, Nagel D, et al. (1976) Metabolism of the pancreatic carcinogens N-nitrosobis(2-oxopropyl)amine and N-nitrosobis(2-hydroxypropyl)amine in the Syrian hamster. J Natl Cancer Inst 57:1175–1178.

Gingell R, Brunk G, Nagel D, Pour P (1979) Metabolism of three radiolabeled pancreatic carcinogenic nitrosamines in hamsters and rats. Cancer Res 39:4579–4583.

Gingell R, Brunk G, Nagel D, et al. (1980) Metabolism and mutagenicity of N-nitroso-2-methoxy-2,6-dimethylmorpholine in hamsters. J Natl Cancer Inst 64:157–161.

Hanis NM, Holmes TM, Shallenberger LG, Jones KE (1982) Epidemiologic study of refinery and chemical plant workers. J Occup Med 24:203–212.

Helgeson AS, Pour P, Lawson T, Grandjean CJ (1980a) Exocrine pancreatic secretion in the Syrian golden hamster *Mesocricetus auratus*. I. Basic values. Comp Biochem Physiol 66:473–477.

Helgeson AS, Pour P, Lawson T, Grandjean C (1980b) Exocrine pancreatic secretion in the Syrian golden hamsters *Mesocricetus auratus* II. Effect of secretin and pancreozymin. Comp Biochem Physiol 66:479–483.

House EL, Nace PF, Tassoni JP (1956) Alloxan diabetes in the hamster: Organ changes during the first day. Endocrinology 59:433–443.

Issenberg P, Conrad EE, Nielsen JW, et al. (1983) Determination of N-nitrosobis(2-hydroxypropyl)amine (BHP) in environmental samples. Eighth International Meeting on N-nitroso compounds: Occurrence and Biologic Effects. Banff, Canada, 4–9 September.

Iwaki Y, Kasai M, Terasaki PI, et al. (1982) Monoclonal antibody against A. Lewis b antigen produced by the hybridoma immunized with a pulmonary carcinoma. Cancer Res 42:409–411.

Kawabata T, Wick DG, Guengerich FP, Baron J (1984) Immunohistochemical localization of carcinogen-metabolizing enzymes with the rat and hamster exocrine pancreas. Cancer Res 44:215–223.

Kodama T, Mori W (1983) Morphological behavior of carcinoma of the pancreas. 2. Argyrophil cells and Langerhans' islets in the carcinomatous tissues. Acta Pathol Jpn 33:483–493.

Kruger FW (1973) Metabolism of nitrosamines *in vivo*. II. On the methylation of nucleic acids by aliphatic di-n-alkyl-nitrosamines *in vivo* caused by β-oxidation: The increased formation of 7-methylguanine after application of β-hydroxypropyl-propyl-nitrosamine compared to that after application of di-n-propyl-nitrosamine. Z Krebsforsch 79:90–97.

Kuhns WJ, Schoentag R (1981) Carcinoma-related alterations of glycosyltransferases in human tissues. Cancer Res 41:2767–2772.

Lawson TA, Gingell R, Nagel D, et al. (1981) Methylation of hamster DNA by the carcinogen N-nitrosobis(2-oxopropyl)amine. Cancer Lett 11:251–255.

Lawson T, Hines L, Helgeson S, Pour P (1982) The persistence of DNA damage in the pancreas of Syrian golden hamsters treated with N-nitrosobis(2-oxopropyl)amine. Chem Biol Interact 38:317–323.

Like A, Orci L (1972) Embryogenesis of the human pancreatic islets: A light and electron microscopic study. Diabetes 21:511–534.

Metzgar RS, Gaillard MT, Levine SG, et al. (1982) Antigens of human pancreatic adenocarcinoma cells defined by murine monoclonal antibodies. Cancer Res 42:601–608.

Monson RR, Fine LJ (1978) Cancer mortality and morbidity among rubber workers. J Natl Cancer Inst 61:1047–1053.

Moore MA, Takahashi M, Ito N, Bannasch P (1983) Early lesions during pancreatic carcinogenesis induced in Syrian hamsters by DHPN and DOPN. II. Ultrastructural findings. Carcinogenesis 4:439–448.

Nace PF, House EL, Tassoni JP (1956) Alloxan diabetes in the hamster: Dosage and blood curves. Endocrinology 58:305–308.

Ogrowsky D, Fawcett J, Althoff J, et al. (1980) The structure of the pancreas in Syrian hamsters: Scanning electron microscopic observations. Acta Anat 107:121–128.

Parsa I, Sutton AL, Chen CK, Delbridge C (1982) Monoclonal antibody for identification of human duct cell carcinoma of pancreas. Cancer Lett 17:217–222.

Pictet RL, Rutter WJ (1972) Development of the embryonic endocrine pancreas. In: Steiner D, Freinkel N, eds., Handbook of physiology, vol. 1. Baltimore: Williams & Wilkins, sect. 7, p. 250.

Pierce GB, Cox WF (1977) Neoplasms as caricatures of tissue renewal. In: Saunders GF, ed., Cell differentiation and neoplasia. New York: Raven Press, p. 57.

Pour PM (1978) Islet cells as a component of pancreatic ductal neoplasms. I. Experimental study: Ductular cells, including islet cell precursors as primary progenitor cells of tumors. Am J Pathol 90:295–316.

Pour PM (1980) Experimental pancreatic ductal (ductular) tumors: In: Fitzgerald PJ, Morrison AB, eds., The pancreas. Baltimore: Williams & Wilkins, pp. 111–139.

Pour PM (1981) The endocrine-exocrine pancreas: Its clinical and morphological aspects and hyperplastic and neoplastic patterns. In: Nagasawa H, Abe K, eds., Hormone related tumors. Tokyo: Japan Scientific Societies Press and Berlin: Springer-Verlag, pp. 103–120.

Pour PM, Donnelly T (1978) The effect of cholecystoduodenostomy and choledochostomy in pancreatic carcinogenesis. Cancer Res 38:2048.

Pour PM, Levitt MH (1979) Pancreatic tumors. In: Animal model of human disease. The Registry of Comparative Pathology. Washington, D.C.: Armed Forces Institute of Pathology, pp. 3–4.

Pour PM, Raha C (1981) Pancreatic carcinogenic effect of N-nitrosobis(2-oxobutyl)amine and N-nitroso(2-oxobutyl) (2-oxopropyl)amine in Syrian hamster. Cancer Lett 12:223–229.

Pour PM, Salmasi SZ (1979) Ductular origin of pancreatic cancer and its multiplicity in man comparable to experimentally induced tumors. A preliminary study. Cancer Lett 6:89–97.

Pour PM, Wilson R (1980) Experimental pancreas tumor. In: Moossa, AR, ed., Cancer of the pancreas. Baltimore: Williams & Wilkins, pp. 37–158.

Pour PM, Krüger FW, Althoff J, Cardesa A, Mohr U (1975a) Effect of beta-oxidized nitrosamines on Syrian hamsters. III. 2,2′-Dihydroxy-di-*n*-propyl-nitrosamine. J Natl Cancer Inst 54:141–146.

Pour PM, Mohr U, Cardesa A, et al. (1975b) Pancreatic neoplasms in an animal model: Morphological, biological, and comparative studies. Cancer 36:379–389.

Pour PM, Mohr U, Cardesa A, et al. (1976) Spontaneous tumors and common diseases in two colonies of Syrian hamsters. II. Respiratory tract and digestive system. J Natl Cancer Inst 56:937–948.

Pour PM, Althoff J, Krüger FW, Mohr U (1977a) A potent pancreatic carcinogen in Syrian hamsters, N-nitrosobis(2-oxopropyl)amine. J Natl Cancer Inst 58:1449–1453.

Pour PM, Althoff J, Nagel DL (1977b) Induction of epithelial neoplasms by local application of N-nitrosobis(2-hydroxypropyl)amine and N-nitrosobis(2-acetoxypropyl)-amine. Cancer Lett 3:109–113.

Pour PM, Salmasi S, Runge RG (1978) Selective induction of pancreatic ductular tumors by single doses of N-nitrosobis(2-oxopropyl)amine in Syrian golden hamsters. Cancer Lett 4:317–323.

Pour PM, Althoff J, Salmasi S, Stepan K (1979a) Spontaneous tumors and common diseases in three hamster strains. J Natl Cancer Inst 63:797–811.

Pour PM, Salmasi SZ, Runge RG (1979b) Ductular origin of pancreatic cancer and its multiplicity in man comparable to experimentally induced tumors. A preliminary study. Cancer Lett 6:89–97.

Pour PM, Salmasi SZ, Runge RG, et al. (1979c) Carcinogenicity of N-nitrosobis(2-hydroxypropyl)amine and N-nitrosobis(2-oxopropyl)amine in MRC rats. J Natl Cancer Inst 63:181–190.

Pour PM, Wallcave L, Gingell R, et al. (1979d) The carcinogenic effect of N-nitroso(2-hydroxypropyl) (2-oxopropyl)amine, a postulated proximate pancreatic carcinogen in Syrian hamsters. Cancer Res 39:3828–3833.

Pour PM, Gingell R, Langenbach R, et al. (1980a) Carcinogenicity of N-nitrosomethyl(2-oxopropyl)amine in Syrian hamsters. Cancer Res 40:3585–3590.

Pour PM, Salmasi S, Helgeson S, Stepan K (1980b) Induction of benign and malignant tumors in Syrian hamsters by topical application of N-nitrosobis(2-oxopropyl)amine and N-nitroso(2-hydroxypropyl)amine. Cancer Lett 10:163–167.

Pour PM, Wallcave L, Nagel D, Salmasi S (1980c) Induction of local epidermal papillomas and carcinoma by selected nitrosamines. Cancer Lett 10:365–373.

Pour PM, Runge RG, Birt D, et al. (1981a) Current knowledge of pancreatic carcinogenesis in the hamster and its relevance to the human disease. Cancer 47:1573–1587.

Pour PM, Wallcave L, Nagel D (1981b) The effect of N-nitroso-2-methoxy-2,6-dimethylmorpholine on endocrine and exocrine pancreas in Syrian hamsters. Cancer Lett 13:233–240.

Pour PM, Birt D, Salmasi SZ, Goetz U (1983a) Modifying factors in pancreatic carcinogenesis in the hamster model. 1. The effect of protein-free diet fed during the early stages of carcinogenesis. J Natl Cancer Inst 70:141–146.

Pour PM, Donnelly K, Stepan K (1983b) Modification of pancreatic carcinogenesis in the hamster model. 2. The effects of partial pancreatectomy. Am J Pathol 110:75–82.

Pour PM, Donnelly K, Stepan K (1983c) Modification of pancreatic carcinogenesis in the hamster model. 3. Inhibitory effect of alloxan. Am J Pathol 110:310–314.

Pour PM, Lawson T (1983d) Pancreatic carcinogenic nitrosamines in Syrian hamsters. Eighth International Meeting on N-nitroso compounds: Occurrence and Biologic Effects. Banff, Canada, 4–9 September.

Pour PM, Sayed S, Sayed G (1982) The hyperplastic, preneoplastic and neoplastic lesions found in 83 human pancreas. Am J Clin Pathol 77:137–152.

Reid JD, Yuh S-L, Metrelli M, Jaffee R (1982) Ductuloinsular tumors of the pancreas. Cancer 49:908–915.

Reznik-Schüller HM, Lijinsky W, Hague BF (1980) Electron microscopic autoradiography of the pancreas in the hamster treated with tritiated N-nitroso-2,6-dimethylmorpholine. Cancer Res 40:2245–2251.

Runge RG, Pour PM (1980) Blood group specificity of pancreatic tumor mucin. Cancer Lett 10:351–357.

Runge R, Takahashi M, Pour PM (1978) Pancreatic ductulitis in Syrian golden hamsters bearing homologous transplantable pancreatic adenocarcinomas. Cancer Lett 5:225–229.

Salmon C, (1979) Blood group precursors in tumor associated antigens. Protides Biol Fluid Proc Colloq 27:85–88.

Scarpelli DG, Rao MS, Subbaro V (1983) Augmentation of carcinogenesis by N-nitrosobis(2-oxopropyl)amine administered during S phase of the cell cycle in regenerating hamster pancreas. Cancer Res 43:611–616.

Scarpelli DG, Rao MS (1978) Pathogenesis of pancreatic carcinoma in hamsters induced by N-nitrosobis(2-oxopropyl)amine (BOP). Fed Proc 37:231.

Scarpelli DG, Rao MS, Subbarao V, et al. (1980) Activation of nitrosamines to mutagens by post mitochondrial fraction of hamster pancreas. Cancer Res 40:67–74.

Schlosnagle DC, Campbell WG (1981) The papillary and solid neoplasms of the pancreas: Report of two cases with electron microscopy, one containing neurosecretory granules. Cancer 47:2603–2610.

Schwentker F (1934) The antibody response of rabbits to injections of immulsions and extracts of homologous brain. J Exp Med 60:559–574

Takahashi M, Pour PM (1978) Spontaneous pancreas alteration in aging Syrian hamsters. J Natl Cancer Inst 60:355–364.

Takahashi M, Pour PM, Althoff J, Donnelly T (1977) The pancreas of the Syrian hamster (Mesocricetus auratus). I. Anatomical study. Lab Anim Sci 27:336–342.

Tannenbaum SR (1981) Endogenous formation of N-nitroso compounds. In: Banbury Report 7. Gastrointestinal cancer: Endogenous factors. Cold Spring Harbor, N.Y.: Cold Spring Harbor Laboratory, pp. 269–283.

Trandaburu T, Ionescu M (1971) Ultrastructural alterations in the pancreatic β-cells of the newt *(Triturus vulgaris)* induced by alloxan. Acta Anat 79:257–269.

Tweedie JH, Reber HA, Pour P (1981) Protective effect of ethanol on the development of pancreatic cancer. APA, NPaCP Joint Meeting, November 5,6, Chicago.

Walters MN-I (1965) The ductular cell in pancreatic cystic fibrosis. J Pathol 90:45–52.

Wilander E, Tjälve H (1975) Diabetogenic effects of N-nitrosomethylurea with special regard to species variation. Exp Pathol 11:133–138.

PATHOPHYSIOLOGY OF ANOREXIA AND DISTURBANCES OF TASTE IN CANCER PATIENTS

WILLIAM D DEWYS, M.D.,
AND FREDDIE ANN HOFFMAN, M.D.

Decreased appetite and decreased food intake lead to weight loss and muscle wasting in cancer patients. In some patients with cancer, mechanical factors may interfere with intake and/or digestion of food. This chapter will focus on decreased food intake, which may occur as a systemic effect of malignancy or as a conditioned aversion to food intake. Conditioned aversions may evolve in relation to the effect of therapy or in relation to local or systemic effects of malignancy.

Weight loss *prior to treatment* is an important prognostic factor in patients with cancer. In a survey of 12 chemotherapy protocols of the Eastern Cooperative Oncology Group (ECOG), using data from 3047 patients with advanced and/or metastatic cancer, the median survival was significantly shorter in patients with weight loss compared with that of patients with no weight loss, as displayed in Table 1 (DeWys et al., 1980). The effect of weight loss on prognosis was independent of the effect of performance status using the ECOG scale, as shown in Table 2. In addition, the prognostic effect of weight loss was independent of tumor extent, as shown in Table 3. In many patients the mechanism of weight loss is enigmatic. In this chapter we will review possible mechanisms, with particular emphasis on anorexia.

PATHOPHYSIOLOGY OF CANCER CACHEXIA

In the patient with malignancy, weight loss or cancer cachexia is caused by decreased caloric intake, increased caloric expenditure, and altered metabolism. A detailed discussion of the pathophysiology of cancer cachexia is beyond the scope of this chapter, so the reader is referred to two recent reviews (DeWys, 1982; Lawson et al., 1982).

From the Division of Cancer Prevention and Control (WDD); and the Cancer Therapy Evaluation Program, Division of Cancer Treatment, National Cancer Institute, Bethesda, Maryland (FAH).

TABLE 1. Effect of Weight Loss on Survival

Tumor type	Median survival (weeks) No weight loss	Weight loss[a]	P value[b]
Favorable non-Hodgkin's lymphoma	[c]	138	<.01
Breast	70	45	<.01
Acute nonlymphocytic leukemia	8	4	N.S.
Sarcoma	46	25	<.01
Unfavorable non-Hodgkin's lymphoma	107	55	<.01
Colon	43	21	<.01
Prostate	46	24	<.05
Lung, small cell	34	27	<.05
Lung, nonsmall cell	20	14	<.01
Pancreas	14	12	N.S.
Nonmeasurable gastric	41	27	<.05
Measurable gastric	18	16	N.S.

[a]All categories of weight loss (0–5%, 5–10%) have been combined.
[b]The P values refer to a test of the hypothesis that the entire survival curves are identical, not merely a test of the medians. However, in all disease sites under study, the median is a representative indicator of the survival distribution; consequently, its use as a summary statistic is acceptable.
[c]Only 20 of 199 patients have died, so median survival cannot be estimated. However, the observed rate of failure predicts that the survival will be significantly longer than for the group with weight loss.
Source: DeWys et al., (1980).

Caloric intake in cancer patients may be low relative to predicted normal caloric requirements (absolute hypophagia) or may fail to increase in response to increased energy expenditure (relative hypophagia) (DeWys and Kisner, 1982). In a study in which observed caloric intake was compared with a prediction of caloric requirement based on body size, age, and sex, 25% of cancer patients had a caloric intake below basal or resting energy requirements, 45% had an intake between resting requirements and the requirements for moderate activity, and 30% had an intake that was sufficient for moderate activity

TABLE 2. Relationship Between Weight Loss, Performance Status, and Median Survival for Colon Cancer

Performance status (ECOG)[a]	Median survival (weeks) No weight loss	Weight loss	P value
0–1	46	31	<.01
2–3	19	15	N.S.

[a]0—Fully active.
1—Ambulatory, capable of light work.
2—In bed < 50% of time, capable of self-care but not of work activities.
3—In bed > 50% of time, capable of only limited self-care.
4—Completely bedridden.

TABLE 3. Effect on Median Survival of Weight Loss Tumor Extent for Colon Cancer.

	No weight loss		Weight loss		
Tumor extent[a]	Median survival (weeks)	Patients (number)	Median survival (weeks)	Patients (number)	*P* value for survival difference
0	52	60	31	51	.05
1	37	75	19	101	.01
2	25	6	14	14	N.S.

[a]Tumor involvement was coded as absent or present for three anatomic sites: liver, lung, and bone. No patient had metastases to all three sites.

(DeWys et al., 1982). However, in many cancer patients energy expenditure is higher than would be predicted based on age, sex, body size, and activity level. Warnold and coworkers (1978) studied caloric expenditure in a group of sedentary cancer patients and compared this data with observations in sedentary noncancer patients. Caloric intake was only slightly lower in the cancer patients compared with that of the controls; however, the caloric expenditure of the cancer patients averaged nearly 50% over their intake. Thus, while their intake was approximately what one would expect for sedentary activity, their expenditure was equivalent to that expected with a moderately high activity level. (DeWys and Kisner, 1982).

The pathophysiology of increased energy expenditure in the cancer patient is only partly understood, but it includes energy expenditure within the tumor and increased energy expenditure within host organs as a remote effect of a tumor. Energy is expended within a tumor for maintenance of vital cellular functions, such as transmembrane ionic gradients, and for synthesis of structural components, such as protein for tumor cell growth and division.

Tumors exert many remote metabolic effects, including stimulation of synthesis of secretory proteins by the liver (acute phase reactants). This increased protein synthesis requires energy (Narendra, 1977) which may be an important component of the increased energy expenditure of the cancer patient.

CONTROL OF FOOD INTAKE

As a background for considering the possible mechanisms of reduced eating in cancer patients, it is instructive to review current understanding of control of food intake in normal subjects and to relate this to physiologic and biochemical observations in cancer patients (DeWys, 1977a). The food intake control mechanism includes a "controller," a controlled system, and feedback elements. The "controller" is a complex system within the brain that includes cortical, subcortical, hypothalamic, and autonomic components. The controlled system encompasses the intake, distribution, and storage of calories. The feedback elements are comprised of the sensory perceptions of food (especially taste and smell); signals from the gastrointestinal tract (for example, sense of fullness); plasma concentrations of glucose, free fatty acids, glycerol, and amino acids; and the peripheral metabolic state. Humoral responses to feedback elements (insulin release, and such) also contribute to controller function.

Since the system is responsive to multiple feedback stimuli, removal or alteration of only one source of stimulation or inhibition may not have detectable long-term effects. For example, persons who have undergone surgical vagotomy, which precludes gastrointestinal stretch signals from reaching the brain, continue to be able to regulate food intake and maintain a stable body weight. It is likely, therefore, that severely anorectic patients may have multiple aberrations in their food intake regulatory system.

The hypothalamic components of the "controller" have been evaluated in the cancer-bearing host with the general conclusion that the function of these centers is not abnormal (Morrison, 1976). These hypothalamic centers are affected by circulating neurotransmitters (Leibowitz, 1976). It is possible that elevations in plasma norepinephrine levels that have been observed in cancer patients may influence hypothalamic centers to suppress appetite; however, this postulation requires further study. In addition, the cortical component of the controller may be altered in cancer patients and will be considered later under the topic "conditioned aversion."

Many of the feedback elements are altered in the cancer patient in directions that would tend to suppress food intake. Alterations of sensory perceptions of food will be discussed in the next section. Other feedback elements that may be altered include elevated plasma concentrations of glucose, free fatty acids, and altered plasma amino acid profiles (DeWys, 1977a).

TASTE ABNORMALITIES IN CANCER PATIENTS

Many cancer patients express symptoms suggestive of alterations in taste perception (DeWys, 1974; DeWys and Walters, 1975). These symptoms include descriptions of a reduction in the pleasant taste of food and a negative or bad taste sensation related to specific foods. Many patients equated reduced taste for foods with reduced appetite, and this reduced appetite could be correlated with reduced caloric intake as measured from diet diaries. The negative taste sensations were most often associated with meat, coffee, and chocolates. These symptoms did not correlate with the histologic type of cancer, but there was a general correlation with tumor extent.

The "detection" and "recognition" thresholds for salt, sweet, sour, and bitter taste sensations were studied in a series of 50 patients with a spectrum of tumor types (excluding oral cancers) (DeWys, 1974; DeWys and Walters, 1975). The results were compared to those of similar testing in normal volunteers and hospitalized patients with diagnoses other than cancer. The most frequent abnormality was an elevation of the recognition threshold for sweet, which occurred in 17 patients. Other abnormalities included increased recognition thresholds for salt (5/50), bitter (3/50), or sour (1/50) and decreased recognition threshold for bitter (8/50). (The recognition threshold is the lowest concentration of solute that was correctly identified as salty, sweet, sour, or bitter.)

The symptom of decreased taste sensation correlated with an elevated threshold for sweet in that 12/25 patients with this symptom had a recognition

TABLE 4. Correlation Between Tumor Extent and a Measured Abnormality of Taste Sensation in Cancer Patients

Tumor extent	Number of patients: Normal taste threshold	Abnormal taste threshold
Limited	9	0
Moderate	18	3
Extensive	5	15

Source: Modified from DeWys and Walters, 1975.

Chi^2 for 3 × 2 table = 19.3; $P < .001$.

threshold for sweet above the normal range and an additional 8/25 had values above the median normal value. The symptom of a bad taste sensation for meat correlated with a lowered recognition threshold (an increased sensitivity) for bitter taste. Eight out of 16 patients with this symptom had recognition thresholds for bitter taste below the normal range, and an additional four patients had values below the median normal value.

The correlation between tumor extent and the presence of a measured abnormality of taste sensation is shown in Table 4. These abnormalities of taste were reversible in patients who responded to antineoplastic therapy (DeWys, 1974). In nine patients, taste sensation was measured before and after reduction in tumor volume. In four patients, an abnormally low bitter threshold normalized; in five patients high normal or elevated thresholds for sweet shifted to lower values.

These results have been confirmed by other clinical studies, as summarized in Table 5. Differences between series are probably a result of differences in case selection, especially differences in tumor extent. For example, the series with the lowest frequency of abnormality (Carson and Gormican, 1977) includes a large number of patients with resected tumors with no apparent metastases. Collectively these studies confirm the observations already noted

TABLE 5. Abnormalities of Taste Recognition Thresholds in Cancer Patients[a]

Reference	Increased for sweet > 90 mmol/L	Increased for salt > 120 mmol/L	Increased for sour > 60 mmol/L	Increased for bitter > 1200 mmol/L	Decreased for bitter < 90 mmol/L
DeWys and Walters (1975)	17/50	5/50	1/50	3/50	8/50
Gorshein (1977)	5/5	0/5	0/5	0/5	1/5
Carson and Gormican (1977)	3/48	8/48	N.R.[b]	N.R.	N.R.
Williams and Cohen (1978)	9/30	6/30	1/30	2/30	3/30
Bolze et al. (1982)	15/35	5/35	9/35	5/35	N.R.

[a]Data shown as number abnormal over number studied.
[b]N.R. = not reported.

here; namely, a correlation between a general decrease in taste pleasurability and elevated sweet threshold, a correlation between low bitter threshold and rejection of meat, a correlation between tumor extent and the occurrence of an abnormality of taste, and reversibility of the abnormality after reduction in tumor burden (DeWys, 1978). The time course of reversal of taste abnormalities after successful treatment of laryngeal cancer has been studied by Kashima and Kalinowski (1979). They noted that recovery occurred progressively over 6 months after treatment. Recurrence of taste abnormalities usually coincided with the documentation of tumor recurrence; but in two patients deterioration of taste occurred 5 to 6 months before clinical proof of recurrence (Kashima and Kalinowski, 1979). In addition, these abnormalities of taste sensation have been correlated with reduced energy intake (DeWys, 1977b; Gorshein, 1977; Carson and Gormican, 1977; Williams and Cohen, 1978) and increased weight loss (Bolze et al., 1982).

The pathophysiology of these changes in taste sensation is not understood. Elevated thresholds may develop as a consequence of nutritional deficiency (Henkin et al., 1971). Cancer patients may develop nutritional deficiencies related to the nutritional demands of tumor growth and/or decreased nutrient intake. Bolze and colleagues (1982) evaluated plasma zinc levels and taste sensation in a series of cancer patients. They reported that plasma zinc levels did not correlate with any particular alteration in taste acuity. However, previous studies suggest that the presence of zinc deficiency causes an elevation of multiple thresholds (Henkin et al., 1971). In the study by Bolze and colleagues, 10 patients had subnormal plasma zinc levels and three of these patients had elevations of three or four thresholds, while among 25 with normal plasma zinc levels only one had three or four abnormal thresholds (Table 6). Although this study does not show a relationship between the presence of any specific taste abnormality and plasma zinc levels, it does suggest a correlation between low plasma zinc levels and the presence of multiple abnormalities of taste sensation.

Mossman and Henkin (1978), in an uncontrolled study, gave zinc supplements to seven cancer patients with elevated taste thresholds and reported a decrease in thresholds following zinc therapy. An anecdotal report of improvement in taste thresholds following parenteral nutrition in a cancer patient is also compatible with correction of a nutritional deficiency, but it does not permit identification of the putative deficiency (Russ and DeWys, 1977).

TABLE 6. Correlation Between Multiple Taste Abnormalities and Plasma Zinc Levels

Number of elevated thresholds	Plasma zinc (μg/dL)[a]	
	< 72	> 72
3–4	3	1
0–2	7	24

Source: Bolze et al. (1982).

Chi^2 = 4.77; P = < .03.

[a]The normal range for plasma zinc is 72–125 μg/dL.

LEARNED FOOD AVERSIONS AND EATING

Psychological mechanisms may also contribute to reduced caloric intake in cancer patients. Garcia and coworkers (1974) reported that animals who ate a particular food before receiving radiation treatment subsequently avoided that food. This "learned aversion" presumably developed from the association of the symptoms of radiation therapy and the eating of the food. Important features of learned aversion are: (1) the learning occurs rapidly, (2) delays of hours between the tasting of the food and the unpleasant experience will still produce an aversion to the taste, (3) aversions are most likely to occur with the most novel foods, and (4) repeated pairings of food and illness can cause even the most pleasant and familiar food to become aversive (Bernstein, 1982). Bernstein and colleagues have studied learned food aversion in cancer patients and in animal tumor models. In one study, an ice cream with a novel flavor was fed to children in an experimental group just before they received chemotherapy that had gastrointestinal toxicity. Comparison groups received either the same chemotherapy without the flavored ice cream or the ice cream with nontoxic chemotherapy. When offered the same flavored ice cream 1 to 4 weeks later, the comparison groups were three times as likely to choose the ice cream as were the patients in the experimental group (Bernstein, 1978; Bernstein et al., 1979). Thus, pairing of the taste of the ice cream with gastrointestinal toxicity resulted in aversion to the ice cream.

These studies were extended to determine whether patients receiving chemotherapy develop aversions to foods in their usual diet (Bernstein, 1982). On follow-up evaluations, foods that had been eaten within 5 hours of gastrointestinal toxic chemotherapy appeared on the patient's lists of disliked foods. Thus, learned aversions may develop to foods in the usual diet if the foods happen to be eaten within several hours of the treatment.

Using an animal tumor model, Bernstein and Sigmundi (1980) have also tested the hypothesis that appetite loss might be based on learned aversions in which tumor-related symptoms are associated with food intake in a learned aversion paradigm. Tumor-bearing rats were fed one diet for 10 days. During this 10-day period food intake declined by about 40%. The rats were then tested as to preference for their current diet or a new diet and showed a striking preference for the new diet (89% versus 52% in nontumor controls). When the tumor-bearing rats were switched to the new diet, they increased their food intake by 85%. The results were essentially similar when the experiment was repeated with the diets given in the opposite sequence, thus excluding explanations related to taste or palatability of the diet. These results suggest that tumor-bearing rats associate their tumor-induced discomfort with their diet and that these aversions contribute to tumor-induced anorexia.

THERAPEUTIC CONSIDERATIONS

Based on the preceding discussion, it is possible to formulate strategies that may increase caloric intake in cancer patients (Bernstein et al., 1980; DeWys and Herbst, 1977; DeWys, 1980; DeWys and Kubota, 1981). Open discussions with a patient that demonstrate the physician's awareness and an understanding of the patient's problem may help to alleviate anxiety and promote a sense of well-being. Patients who note that food has "lost its taste" may benefit from the use of increased seasoning and flavoring of food. Patients reporting "a bad taste" from meat may be able to mask the unpleasant taste by using sauces or such or may be advised to use alternate sources of protein for their diet. Some patients with this symptom may dislike beef or pork, but they may be able to eat poultry or fish. Others may also develop a dislike for poultry or fish, but they may be able to eat eggs and cheese as a protein source.

The taste preferences of a cancer patient should also be considered when one prescribes commercially available meal-replacement nutritional supplements (DeWys and Herbst, 1977). Overall, the taste evaluation of a specific nutritional supplement by a cancer patient may differ significantly from the evaluation of the same supplement by a healthy person. A product that is judged favorably by healthy people may receive an indifferent or negative rating by a cancer patient. Patients with cancer may differ widely in their reactions to any given product. We therefore suggest that patients be encouraged to taste a variety of these supplements so that one that has an acceptable taste can be prescribed. This tasting process may have to be repeated over time as the patients develop a dislike of their current prescriptions. This sequence has been termed "taste fatigue," but it may in fact be a consequence of a tumor-related learned aversion.

Animal models have been studied to evaluate strategies for reducing or eliminating food aversions (Bernstein et al., 1980; Smith and Blumsack, 1981). The administration of antihistamines to rats prior to treatment will block radiation-induced, but not drug-induced, taste aversions (Smith and Blumsack, 1981). In a drug-treatment model, withholding food for 6 hours before and after each treatment did not reduce the magnitude of diet aversion (Bernstein et al., 1980). A blocking strategy involving the introduction of a novel flavor into the water around the time of treatment was also unsuccessful. However, replacing the standard diet with a novel diet on the treatment days reduced the aversion to the standard diet. As noted earlier, changing from the standard diet to a new diet in the rat model of tumor-related food aversion resulted in an 85% increase in food intake (Bernstein, 1982).

The durability of this improvement, however, was not reported. One might expect that a learned aversion to the new diet would develop, perhaps even more rapidly than the aversion for the initial diet. The phenomenon seen in this animal model may explain a clinical observation. Patients who were having difficulty eating a standard American diet have been able to increase their food intake by switching to novel diets, especially to Chinese or Japanese diets. Over time however, their ability to eat the new diet also declined, suggesting learned aversion to the novel diet.

In some patients, these strategies will fail. Enteral or parenteral nutritional intervention should be considered if the patient's disease is at a treatable point in its natural history (DeWys and Kubota, 1981). The goal of nutritional intervention should be to maintain or replete the patient's nutritional status, particularly when attention to nutritional status will assist in the administration of definitive anticancer therapy.

REFERENCES

Bernstein IL (1978) Learned taste aversions in children receiving chemotherapy. Science (Washington) 200:1300–1303.

Bernstein IL (1982) Physiological and psychological mechanisms of cancer anorexia. Cancer Res 42:715s–720s.

Bernstein IL, Sigmundi R (1980) Tumor anorexia: a learned food aversion? Science (Washington) 209:416–418.

Bernstein IL, Wallace MJ, Bernstein ID, et al. (1979) Learned food aversions as a consequence of cancer treatment. In: van Eys J, Seelig MS, Nichols BL, eds., Nutrition and cancer. New York: Spectrum Publications, pp. 159–164.

Bernstein IL, Vitiello MV, Sigmundi RA (1980) Effects of interference stimuli on the acquisition of learned aversions to foods in the rat. J Comp Physiol Psychol 94:921–931.

Bolze MS, Fosmire GJ, Stryker JA, et al. (1982) Taste acuity, plasma zinc levels and weight loss during radiotherapy: A study of relationships. Radiology 144:163–169.

Carson JAS, Gormican A (1977) Taste acuity and food attitudes of selected patients with cancer. J Am Diet Assoc 70:361–364.

DeWys WD (1974) Abnormalities of taste as a remote effect of malignancy. Ann NY Acad Sci 230:427–434.

DeWys WD (1977a) Anorexia in cancer patients. Cancer Res 37:2354–2358.

DeWys WD (1977b) Changes in taste sensation in cancer patients: Correlation with caloric intake. In: The chemical senses and nutrition. Kare M, ed., New York: Academic Press, pp. 381–391.

DeWys WD (1978) Changes in taste sensation and feeding behavior in cancer patients: A review. J Hum Nutr 32:447–453.

DeWys WD (1980) Nutritional care of the cancer patient. JAMA 244:374–376.

DeWys WD (1982) Pathophysiology of cancer cachexia: Current understanding and areas for future research. Cancer Res 42:721s–726s.

DeWys WD, Herbst SH (1977) Oral feeding in the nutritional management of the cancer patient. Cancer Res 37:2429–2431.

DeWys WD, Kisner D (1982) Principles of nutritional care of the cancer patients. In: Carter S, Glastein E, Livingston RB, eds., Principles of cancer treatment. New York: McGraw-Hill, pp. 252–259.

DeWys WD, Kubota T (1981) Enteral and parenteral nutrition in the care of the cancer patient. JAMA 246:1725–1727.

DeWys WD, Walters K (1975) Abnormalities of taste sensation in cancer patients. Cancer 36:1888–1896.

DeWys WD, Begg C, Lavin PT, et al. (1980) Prognostic effect of weight loss prior to chemotherapy in cancer patients. Am J Med 69:491–497.

DeWys WD, Costa G, Henkin R (1982) Clinical parameters related to anorexia. Cancer Treatm Rep (suppl.) 65:49–52.

Garcia J, Hankins WG, Rusiniak KW (1974) Behavioral regulation of the milieu interne in man and rat. Science (Washington), 185:823–831.

Gorshein D (1977) Posthyspophysectomy taste abnormalities: Their relationship to remote effects of cancer. Cancer 39:1700–1703.

Henkin RI, Schechter PJ, Hoye R, Mattern FCT (1971) Idiopathic hypoguesia with dysguesia, hyposmia and dysosmia: A new syndrome. JAMA 217:434–440.

Kashima HK, Kalinowski B (1979) Taste impairment following laryngectomy. Ear Nose Throat 58:88–92.

Lawson DH, Richmond A, Nixon DW, Rudman D (1982) Metabolic approaches to cancer cachexia. Annu Rev Nutr 2:277–301.

Leibowitz SF (1976) Brain catecholaminergic mechanisms for control of hunger. In: Novin D, Wyrwicki W, Bray G, eds., Hunger: Basic mechanisms and clinical implications. New York: Raven Press, pp. 1–18.

Morrison SD (1976) Control of food intake in cancer cachexia: A challenge and a tool. Physiol Behav 17:705–714.

Mossman KL, Henkin RI (1978) Radiation-induced changes in taste acuity in cancer patients. Int J Radiat Oncol Biol Phys 4:663–670.

Narendra GM (1977) The site of synthesis and functions of acute plasma proteins: close relationships with the reticuloendothelial system. Med Hypoth 3:63–70.

Russ J, DeWys WD (1977) Correction of taste abnormality of malignancy with intravenous hyperalimentation. Arch Intern Med 138:799–800.

Smith JC, Blumsack JT (1981) Learned taste aversion as a factor in cancer therapy. Cancer Treatm Rep (suppl.) 65:37–42.

Warnold I, Lundholm K, Schersten T (1978) Energy balance and body composition in cancer patients. Cancer Res 38:1801–1807.

Williams LR, Cohen MH (1978) Altered taste thresholds in lung cancer. Am J Clin Nutr 31:122–125.

ANTITUMOR EFFECT OF INDOMETHACIN IN RATS WITH AUTOCHTHONOUS INTESTINAL TUMORS

MORRIS POLLARD, D.V.M., PH.D.

The publications of Laqueur (1964) and Druckrey and coworkers (1967) provided the initiative for significant progress in experimental cancer of the intestines. Their demonstrations of cancer induction by hydrazine-related compounds provided investigators with the means to examine many facets of the problem through development of model tumor systems in rats and mice (Haase et al., 1973; Newberne and Rogers, 1973; Nigro et al., 1973; Reuber and Hill, 1973; Ward, 1974). Intestinal carcinogens, in addition to 1,2 dimethylhydrazine (DMH), attracted the attention of investigators: they included metabolites of DMH (azoxymethane, methylazoxymethanol), N-methylnitrosourea, N-nitro-N-nitrosoguanidine, aflatoxin, and bracken fern. Most of the model systems reported subsequently were derived from those listed here. The model tumor systems have yielded information on the chemistry of carcinogenesis and subsequent pathogenesis of the disease, on genetic susceptibility, prevention, promotion, therapy, and epidemiology of intestinal cancer. Such studies could not be performed without test animals.

MODEL TUMOR SYSTEMS

The development of animal model tumor systems as a counterpart to human disease has been the subject of intense investigation. These studies were based on judicious selection of the most appropriate initiator, of the best animal species and strains, and of the ancillary factors, such as diet and microbial flora, which might modulate host responses to tumorigenesis. An ideal model system in animals should resemble the counterpart disease in humans. Tumors should be autochthonous, they should occur in high incidence in the natural anatomic site, and they should show some evidence of phenotypic diversity, especially

From the Lobund Laboratory, University of Notre Dame, Notre Dame, Indiana.

in the intestine. The tumors should grow progressively and spread to other sites by metastasis. The results of the standard experimental protocol should be reproducible. Control animals should be free of "spontaneous" tumors. In most respects, the tumor models that have been developed for intestinal cancer in rats and mice comply with these criteria except for metastasis. However, one strain of rats has developed intestinal tumors "spontaneously" (Miyamoto and Takizawa, 1975).

Investigators now have a wide choice of carcinogenic agents that induce tumors predictably in the intestinal tract (Pozharisski et al., 1979). Some of them act directly on the target cells, and others must be activated metabolically to active electrophilic forms that manifest their effects in distant organs (Miller, 1978). For example, DMH is not carcinogenic but must be metabolized (presumably in the liver) through azoxymethane to methylazoxymethanol (MAM), which is considered the active form (Druckrey, 1972; Fiala, 1977). As applied here, the initiator (DMH) is fed or inoculated parenterally, and mucosal cells in the large and small intestines are transformed. The resultant neoplasms, in many respects, resemble those observed in humans.

STAGES OF CARCINOGENESIS

The subjects of prevention, diagnosis, and therapy of human intestinal cancer have been examined using tumor model systems. Three stages of tumorigenesis have been described: (a) carcinogenic agents that induce intestinal tumors have been inactivated in vivo when administered coincidently with compounds classified as antioxidants or those that induce mixed function oxidase activity. The procedure is called *chemoprevention* (Wattenberg, 1978). (b) Following exposure to an initiating agent, the transformed cells can remain dormant for long periods; however, by subsequent administrations of chemical agents called *promotors*, the appearance of tumors can be accelerated (Berenblum, 1941; Rous and Kidd, 1941). The promotion of intestinal carcinogenesis has been demonstrated by feeding cholestyramine (Nigro et al., 1973; Asano et al., 1975), sodium barbiturate (Pollard and Luckert, 1979), high fat diets (Bull et al., 1979; Carroll, 1980), or cholesterol metabolites (Reddy and Watanabe, 1979) to carcinogen-exposed rats. The mechanisms of tumor promotion are as yet uncertain, but they have been associated with enzymes such as ornithine decarboxylase (Verma and Boutwell, 1977) and with prostaglandins (Levine, 1981). In the third stage of tumorigenesis, active tumors appear that enlarge and spread in autonomous fashion. For use at this stage of disease, oncolytic and other antitumor agents, such as retinoids (Sporn, 1976), are under investigation. However, negative reports concerning retinoids have appeared recently (Wenk et al., 1981; Silverman et al., 1981). The third stage is being investigated in the Lobund Laboratory in regard to the blocking of prostaglandin synthesis (arachidonic acid transformation) in the model tumor system that is described following.

THE LOBUND EXPERIMENTAL PROTOCOL FOR INTESTINAL CANCER

In the course of 5 years, we have developed and used a unique model tumor system in Lobund strain Sprague-Dawley (S-D) rats. The experimental protocol is based on several premises: (a) the male S-D rat is unusually susceptible to minimal doses of DMH, MAM, and methylacetoxymethyl nitrosamine DMN Oac; (b) demonstrable tumors appear in S-D rats within 20 weeks after exposure to the carcinogen; (c) the number of tumors per rat is related to the amount of carcinogen administered to each rat; (d) S-D rats do not develop intestinal tumors "spontaneously"; and (e) the S-D rat is free of complicating infectious agents. In contrast, the Lobund strain of Wistar rat (L-W) is uniquely resistant to the carcinogenic effects of DMH and of DMN Oac (Asano and Pollard, 1978; Pollard and Luckert, 1981a). The investigations with this model system have revealed that the development of intestinal tumors can be inhibited by a drug (indomethacin) that blocks the production of prostaglandins and is classified as a nonsteroidal, antiinflammatory agent (Vane, 1972).

Animals

Conventional male S-D rats were random-propagated in a closed colony and maintained in Lobund Laboratory through 36+ generations. They accepted reciprocal skin grafts. They were fed, ad libitum, diet L-485 (Kellogg and Wostmann, 1969) and unchlorinated water from deep wells and held in plastic boxes on granulated corncob bedding. The animal rooms were air-conditioned (22°C), humidified (60%), and provided with 12-hour cycles of light and darkness. No "spontaneous" tumors of the intestine have been observed in S-D rats when examined up to age 36 months.

After exposure to a carcinogenic agent, the rats were held in flexible plastic isolators that were vented to the roof of the building; and all waste was removed aseptically and incinerated. After 1 week, they were moved to isolated animal rooms in which they were maintained in laminar flow units until completion of the experimental period.

Dose Responses to Carcinogens

In the basic protocol, conventional male weanling S-D rats (approximately 150 g) were administered 1, 5, or 10 doses of 1,2 dimethylhydrazine dihydrochloride (DMH)[1] by gavage (30 mg/kg body wt) at weekly intervals, in order to determine sensitivity of the test system. MAM was inoculated subcutaneously (30 mg/kg body wt) and DMN Oac was inoculated intraperitoneally (13 mg/kg body wt). The drugs were dissolved in sterile distilled water just prior to administration to the rats. The rats were killed at 20 weeks after initial exposure to the carcinogen and examined for gross and microscopic evidence of disease.

In response to 5 or 10 doses of DMH, all the S-D rats developed an average of 4.8 and 14 tumors/rat, respectively. A single dose of DMH induced tumors in 21/30 (70%) of the rats, with an average of 1.0 tumor/rat. In response to 10 doses of MAM, tumors developed in all rats, with an average of 20.4 tumors/

[1]1,2 dimethylhydrazine (DMH) was purchased from Aldrich Chemical Co., Milwaukee, WI. Methylazoxymethanol acetate (MAM) was purchased from Schwarz/Mann Co., Orangeburg, NY. Methyl(acetoxymethyl)nitrosamine (DMN Oac) was received as a gift from Dr. J. R. Rice, National Cancer Institute, Bethesda, MD. N-Methylnitrosourea (NMU) was purchased from Stark Associates, Inc., Buffalo, NY. Indomethacin [99.7% pure 1-(p-chlorobenzoyl)-5-methoxy-2-methyl-indole 3-acetic acid] was a gift from Merck Sharp and Dohme, Rahway, NJ.

TABLE 1. Dose Response of Lobund Sprague-Dawley Rats to DMH, MAM, or DMN Oac[a]

No. doses	No. rats with tumors/ No. rats inoculated (%)	Total no. tumors	Average no. tumors/ Tumor-bearing rat	Average no. tumors/ No. rats inoculated
DMH				
1	21/30 (70)	30	1.4	1.0
5	69/69(100)	338	4.8	4.8
10	23/23 (100)	323	14.0	14.0
MAM				
1	47/58 (82)	117	2.5	2.0
10	10/10 (100)	204	20.4	20.4
DMN Oac				
1	36/48 (75)	72	2.0	1.5

[a]Weanling male Lobund Sprague-Dawley rats were each administered 1,2-dimethylhydrazine by gavage at weekly intervals (30 mg/kg body wt/week), or methylazoxymethanol acetate (MAM), same dosage by subcutaneous inoculation, or methyl(acetoxymethyl)nitrosamine (DMN Oac), 13 mg/kg body wt., intraperitoneally. At week 20 after the first dose of carcinogen, each rat was killed and examined for tumors in the intestines.

rat. In response to 1 dose of MAM, 47/58 (82%) of the rats developed an average of 2.0 tumors each. Following a single dose of DMN Oac, 36/48 (75%) of the rats developed an average of 1.5 tumors/rat (Table 1).

The tumors were polypoid or sessile; some were extensive and invaded the serosa of the intestine. Some of the large tumors were mucinous and so extensive as to obstruct the lumen. Metastatic lesions were observed infrequently. The histologic patterns of the tumors agreed with those observed by Ward (1974).

Strain Susceptibility to DMH

Male weanling rats, representing several strains, were inoculated with 10 doses of DMH (30 mg/kg body wt/week): they were identified as S-D, Fischer 344, Buffalo, and Lobund Wistar (L-W) strains. They were killed for examinations at week 20 after first exposures to DMH. Lobund strain S-D rats were most susceptible to DMH, if judged by numbers of tumors in the intestines, with 16.7/rat. Numbers of tumors/rat (5.1/rat) were lower in the Fischer strain; however, all of them developed tumors. The Buffalo rat was intermediate in susceptibility to DMH (average 1.3 tumors/rat) and the L-W rats were resistant to the carcinogenic effects of DMH (Table 2). L-W rats were resistant also to DMN Oac (Pollard and Luckert, 1981a). MAM induced intestinal tumors in L-W rats (Pollard and Zedeck, 1978), which suggests that the resistance to DMH may have been due to failure to activate DMH.

TABLE 2. Susceptibilities of Rat Strains to the Carcinogenic Effects of Dimethylhydrazine[a]

Rat strain	Rats with tumors/ Rats inoculated (%)	Tumors			
		Colon	Duodenum	Per tumor-bearing rat	Per rat inoculated
Sprague-Dawley I	13/13 (100)	111	108	16.7	16.7
Fischer (F344)	10/10 (100)	35	16	5.1	5.1
Buffalo	10/15 (66)	17	2	1.9	1.3
Wistar	0/14	0	0	0	0

[a]Weanling male rats were administered DMH by gavage (30 mg/kg body wt) once a week for 10 weeks. At 20 weeks after onset of trial, each rat was examined at autopsy for tumors in the intestines and elsewhere. Control uninoculated rats were negative for tumors.

APPLICATIONS OF THE MODEL TUMOR SYSTEM

At intervals after administration of a carcinogen, groups of the rats were treated with a putative modulating agent, administered daily by gavage, or continuously in the drinking water. The treated rats (and carcinogen-inoculated controls) were examined for disease at 20 weeks after initial exposure to the carcinogenic agent. Each rat was weighed, anesthetized with diethyl ether, and exsanguinated from the exposed heart. The thorax and abdominal cavities were opened and examined for gross evidence of disease. The intestinal tract was excised from the anus to the stomach, opened longitudinally, washed free of contents, and examined visually for tumors with a duoloupe (3 × magnification). The numbers and locations of tumors were recorded. The intestinal tract was fixed in Bouin's solution for 18 hours, changed twice with 70% ethanol, and then examined again for tumors (3 × magnification). Tumors or other lesions of uncertain nature were embedded, sectioned, and stained with hematoxylin and eosin and examined microscopically.

The basic protocol was modified by administrations of other carcinogenic agents: methylazoxymethanol acetate (MAM,[1] methyl(acetoxymethyl)nitrosamine (DMN Oac),[1] and N-methyl nitrosourea (MNU).[1] While the basic protocol was usually terminated at week 20, individual experiments were extended to 40 weeks. The results were analyzed by Student's *t* test.

Prostaglandin-blocking Agents

It should be no surprise that for many years cancers have been associated with prostaglandin (PG) activities. Early publications by Jaffe (1974), by Bennett and del Tacca (1975), and by Hokama et al. (1981) reported that intestinal tumors produced high levels of PGs compared with levels in the normal mucosa around the tumors. Reviews have been published on the relationshp of PGs to cancer (Bennett, 1979; Goodwin et al., 1980; Karim and Rao, 1976). Investigators have demonstrated that PG-blocking drugs interfered with propagation of

TABLE 3. Effect of Indomethacin on Development of DMH-induced Intestinal Tumors[a]

Exp. no.	No. rats	Interval/ days[b]	Indomethacin	Weights avg./g Body wt	Liver (% body wt)
I	10	3	+	402	11.2 (2.7)
	10		−	397	10.7 (2.6)
				0.8501[c]	
II	10	12	+	390	12.3 (3.1)
	10		−	402	13.0 (3.2)
				0.4274[c]	
III	10	35	+	436	14.4 (3.3)
	9		−	415	14.2 (3.4)
				0.9342[c]	

Source: Pollard and Luckert (1980).

[a]Weanling male Sprague-Dawley rats were administered 1,2 dimethylhydrazine dihydrochloride by gavage (30 mg/kg body wt/week) for 5 weeks. At intervals, after the fifth dose of DMH, a group of the rats were given, ad libitum, water with indomethacin (20 mg/L) and the control rats were given drug-

tumor cells in vivo and in vitro (reviewed by Levine, 1981). Experiments with transplanted prostate adenocarcinoma cells in rats demonstrated that administrations of aspirin or of indomethacin interfered with the predictable spread pattern of tumor cells to other organs (Pollard et al., 1977). Most investigations on effects of indomethacin on cancer in animals involved transplanted tumor cells. The present report deals with the effects of indomethacin[1] on autochthonous intestinal tumors that were induced in rats by DMH, MAM, DMN Oac, and MNU. In our judgment, the results of the study are relevant to the human disease.

Following 10 doses of DMH, aspirin was administered in the drinking water (625 mg/L) to S-D rats until week 20, when they were killed for examinations. The aspirin was replaced with freshwater at daily intervals. When the rats were examined at autopsy, the drug-treated rats showed no evidence of drug-related toxicity. Despite this large dose of aspirin, the patterns of intestinal tumors were not modified significantly in the rats that consumed the aspirin-supplemented water, compared with control rats on drug-free water.

It was our judgment that the tumor burden resulting from 10 doses of DMH or of MAM may have been excessive and unrealistic; so further trials were conducted in rats that had received 1 or 5 doses of the carcinogenic agents. At intervals of 3, 12, or 25 days following the fifth dose of DMH, groups of rats were administered indomethacin in 1% cornstarch (a) by daily gavage or (b) by feeding this drug ad libitum in drinking water (20 mg/L). In the latter instance, indomethacin was dissolved in absolute ethanol, which was then added to the drinking water. In one trial, ethanol alone was added to the drinking water, without effect on the tumor response to DMH. Fresh indomethacin was provided at 3-day intervals.

TABLE 3. *(continued)*

No. rats with tumors	No. tumors		Avg. tumor/ rat	Avg. tumor/ tumor-bearing rat
	Colon	Duodenum		
6	7	1	0.9	1.3
10	38	15	5.3	5.3
			0.002[c]	
5	7	2	0.9	1.8
10	21	5	2.6	2.6
			0.0065[c]	
4	5	0	0.5	1.2
9	11	9	2.2	2.2
0.0016[c]			0.007[c]	

free water. The indomethacin was changed at 3-day intervals. All rats were killed and examined at 20 weeks after onset of the experiment. Average consumption of indomethacin per rat was 0.55 mg/kg body wt/day.

[b]Interval in days between last dose of DMH and onset of indomethacin therapy.

[c]Test is significant at level indicated.

Effect of Indomethacin Following Five Doses of DMH

Rats that consumed indomethacin by gavage consumed 0.25 mg indomethacin/kg body wt/day. Rats that consumed the drug in drinking water ingested an average of 0.55 mg/kg body wt/day, and the antitumor effects of the latter regime were much more significant. The numbers of rats with tumors were reduced by 40% ($P < .0016$) among those that received indomethacin in the drinking water (Pollard and Luckert, 1980) (Table 3); and the number of tumors per indomethacin-treated rat was lower than in the control rat ($P < .002$, .0065, .007). There was no obvious toxic manifestation as judged by body weights or liver weights; however, noteworthy lesions were observed in the intestines of rats that consumed indomethacin. This was in the form of distinct "knobs" protruding on the serosal surfaces of the small intestines. They were granulomatous lesions, suggestive of a reparative process, over areas of mucosal damage. At 10 mg indomethacin/L drinking water (0.27 mg/kg body wt/day), no antitumor effect was demonstrable in DMH-treated rats. At 40 mg indomethacin/L drinking water (1.10 mg/kg body wt/day), many of the rats developed intestinal perforations and lethal peritonitis.

Effect of Indomethacin Following One Dose of DMH or MAM

Groups of rats were administered 1 dose of DMH or of MAM. Thirty-four days later (DMH), or at 7 and 35 days later (MAM), groups of rats were administered indomethacin (20 mg/L) in the drinking water. When examined at week 20, in those that consumed indomethacin there was a significant reduction in numbers of rats with intestinal tumors and in numbers of tumors/rat, compared

TABLE 4. Effect of Indomethacin on Intestinal Tumors Induced in Rats by 1,2-Dimethylhydrazine or Methylazoxymethanol[a]

Interval	Treatment	Rats with tumors/ rats inoculated	Body weight (Avg/g)	Tumors: Colon	Tumors: Duodenum	Average (tumors/ rat)
I. DMH-induced						
34 days	Indomethacin	2/9	403	1	1	0.22
	No drug	9/10	436	11	2	1.30
	Significance[b]	.0019	.0248			.0102
II. MAM-induced						
7 days	Indomethacin	1/7	415.4	0	1	0.14
	No drug	7/9	427	4	8	1.3
	Significance[b]	.0085	.57			.0075
35 days[c]	Indomethacin	0/5	237.2	0	0	0
	No drug	3/5	229.2	4	3	1.4
	Significance[b]		.6573			

Source: Pollard and Luckert (1981a).

[a]Weanling male Sprague-Dawley rats were administered one dose of DMH by gavage (30 mg/kg body wt), or MAM acetate subcutaneously (30 mg/kg body wt.) Thirty-four days later (DMH), and 7 and 35 days later (MAM), groups of rats were given water to which indomethacin was added (20 mg/L). The average consumption of indomethacin was 0.55 mg/kg body wt/day. Control rats received water without the drug. The rats were killed for examinations at 20 weeks after exposures to the carcinogens.

[b]Student's *t* test.

[c]Female rats.

with control rats (Pollard and Luckert, 1981a) (Table 4). One group of rats (II-35 days) consisted of females, and the incidence of tumors/rat was similar to that among male rats.

Effect of Indomethacin in Rats Following One Dose of DMN Oac

Preliminary dose-response trials with male weanling S-D and L-W rats were determined with a single intraperitoneal dose of DMN Oac (13 mg/kg body wt) (Joshi et al., 1977). When examined after 20 weeks, 36/48 (75%) of S-D rats had

TABLE 5. Effect of Indomethacin on Induction of Intestinal Tumors by DMN Oac

Treatment	Rats with tumors	Tumors in colon	Tumors in small intestine	Mean number of tumors per rat
Indomethacin	1 of 7	0	1	0.14[a]
Control	6 of 8	5	7	1.5
Indomethacin	0 of 5	0	0	
Control	8 of 10	7	7	1.4

Source: Pollard and Luckert (1981b). Science 214: 558–559. Copyright 1981 by the American Association for the Advancement of Science.

[a]$P < .05$, Student's *t* test.

developed intestinal tumors, an average of 1.5/rat. No tumor was found among 21 male L-W rats. Thereafter, S-D rats were inoculated once with DMN Oac at same dose; after 14 days, groups were administered indomethacin in the drinking water (20 mg/L). Fresh indomethacin was provided at intervals of 3 days. As indicated in Table 5, few of the rats that consumed the indomethacin had tumors (1 of 12) compared with controls (14 of 18); also, the numbers of tumors in rats that consumed indomethacin manifested a marked reduction of tumors/ rat (Pollard and Luckert, 1981b).

Effect of Indomethacin in Rats Following Inoculation with N-Methylnitrosourea (NMU)

Narisawa and coworkers (1981) inoculated Fischer rats intrarectally with NMU (2 mg 3 ×/week for 5 weeks). At 11 weeks, groups of rats were administered indomethacin, suspended in methylcellulose, intraperitoneally (2.5 mg/kg) three times per week for 15 weeks. When examined at autopsy, 9/29 (31%) of indomethacin-treated rats had tumors, an average of 0.45/rat; and among control rats, 14/20 (70%) had tumors, an average of 1.1/rat.

In our assessment of indomethacin on MNU-induced tumors, male weanling S-D rats were inoculated intrarectally with MNU,[1] 4 doses of 2 mg at intervals of 3 days. Three weeks later indomethacin was administered in the drinking water (20 mg/L) to a group of the rats. When examined at 28 weeks after the last dose of MNU, 2/7 (28%) of the indomethacin-treated rats had tumors, an average of 0.4/rat; and 6/8 (75%) of the control rats had tumors, an average of 1.4/rat. Also, the indomethacin-treated rats had developed one tumor in the kidney, and the controls had developed four tumors in other organs (Table 6).

DISCUSSION

From the data just presented, it appears that tumors induced in the intestines of S-D rats by DMH were sensitive to the effects of indomethacin, a drug whose principal activities have been ascribed to blockage of PG synthesis. As the dosage of the initiating agent (DMH) was reduced, the demonstrable antitumor effect of indomethacin increased. As dosage of indomethacin was reduced, an antitumor effect was not manifested; and as dosage was increased, it resulted in lethal damage to the host. Indomethacin was effective on tumors induced in

TABLE 6. Effect of Indomethacin on Tumors Induced in Rats by N-Methylnitrosourea

Treatment	Number	Interval after MNU/ weeks	Rats with tumors/ rats inoculated	Tumors: Colon	Tumors: Small intestine	Tumors: Other organs[b]	Tumors: Tumors/ rat
Control	10	—	6/8 (75%)	7	3	4	1.4
Indomethacin	10	3	2/7 (28%)	3	0	1	0.4

[a]Male Sprague-Dawley rats were inoculated intrarectally with N-methylnitrosourea: 4 doses of 2 mg at intervals of 3 days. They were fed indomethacin in drinking water (20 mg/L) ad libitum.

[b]Tumors were carcinomas in the breast (1), liver (1), kidney (2), and sarcoma in the spleen (1).

rats by MAM, DMN Oac, and MNU, as well as DMH, which suggests that the tumors have a common indomethacin-sensitive biologic factor(s).

The growth of tumors may be promoted as a consequence of immunosuppression, caused by the PGs that they produce. The immune status has been enhanced when PG synthesis was blocked (Grinwich and Plescia, 1977; Pelus and Strausser, 1977). Prostaglandins may be an essential product of tumor cells whose function is as yet obscure.

Treatment of tumor cells in vitro with indomethacin reduced the rate of propagation of the cells without evidence of cytotoxicity or of thymidine uptake. While indomethacin interferes with the propagation of many tumor cell types, it also interferes with other biosynthetic processes. In addition, it interferes with the production of phospholipase A_2, phosphodiesterase, acylhydrolase, and cAMP-dependent protein kinase. Thus, effects of indomethacin may not be attributed alone to blockage of PG biosynthesis (reviewed by Levine, 1981). Although aspirin is not as powerful as indomethacin in blocking the synthesis of PG, it has not manifested an antitumor effect on DMH-induced intestinal tumors. Possibly, this may be due to inadequate dosage or to a level of activity far below that of indomethacin (Levine et al., 1976).

The antitumor effect of indomethacin cannot be interpreted as chemoprevention, since the intervals between exposures to carcinogens and onset of indomethacin treatment were beyond the time period of initiation activity (48 hours) in rats (Fiala, personal communication, 1981; Rice, personal communication, 1981).

Why have we concentrated our attention on indomethacin? Tumor cells, in general, produce more PGs than "normal" cells (Levine, 1981). Of the PG-blocking agents that have been examined in rats, indomethacin interfered most consistently with growth of autochthonous intestinal tumors. Since this drug was judged to be the most powerful of the nonsteroidal antiinflammatory agents (Robinson and Vane, 1974; Levine et al., 1976), this high level of activity may be required for the antitumor effect to be manifested. Indomethacin blocked PG synthesis at the cyclooxygenase level, which thus blocked the synthesis of prostaglandins, prostacyclin, and thromboxanes. Other agents (5, 8, 11, 14-eicosatetranoic acid and antiinflammatory steroids) also block the synthesis of cyclooxygenase products. At this time we cannot identify the arachidonic acid transformation product that is related to tumor growth. This subject is examined extensively by Levine (1981).

Except for surgical intervention, there is little that can be done clinically to interfere with the growth and spread of intestinal cancer in humans. Except for therapeutic benefit against desmoid tumors in humans (Waddell and Gerner, 1980), there is no evidence that indomethacin can serve as a therapeutic drug for early or advanced cancer in humans. Based on data thus far acquired through the model tumor system used here, the best assessment indicates that indomethacin slows the growth of autochthonous intestinal tumors. For example, when onset of indomethacin treatment was delayed, the actual number of tumors/rat was increased with time; but, compared with untreated control animals, tumor sizes and numbers remained significantly reduced.

In preliminary trials, indomethacin has interfered with tumorigenesis when administered as late as 80 days after exposure to MAM, and the antitumor effect has been manifested in the rats for as long as 10 months after onset of the experiment (Pollard and Luckert, 1983). The major limitation of indomethacin administration is its damage to the intestinal mucous membrane in rats, which warrants the search for another less toxic drug with the same antitumor effects. In this respect, with judicious attention, indomethacin is used extensively in humans as an effective antiinflammatory drug.

We share the viewpoint with others that therapeutic benefits demonstrated by drugs on model tumor systems in animals are significant as putative therapeutic agents in humans. It depends to a great extent on the accurate representation of the animal disease as a counterpart of the disease in humans.

ADDENDUM

After completion of this chapter, additional investigations revealed that a new class of nonsteroid antiinflammatory agent (NSAID), piroxicam, demonstrated an antitumor effect in MAM-treated rats that was highly significant with no evidence of toxicity (Pollard et al., 1983). Evidence that indomethacin also blocks the initiation effect of MNU was presented by Narisawa et al. (1983). It is of significance to note that administration of Sulindac, an NSAID, was of therapeutic benefit to patients with intestinal polyposis (Waddell and Loughry, 1983).

This research program was supported in part by PHS grant CA 15957 through the Large Bowel Cancer Project, PHS grant CA 00295, and the Ambrose and Gladys Bowyer Foundation and a grant from the Xerox Foundation.

REFERENCES

Asano T, Pollard M (1978) Strain susceptibility and resistance to 1,2 dimethylhydrazine-induced enteric tumors in germfree rats. Proc Soc Exp Biol Med 158:89–91.

Asano T, Pollard M, Madsen DC (1975) Effects of cholestyramine on 1,2-dimethylhydrazine-induced enteric carcinoma in germfree rats. Proc Soc Exp Biol Med 150:780–785.

Bennett A (1979) Prostaglandins and cancer. In: Karim SMM, ed., Practical applications of prostaglandins and their synthesis inhibitors. Lancaster, U.K.: MTP Press Ltd, pp. 149–188.

Bennett A, del Tacca M (1975) Prostaglandins in human colonic carcinoma. Gut 16:409.

Berenblum I (1941) The cocarcinogenic action of croton resin. Cancer Res 1:44–48.

Bull AW, Soullier BK, Wilson PS, et al. (1979) Promotion of azoxymethane-induced intestinal cancer by high-fat diet. Cancer Res 39:4956–4959.

Carroll KK (1980) Lipids and carcinogenesis. J Environ Pathol Toxicol 3:253–271.

Druckrey H (1972) Organospecific carcinogenesis in the digestive tract. In Nakahara W, et al., eds., Topics in chemical carcinogenesis. Baltimore: University Park Press, pp. 73–101.

Druckrey H, Preussmann R, Matkies F, Ivankovic S (1967) Selective erzeugung von darmkrebs by ratten durch 1,2 dimethylhydrazine. Naturwissenschaften 54:285.

Fiala ES (1977) Investigations into the metabolism and mode of action of the colon carcinogens 1,2-dimethylhydrazine and azoxymethane. Cancer 40:2436–2445.

Goodwin JS, Husby G, Williams RC Jr. (1980) Prostaglandin E and cancer growth. Cancer Immunol Immunother 8:3–8.

Grinwich KD, Plescia OJ (1977) Tumor-mediated immunosuppression: Prevention by inhibitors of prostaglandin synthesis. Prostaglandins 14:1175–1182.

Haase P, Cowen DM, Knowles JC, et al. (1973) Evaluation of dimethylhydrazine-induced tumours in mice as a model system for colorectal cancers. Br J Cancer 28:530–543.

Hokama Y, Cripps C, Sumida K, et al. (1981) Significant increase of plasma prostaglandins in cancer patients. Res Commun Chem Pathol Pharmacol 31:379–382.

Jaffe BM (1974) Prostaglandins and cancer: An update. Prostaglandins 6:453–461.

Joshi SR, Rice JR, Wenk ML, et al. (1977) Selective induction of intestinal tumors in rats by methylacetoxymethyl nitrosamine, an ester of the presumed reactive metabolite of dimethylnitrosamine. J Natl Cancer Inst 58:1531–1535.

Karim SMM, Rao B (1976) Prostaglandins and tumours. In: Karim SMM, ed., Prostaglandins: Physiological, pharmacological and pathological aspects. Baltimore: University Park Press, pp. 303–325.

Kellogg TF, Wostmann BS (1969) Stock diet for colony production of germfree rats and mice. Lab Anim Care 19:812–814.

Laqueur GL (1964) Carcinogenic effects of cycad meal and cycasin, methylazoxy-methanol glycoside, in rats and effects of cycasin in germfree rats. Fed Proc 23:1386–1387.

Levine L (1981) Arachidonic acid transformation and tumor production. Adv Cancer Res 35:49–79.

Levine L, Pong S-S, Robinson D, Kantrowitz ER (1976) Prostaglandins: Biosynthesis, metabolism, and synthesis inhibitors. J Invest Dermatol 67:665–666.

Miller EC (1978) Some current perspectives on chemical carcinogenesis in humans and experimental animals. Cancer Res 38:1479–1496.

Miyamoto M, Takizawa S (1975) Colon carcinoma in highly inbred rats. J Natl Cancer Inst 55:1471–1472.

Narisawa T, Sato M, Tani M, et al. (1981) Inhibition of development of methylnitrosourea-induced rat colon tumors. Cancer Res 41:1954–1957.

Narisawa T, Satoh M, Sano M, Tokahashi T (1983) Inhibition of initiation and promotion on n-methylnitrosourea-induced colon carcinogenesis in rats by nonsteroid anti-inflammatory agent indomethacin. Carcinogenesis 4:1225–1227.

Newberne PM, Rogers AE (1973) Rat colon carcinomas associated with aflatoxin and marginal vitamin A. J Nat Cancer Inst 50:439–448.

Nigro ND, Bhadrachari N, Chomchai C (1973) A rat model for studying colonic cancer: Effect of cholestyramine on induced tumors. Dis Colon Rectum 16:438–443.

Pelus LM, Strausser HR (1977) Minireview. Prostaglandins and the immune response. Life Sci 20:903–914.

Pollard M, Luckert PH (1979) Promotional effect of sodium barbiturate on intestinal tumors induced in rats by dimethylhydrazine. J Natl Cancer Inst 63:1089–1092.

Pollard M, Luckert PH (1980) Indomethacin treatment of rats with dimethylhydrazine-induced intestinal tumors. Cancer Treatm Rep 64:1323–1327.

Pollard M, Luckert PH (1981a) Treatment of chemically-induced intestinal cancer with indomethacin. Proc Soc Exp Biol Med 167:161–164.

Pollard M, Luckert PH (1981b) Effect of indomethacin on intestinal tumors induced in rats by the acetate derivative of dimethylnitrosamine. Science 214:558–559.

Pollard M, Luckert PH (1983) Prolonged antitumor effect of indomethacin on autochthonous intestinal tumors in rats. J Natl Cancer Inst 70:1103–1105.

Pollard M, Zedeck MS (1978) Induction of colon tumors in dimethylhydrazine-resistant Wistar rats by methylazoxymethanol. Nat Cancer Ins 61:493–494.

Pollard M, Chang CF, Luckert PH (1977) Investigations on prostate adenocarcinomas in rats. Oncology 34:129–132.

Pollard M, Luckert PH, Schmidt MA (1983) The suppressive effect of piroxicam on authchthonous intestinal tumors in the rat. Cancer Lett 21:57–61.

Pozharisski KM, Likkachev AJ, Klimashewski VF, Shaposhnikov JD (1979) Experimental intestinal cancer research with special reference to human pathology. Adv Cancer Res 30:165-237.

Reddy BS, Watanabe K (1979) Effect of cholesterol metabolites and promoting effect of lithocholic acid in colon carcinogenesis in germfree and conventional F344 rats. Cancer Res 39:1521-1524.

Reuber MD, Hill TA (1973) A biologic model for large bowel carcinogenesis. Proc Am Assoc Cancer Res No. 220.

Robinson HJ, Vane JR (1974) Prostaglandin synthesis inhibitors. New York: Raven Press.

Rous P, Kidd JC (1941) Conditional neoplasms and subthreshold neoplastic states: A study of the tar tumors of rabbits. J Exp Med 73:365-390.

Silverman J, Katayama S, Zelenakas K, Lauber J, Musser TK, Reddy M, Levenstein MJ, Weisburger JH (1981) Effect of retinoids on the induction of colon cancer in F344 rats by N-methyl-N-nitrosourea or by 1,2 dimethylhydrazine. Carcinogenesis 2:1167-1172.

Sporn MB, Dunlap NM, Newton DL, Smith JM (1976) Prevention of chemical carcinogenesis by vitamin A and its synthetic analogs (retinoids). Fed Proc 35:1332-1338.

Vane JR (1972) Prostaglandins in the inflammatory response. In Lepow IH, Ward PA, eds., Inflammation, mechanisms and control. New York: Academic Press.

Verma AK, Boutwell RK (1977) Vitamin A acid (retinoic acid), a potent inhibitor of 12-0-decarboxylase activity in mouse epidermis. Cancer Res 37:2196-2201.

Waddell WR, Gerner RE (1980) Indomethacin and ascorbate inhibit desmoid tumors. J Surg Oncol 15:85-90.

Waddell WR, Loughry RW (1983) Sulindac for polyposis of the colon. Surg Oncol 24:83-87.

Ward JM (1974) Morphogenesis of chemically induced neoplasms of the colon and small intestine in rats. Lab Invest 30:505-513.

Wattenberg LW (1978) Inhibitors of chemical carcinogenesis. In: Klein G, Weinhouse S, eds., Advances in cancer research. New York: Academic Press, 26:197-226.

Wenk ML, Ward JM, Reznik G, Dean J (1981) Effects of three retinoids on colon adenocarcinomas, sarcomas and hyperplastic polyps induced by intrarectal N-methyl-N-nitrosourea administration in male F344 rats. Carcinogenesis 2:1161-1166.

LARGE BOWEL CARCINOMA: SIGNIFICANCE OF LYMPH NODE REACTIONS

RICHARD C NAIRN, M.D., AND ERIC PIHL M.D.

The major functions of regional lymph nodes is well known (Bellanti, 1978). However, the role of the regional lymph nodes in clinically overt human cancer is still poorly understood. The management of the lymph nodes regional to resected tumors has created one of the most controversial problems in clinical surgery (Fisher, 1975) ever since Virchow (1860) ascribed them a filtering function. With the advent of modern tumor immunology, it has become obvious that their functions are much more complex.

Working with a transplantable rabbit carcinoma, Hall and colleagues (1973) claimed that concomitant removal of lymph nodes leads to shorter survival in comparison with nodes left in situ. In patients without evidence of lymphatic spread at the time of operation, a case could be made for preservation of the lymph nodes (Crile, 1969), at least in tumors at sites where operation for lymph node "recurrence" is easily performed. In colorectal cancer, operations for recurrence are more difficult, and lymph node assessment by palpation at operation has little predictive value. At present, we cannot see any means of improving the accuracy of clinical tumor staging, mainly because approximately one quarter of patients with subsequently histologically confirmed regional (stage C) disease do not have palpable nodes, whereas about half of those with "localized" tumors (stages A and B) do. However, we are unable to test the hypothesis that uninvolved lymph nodes regional to human colorectal carcinomas if left in situ could inhibit postoperative recurrence.

The prognostic significance of lymph node involvement in colorectal cancer is complex; in its assessment, site of origin of the primary tumor and depth of local invasion are also of major importance (Pihl et al., 1983). In colonic primary tumors that have not invaded through the wall, the presence of lymph node

Supported by a grant from the Anti-Cancer Council of Victoria.

From the Department of Pathology and Immunology, Monash University, and Alfred Hospital, Melbourne, Australia.

spread does not itself appear materially to affect long-term survival, whereas in the corresponding rectal tumors and in those of either site invading beyond the muscle, survival is reduced by approximately 30 to 60% in cases with lymphatic spread (Pihl et al., 1984). Thus, at this stage of the natural history, the lymph nodes appear to be an ineffective barrier to spread and may even provide a source for further tumor dissemination. At the preclinical stage, hardly anything is known about the role of the regional lymph node, and experimental animal colorectal cancer data in this connection are scanty.

LYMPH NODE IMMUNOMORPHOLOGY

The topographic distribution of thymus-dependent (T) and thymus-independent (B) lymphocyte areas in the human lymph node is well known (reviewed by Turk, 1977). These areas are easily identified in routine histologic sections of human pericolic, perirectal, and mesenteric lymph nodes (Figure 1).

T-Lymphocyte Distribution

Lymph nodes regional to the normal human large bowel are small, difficult to find, and rarely available to the pathologist. Immunomorphologically, such lymph nodes may be referred to as showing an "unstimulated" pattern (Tsakraklides et al., 1975); namely, there are few germinal centers and paracortical areas are small. T-lymphocytes from the thoracic duct enter the lymphoid tissue in the postcapillary venule and accumulate in the paracortical area. On antigenic stimulation, a massive paracortical T-cell proliferation takes place and numerous large pyroninophilic blast cells are easily recognized. In stimulated human mesocolic lymph nodes, the paracortical areas most often have a discrete irregular nodular appearance (Figure 1), although sometimes the paracortex is dispersed around the subcapsular area. A small number of T-lymphocytes may also be found within cortical follicles, but we are unaware of their significance.

B-Lymphocyte Distribution

Circulating B-cells are known to enter the lymph node in the same way as T-lymphocytes, through the postcapillary venule in the paracortex to localize in the follicular (cortical) area. The role of the germinal centers (Figure 1) is incompletely known. On antigenic stimulation of a lymph node, the number of lymphoid follicles and germinal centers (B-immunoblasts) increases. Following massive stimulation, these structures are found in the cortex, deep cortex, and medulla; this pattern is commonly seen in lymph nodes regional to large bowel cancer as well as in inflammatory bowel disease. A varying proportion of immunoglobulin-producing B-cells eventually differentiate into plasma cells that localize in the medullary cords.

Macrophage-Histiocyte Distribution

Monocytes enter the lymph nodes via afferent lymphatics and may infiltrate the medullary sinuses or the paracortical area. If the sinus distribution is conspicuous, it is commonly referred to as sinus histiocytosis (Black et al., 1953).

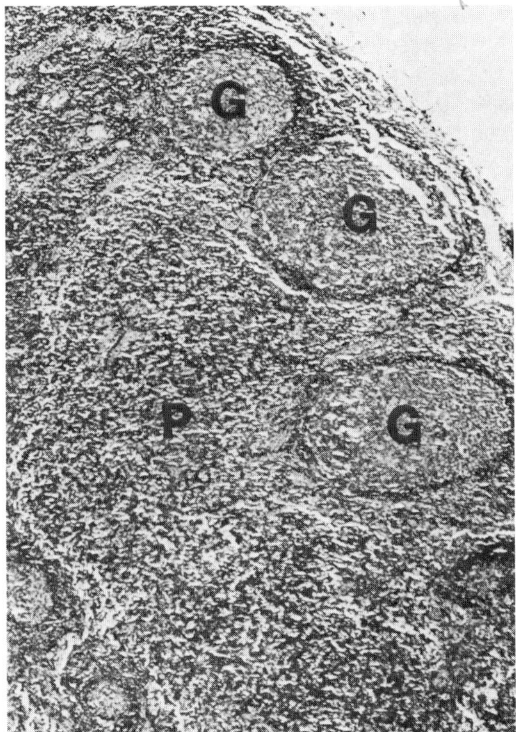

FIGURE 1. Section of a lymph node regional to a stage B colonic adenocarcinoma. Three germinal centers (G, thymus-independent) and a prominent paracortical area (P, thymus-dependent) are seen. (Hematoxylin alone, × 50) *Source:* Pihl et al. (1980c).

Immunomorphologic Analysis

The knowledge that the two major lymphocyte populations, namely, T- and B-cells, occupy distinctive, histologically identifiable areas in the lymph nodes led Cottier and coworkers (1973) to propose a standardized system of reporting human lymph node morphology in relation to inferred immunologic function. This system permits semiquantitative comparisons between lymph nodes, but it has not been widely accepted mainly because its numerous variables demand large samples before the clinical significance of any particular pattern can be established. However, these workers' paper stimulated immunopathologists to investigate further the prognostic implications of regional lymph node patterns in terms of immunologic function. A simplified approach by Tsakraklides and coworkers (1974) distinguished four different lymph node patterns modeled on those commonly used by pathologists for grading Hodgkin's disease: (1) lymphocyte predominance; (2) germinal center predominance; (3) unstimulated; (4) lymphocyte depletion. "Lymphocyte predominance" signifies mainly paracortical (T-lymphocyte) proliferation, and "germinal center predominance," B-lymphocyte proliferation; the unstimulated and lymphocyte depletion patterns are self-explanatory.

We find this terminology useful in routine reporting of cancer regional lymph node immunomorphology. However, the system is based on subjective pattern recognition assessment of the majority of lymph nodes examined and does not lend itself to precise quantification; for example, large lymph nodes classified as showing germinal center predominance could still have a total paracortical area far exceeding that of smaller nodes with a lymphocyte predominance pattern. We have tackled this problem by using a point-counting system of morphologic measurement (Chalkley, 1943; Pihl et al., 1977). This could now be advantageously replaced by modern electronic image analysis (van de Velde et al., 1978), of which we ourselves have so far no practical experience.

The rationale of the labor intensive but otherwise inexpensive point-counting approach is that a square graticule with exactly defined intersections ("points") is mounted in the eyepiece plane of the microscope. If a sufficient number of such points of a particular histologic image is counted, the relative size or distribution of the germinal centers or the paracortex can easily be calculated and expressed as a percentage of the total sectioned lymph node area. Furthermore, the microscope can also be calibrated so that the absolute size of the germinal centers can be expressed in absolute terms as a mm^2 measurement per lymph node section. By this method, or computerized image analysis, the median relative size or median absolute size per lymph node section of a defined lymph node area can be defined. In a series of patients, it could be used to provide prognostic information.

The method tends to underestimate absolute sizes in individual cases, unless care is taken that all lymph nodes examined are embedded and cut in the equatorial plane. The subjective error in the individual immunopathologist's assessment of different lymph node compartments could be overcome by the use of EAC-rosetting on frozen sections: only complement-receptor-bearing lymphocytes in the cortex bind EAC while the paracortex remains clear (Pihl et al., 1976). Indeed, with the introduction of monoclonal antibodies against lymphocyte subclasses, immunofluorescence or immunoenzyme histochemistry will permit even more precise cell identification. Generally, however, such sophistication adds little of practical significance for the experienced pathologist to the information available from routine hematoxylin-eosin stained sections.

PROGNOSTIC SIGNIFICANCE OF LYMPH NODE PATTERNS

The literature on the prognostic significance of lymph node patterns in colorectal cancer is contradictory, perhaps because most studies have been based on pattern recognition ("subjective scoring") by histopathologists.

Paracortex

Patt and coworkers (1975) assessed the approximate concentration of paracortical immunoblasts in lymph nodes regional to cancers of the sigmoid colon in 36 patients and found that those with abundant immunoblasts survived significantly longer and that the better survival could not be attributed to tumor stage. We (Pihl et al., 1977) studied sections of regional lymph nodes from 134 patients with stage B colorectal carcinomas and defined paracortical hyperplasia as a paracortical area exceeding approximately 15% of the lymph nodes in each patient. Our findings were in accord with those of Patt and coworkers (1975) of a prognostically favorable significance of paracortical (T-lymphocyte) hyperplasia, a feature that, on its own, was of relatively small survival significance in that it was associated with approximately one-third fewer recurrences (P = .09) and deaths (P = .04). However, when accompanied by perivascular lymphocytic cuffing in the primary tumor, it defined a subgroup of patients with an estimated survival in excess of 85% at 5 years. A favorable prognostic significance of the lymphocyte predominance (T-lymphocyte) pattern has also been reported by Nacopoulou and coworkers (1981).

Two groups of workers using subjective pattern recognition assessment of lymph node compartments found no correlation between lymph node paracortex and survival: Tsakraklides and coworkers (1975), applying their grading system referred to earlier, found similar survival in patients with lymphocyte predominance and with unstimulated patterns even when Dukes' stages A, B, and C were analyzed separately. Thynne and coworkers (1980) examined the regional lymph nodes of stage C colonic carcinomas uninvolved by metastasis and found no correlation between survival and paracortical immunoblasts scored subjectively as moderately or markedly increased in number.

We (Pihl et al., 1980a), have shown quantitatively, in more than 500 patients that the paracortex (Figure 1) is significantly larger in absolute measurements (mm^2/"mean" lymph node section) in stage A carcinomas than in noninvasive adenomas; that its size reaches a peak in stage B, and that it is significantly smaller in stage C tumors (Table 1). Similar, although less significant, differences were found in relation to relative (%) measurements. We have also shown that the absolute size of the paracortex tends to be smaller in lymph nodes of patients with mucinous carcinomas, which may stimulate less or even

TABLE 1. Regional Lymph Node Immunomorphology in Relation to Tumor Staging

		Paracortex		Germinal centers	
Stage	Number	%/total	Area/node (mm^2)	%/total	Area/node (mm^2)
Benign adenomas	17	15.1	2.2	2.9	0.6
		—	*	*	—
A	73	21.6	2.9	4.8	0.7
		—	—	—	*
B	206	20.6	3.3	6.4	1.3
		*	***	*	**
C	154	18.0	2.2	5.0	0.7
		—	—	—	—
D	76	14.8	1.7	5.7	0.7

Source: Modified from Pihl et al. (1980a).
Wilcoxon analysis of differences between means: — $P > .05$, * $P < .05$, ** $P < .01$, *** $P < .001$.

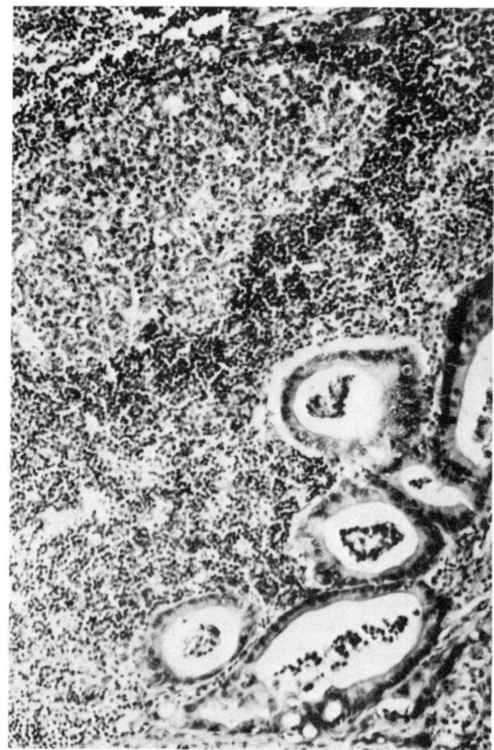

FIGURE 2. Lymph node containing metastasis from a well-differentiated sigmoid colonic adenocarcinoma. The carcinomatous acini (bottom right) are present in a paracortical area. Top left is a prominent germinal center. (Hematoxylin alone, × 130) *Source:* Pihl et al. (1980c).

inhibit cell-mediated immunity (Pihl et al., 1980b). In another study (Pihl et al., 1980c), we showed that lymph node paracortical hyperplasia, exceeding the median in mm^2/"mean" lymph node section within the individual stage, correlated favorably with survival in stages B and C. A paracortical response was very uncommon in tumor-involved nodes (stage C; Figure 2), as evidenced by a median size of 0.2 mm^2; that is, one eighth the corresponding stage B value. A poor paracortical response in tumor-involved lymph nodes has also been reported by Syrjanen and Hjelt (1978). Our patients whose tumor-involved lymph nodes showed paracortical hyperplasia had a highly significant survival advantage; no attempt was made to assess whether paracortical hyperplasia was dependent on actual numbers of involved nodes or the size of the metastases. No significant correlations between lymph node paracortex and survival were found in stages A and D. Moreover, when hyperplasia was defined only as a percentage exceeding the median, correlation with survival could seldom be recognized.

We conclude from these studies that the size of the paracortex is stage

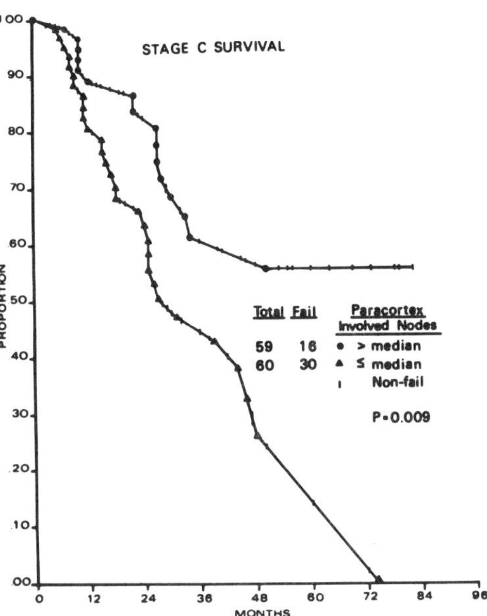

FIGURE 3. Survival time from surgery to death in stage C colorectal cancer. Patients unmatched for age and sex, with tumor-involved lymph nodes and a paracortical response exceeding the median (0.2 mm^2/ node section) survived significantly longer (upper curve), than those without. Survival in the latter patients is nil at 74 months (lower curve). *Source:* Pihl et al. (1980c).

related, reaching a peak in stage B tumors. The assessment should be made by absolute quantification rather than by relative, or subjective assessment, and hypoplasia/hyperplasia should be defined in statistical terms. Under these circumstances, paracortical lymph node hyperplasia on its own lacks survival significance in stages A and D; it is of small favorable significance ($P < .05$) in stage B tumors and in uninvolved lymph nodes of stage C tumors; it is of major favorable significance ($P = .009$) when present in lymph nodes with metastatic deposits (Figure 3). These data need refinement, preferably in a prospective series aimed at minimizing the sampling error.

Germinal Centers

The literature on the possible prognostic significance of follicular (B-cell) response in lymph nodes regional to malignant tumors is equivocal. Black and coworkers (1971) reported a favorable association with survival in gastric carcinoma. In our studies, follicular (i.e., cortical) hyperplasia per se, without independent assessment of germinal centers, does not seem to correlate with survival in colorectal cancer (Pihl et al., 1977). Subjective scoring of regional lymph node germinal center response and its relationship to survival has given conflicting data: Patt and coworkers (1975) reported that patients with few or no active germinal centers tended to do worse; Thynne and coworkers (1980) found no correlation in stage C cancers; Tsakraklides and coworkers (1975) reported a favorable trend; Nacopoulou and coworkers (1981) found a favorable association in stages A and B. These conflicting data clearly indicate the need for more precise studies.

Our quantitative studies of germinal centers (Pihl et al., 1980a) have shown

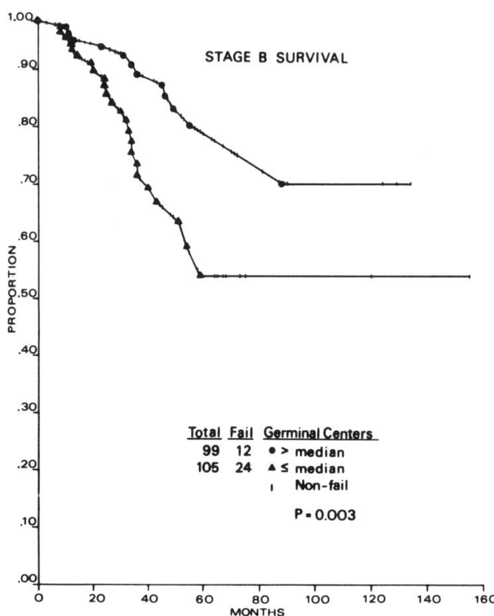

FIGURE 4. Survival in patients with stage B colorectal cancer in relation to regional lymph node germinal center response. Patients with hyperplasia, defined as exceeding the median for the stage (0.7 mm^2/lymph node section), survived significantly longer (upper curve). *Source:* Pihl et al. (1980c).

that their area per mean lymph node section increased significantly from benign lesions to stage A, reaching a peak in stage B and being significantly smaller in stage C; that is, the germinal centers related to staging similarly to the paracortex (Table 1). In contrast, the germinal center reactivity was unrelated to tumor mucin production (Pihl et al., 1980b). When expressed as size in mm^2/mean lymph node section, germinal center hyperplasia, defined as exceeding the median for the stage, was a significantly (P = .003) favorable prognostic finding in stage B (Figure 4). Relative (%) size did not correlate significantly with survival. In stage C, germinal centers correlated (P = .04) favorably with survival only when present in lymph nodes with metastatic deposits. Germinal center hyperplasia did not correlate with survival in stages A and D.

Sinus Histiocytosis

As defined by Black and coworkers (1953), sinus histiocytosis has been controversial because of the difficulty in distinguishing proliferation of histiocytic cells in the lymph node sinuses from a relative increase in macrophages in nodes with paracortical lymphocyte depletion. Patt and coworkers (1975), defining "abundant sinus histiocytosis" as large sinuses almost completely filled with histiocytes, found that this pattern and even smaller numbers of sinus histiocytes correlated significantly ($P < .05$) with favorable survival data in cancer of the sigmoid colon. Similar findings were made independently by Murray and coworkers (1975). Sinus histiocytosis is rarely encountered in nodes with metastatic tumor deposits, the inference being that sinus histiocytosis may resist tumor growth within lymph nodes (Syrjanen and Hjelt, 1978).

We are not aware of any quantitative attempts at evaluating the prognostic implications of sinus histiocytosis, the quantitative significance of which needs to be confirmed by point-counting or image analysis.

HUMORAL ANTIBODY PRODUCTION BY REGIONAL LYMPH NODES

The clinicopathologic significance of the humoral response in the regional lymph nodes in colorectal cancer is unclear. The antigens stimulating germinal center formation and medullary plasma cell proliferation are poorly characterized. We reported serum autoantibodies with specificity for colorectal carcinoma cell membranes and cytoplasm in 13% and 17% of cases, respectively (Nairn et al., 1971), but it is not certain whether these are produced, as seems likely, in the regional lymph nodes or by tumor stroma lymphocytes or by any other lymphoid tissue. We envisage that the use of monoclonal antibodies utilizing regional node lymphocytes might identify putative tumor-associated antigens.

CELL-MEDIATED IMMUNITY (CMI)

There is strong reactivity of lymphocytes from regional nodes after in vitro stimulation by mitogenes. However, comparisons with blood lymphocytes have given conflicting data. The evidence for specific CMI is equivocal, and the identity of corresponding tumor antigens is unknown.

Nonspecific Immunity

Fisher and coworkers (1972) reported that most regional lymph nodes contained cells responding to *phytohemagglutinin* (PHA) stimulation, a finding subsequently confirmed by Ambus and coworkers (1974), who also found an inverse relationship with the response of peripheral blood lymphocytes. In our laboratories, Werkmeister and coworkers (1981) found similar response to PHA stimulation whether or not the lymphoid cells of the nodes were cytotoxic against colon cancer cells. Jubert and coworkers (1977a), using mixed lymphocyte reactivity, found significantly stronger response in mesenteric node lymphocytes than in those from peripheral blood, the reactivity being unrelated to tumor staging (Jubert et al., 1977b). Kojima and colleagues (1980) found that the ability of lymphocytes to be stimulated by PHA was associated with the lymphocyte predominance pattern.

Specific Immunity

In our early in vitro studies of regional lymph nodes, we found, in a microcytotoxicity system, lack of reactivity by nodes from four cases (Nairn et al., 1971). Jubert and coworkers (1977a) reported node lymphocyte blastogenic response to autologous tumor cells in 4 of 26 (15%) cases, the responding nodes being regional to stage B tumors. Ambus and colleagues (1974) also reported a significant blastogenic response to autologous tumor cells by node lymphocytes in 15 of 32 (47%) cases. Guillou and coworkers (1975), using a two-stage inhibition of leucocyte migration technique, observed that the degree of sensitization to a colorectal tumor extract was similar in mesenteric and paracolonic nodes, although their figures indicate a significant sensitization by the former in comparison with control patients' mesenteric lymph nodes.

Microcytotoxicity studies in our laboratories (Pihl et al., 1976) showed that cytotoxicity to autologous tumor cells, demonstrated in 23% of cases, related significantly to combined hyperplasia of B- and T-cell areas and to sinus histiocytosis; cytotoxicity when present was a function of E-rosetting lymphocytes in most cases.

Comment

Most data suggest that the majority of lymph nodes, especially those with tumor involvement, are capable of responding to T-cell stimulators. The response is unrelated to "specific" antitumor cytotoxicity, which can be detected in only one quarter of cases. The sensitizing antigens are unknown, and the possibility that antibody-dependent cellular cytotoxicity (ADCC) mechanisms may have been active in some of the microcytotoxicity studies cannot be excluded. The prognostic significance of in vitro lymph node CMI is unknown.

ANTIBODY-DEPENDENT CELLULAR CYTOTOXICITY (ADCC)

Studies on lymph node ADCC in colorectal carcinoma are few, presumably because of lack of lymph node-derived tumor autoantibody and uncertainty concerning the validity of using colorectal cell lines on which specific tumor antigens have not been demonstrated. We showed (Werkmeister et al., 1981) that cells capable of mediating cytotoxicity against antibody-coated target cells were present in about half the regional lymph nodes assessed. The finding of significant cytotoxicity dependent on both E and non-E rosetting cells in 3 of 25 cytotoxic samples suggest that an ADCC mechanism may have been operating. Such a mechanism cannot be ruled out in any long-term microcytotoxicity study where the target cells contain stromal lymphocytes or where the effector lymphocytes are contaminated by specific antibody-producing cells. The prognostic significance of lymph node ADCC reactivity is unknown.

NATURAL KILLER (NK) CELL CYTOTOXICITY, HISTIOCYTES, AND MACROPHAGES

The incidence and significance of NK-cell activity in regional lymph nodes is difficult to assess, mainly because it has to be tested against arbitrarily selected NK-sensitive targets that may have little if any relevance to the in vivo situation. Generally, human lymph nodes have few NK-cells (Herberman and Holden, 1978). Regional lymph nodes are no exception to this, as demonstrated by testing against the NK-sensitive cell line NC37 (Werkmeister et al., 1981), or against the erythroleukaemic K562 cell line with or without interferon stimulation of the effector cell population (Moore and Vose, 1981).

It would thus appear that regional lymph nodes do not contain NK-cells in significant numbers. Nor do the human lymph nodes in general contain a significant migrating cell population (Guillou et al., 1975), although we feel that the possibility of macrophages sometimes mediating ADCC (Werkmeister et al., 1981) or exerting direct cytotoxicity should be investigated further in relationship to sinus histiocytosis.

CONCLUSIONS AND OUTLOOK ON THE FUTURE

Regional lymph nodes in colorectal cancer commonly contain lymphoreticular cells capable of mediating in vitro cytotoxicity against tumor cells. Several different cytotoxic mechanisms are concerned, including T-cell CMI, ADCC, and macrophage killing. The prognostic significance of these varying activities is not yet adequately explored, and much further work is required in this respect.

Immunomorphologic studies have shown that the in vivo expressions of these reactions, especially hyperplasia of germinal centers and of the paracortex, relate to favorable survival data within Dukes' stages B and C. The survival advantages of hyperplasia in the regional lymph nodes do not necessarily mean restraining activity by the lymph nodes themselves; the favorable patterns observed may merely be a reflection of beneficial handling of the tumor by some other bodily mechanism. This seems to be the case in relationship to the favorable association between autologous serum antitumor cytoplasmic antibody and recurrence-free survival in colorectal cancer as previously demonstrated by us (Nind et al., 1980). Whatever the mechanisms and antigens concerned in regional lymph node hyperplasia, the most likely common denominator in terms of antitumor immunoreactivity would seem to be antibody-mediated cellular cytotoxicity (ADCC).

Modern immunomorphological techniques, including the use of monoclonal antibodies, and careful analysis of survival data will help to elucidate the prognostic significance of these in vitro reactions. Large series of patients will be necessary using maximum numbers of lymph nodes and recording of their distances and relationships to the tumor. Since many of the immune features reviewed here are of prognostic significance only within conventionally defined tumor stages, detailed, accurate staging information must also be available.

What measures should be taken at operation to deal with the regional lymph nodes in colorectal carcinomas? Our recommendations to surgical colleagues would be

1. All lymphoid tissue suspected or known to contain metastatic tumor should be removed.
2. The much harder question of what to do with regional lymph node tissue believed free of tumor is hardly amenable to any scientific answer. Currently, microscopic deposits of metastatic tumor can only be determined histologically. Thus the only logical approach must be to remove regional lymph nodes with the tumor specimen for such examination. Although this may not improve a particular patient's survival, it will aid prognostically and enhance the accuracy of tumor staging. The surgeon's judgment regarding lymphatic excision must weigh possible advantages of extir-

pating microscopic tumors and thus refining prognostic knowledge against the disadvantages of more extensive surgery. Adopting such guidelines and given careful records by individual surgeons, it should therefore be possible to be more specific about optimal resection procedures.

For the near future, survival studies by surgeons with uniform data accrual should provide a policy for lymphatic resection whether radical or conservative. It is the authors' view that more radical lymph node resection should be preferred. The hypothetical advantages of leaving normal, uninvolved lymph node tissue behind are probably negligible at the late symptomatic stage in the natural history of colorectal carcinoma.

REFERENCES

Ambus U, Mavligit GM, Gutterman JU, et al. (1974) Specific and non-specific immunologic reactivity of regional lymph-node lymphocytes in human malignancy. Int J Cancer 14:291–300.

Bellanti JA (1978) Immunology II. Philadelphia: Saunders, pp. 52–57.

Black, MM, Kerpe S, Speer FD (1953) Lymph node structure in patients with cancer of breast. Am J Pathol 29:505–521.

Black MM, Freeman C, Mork T, et al. (1971) Prognostic significance of microscopic structure of gastric carcinomas and their regional lymph nodes. Cancer 27:703–711.

Chalkley HW (1943) Method for the quantitative morphologic analysis of tissues. J Natl Cancer Inst 4:47–53.

Cottier H, Turk J, Sobin LA (1973) A proposal for a standardized system of reporting human lymph node morphology in relation to immunological function. J Clin Pathol 26:317–331.

Crile G (1969) Possible role of uninvolved regional nodes in preventing metastasis from breast cancer. Cancer 24:1283–1285.

Fisher B (1975) Immune parameters in the surgery of cancer. In: Reit AE, ed., Immunity and cancer in man. New York: Marcel Dekker, pp. 81–90.

Fisher B, Saffer EA, Fisher ER (1972) Studies concerning the regional lymph node in cancer. III. Response of regional lymph node cells from breast and colon cancer patients to PHA stimulation. Cancer 30:1202–1215.

Guillou PJ, Brennan TG, Giles GR (1975) A study of lymph nodes draining colorectal cancer using a two-stage inhibition of leucocyte migration technique. Gut 16:290–297.

Hall MG, Chung EB, Leffall LSD (1973) The probable immunological role of regional lymph node in simulated colon carcinoma in the rabbit. Rev Surg 30:220–222.

Herberman RB, Holden HT (1978) Natural cell-mediated immunity. In: Klein G, Weinhouse S, eds., Advances in cancer research. New York: Academic Press, 27:305–377.

Jubert, AV., Talbott TM, Mazier WP, et al. (1977a) Lymphocyte blastogenic responses to allogeneic leucocytes and autochthonous tumor cells in colorectal carcinoma. J Surg Oncol 9:171–178.

Jubert AV, Talbott TM, Mazier WP, et al. (1977b) Correlation of immune responses with Dukes classification in colorectal carcinoma. Surgery 82:452–459.

Kojima O, Fujita Y, Oh A, et al. (1980) Immunomorphologic study of regional lymph nodes in cancer: Response of regional lymph node cells from gastric and colorectal cancer to PHA stimulation. Jpn J Surg 10:212–220.

Moore M, Vose BM (1981) Extravascular natural cytotoxicity in man: Anti-K562 activity of lymph-node and tumor-infiltrating lymphocytes. Int J Cancer 27:265–272.

Murray D, Hreno A, Dutton J, Hampson LG (1975) Prognosis in colon cancer. A pathologic reassessment. Arch Surg 110:908–913.

Nacopoulou L, Azaris P, Papacharalampous N, Davaris P (1981) Prognostic significance of histologic host response in cancer of the large bowel. Cancer 47:930–936.

Nairn RC, Nind APP, Guli EPG, et. al. (1971) Immunological reactivity in patients with carcinoma of colon. Br Med J 4:706–709.

Nind, APP, Nairn RC, Pihl E, et al. (1980) Autochthonous humoral and cellular immunoreactivity to colorectal carcinoma: Prognostic significance in 400 patients. Cancer Immunol Immunother 7:257–261.

Patt DJ, Brynes RK, Vardiman JW, Coppleson LW (1975) Mesocolic lymph node histology is an important prognostic indicator for patients with carcinoma of the sigmoid colon: An immunomorphologic study. Cancer 35:1388–1397.

Pihl E, Nairn RC, Muller HK, et al. (1976) Correlation of regional lymph node histology with *in vitro* antitumour immunoreactivity in colorectal cancer. Cancer Res 36:3665–3671.

Pihl E, Malahy MA, Khankhanian N, et al. (1977) Immunomorphological features of prognostic significance in Dukes' class B colorectal carcinoma. Cancer Res 37:4145–4149.

Pihl E, Nairn RC, Hughes ESR, et al. (1980a) Regional lymph node and stromal immunomorphology in colorectal carcinoma and relation to tumour spread. Pathology 12:15–21.

Pihl E, Nairn RC, Hughes ESR, et al. (1980b) Mucinous colorectal carcinoma: Immunopathology and prognosis. Pathology 12:439–447.

Pihl E, Nairn RC, Milne BJ, et al., (1980c) Lymphoid hyperplasia. A major prognostic feature in 519 cases of colorectal carcinoma. Am J Pathol 100:469–480.

Pihl E, Hughes ESR, McDermott FT, et al. (1983) Clinicopathological correlation of lymph node enlargement, tumour spread and survival in 1505 colorectal cancer patients treated with curative resection. Am J Proct Gastroenterol Col Rect Surg 34:5–8, 26–27.

Syrjanen KJ, Hjelt LH (1978) Tumor-host relationships in colorectal carcinoma. Dis Colon Rectum 21:29–36.

Thynne GS, Weiland LH, Moertel CG, Silvers A (1980) Correlation of histopathologic characteristics of primary tumor and uninvolved regional lymph nodes in Dukes' class C colonic carcinoma with prognosis. Mayo Clin Proc 55:243–245.

Tsakraklides V, Olson P, Kersey JH, Good RA (1974) Prognostic significance of the regional lymph node histology in cancer of the breast. Cancer 34:1259–1267.

Tsakraklides V, Wanebo HJ, Sternberg SS, et al. (1975) Prognostic evaluation of regional lymph nodes morphology in colorectal cancer. Am J Surg 129:174–180.

Turk JL (1977) The organization of lymphoid tissue in relation to function. Lymphology 10:46–53.

Van de Velde CJH, Meyer CJLM, Cornelisse CJ, et al. (1978) A morphometrical analysis of lymph node responses to tumors of different immunogenicity. Cancer Res 38:661–667.

Virchow R (1860) Cellular pathology. Translated by Frank Chance. Philadelphia: J.B. Lippincott Co.

Werkmeister JA, Pihl E, Flannery GR (1981) Lymph node anti-tumour effector cell mechanisms in colorectal carcinoma. Aust J Exp Biol Med Sci 59:115–124.

EXPERIMENTAL CHEMOTHERAPY IN COLON CANCER

JANET A HOUGHTON, Ph.D., AND PETER J HOUGHTON, Ph.D.

Cancer of the large bowel is refractory to treatment with chemotherapeutic agents whether administered singly (Carroll et al., 1979, 1980; Carter and Friedman, 1974; Isacoff et al., 1978; Michaelson et al., 1982; Moertel, 1978; Saiers et al., 1982) or in combination (Bearden et al., 1977; Cantrell et al., 1982; Haller et al., 1978; Moertel, 1978; Presant et al., 1978; Richards et al., 1975; Taylor et al., 1978; Weiss et al., 1982; White et al., 1979). One explanation for this phenomenon may be a general lack of sensitivity of such tumors to cytotoxic agents that are diverse in their mechanisms of action. Alternatively, the response of this class of carcinoma may be very similar to the sensitivity of the normal epithelium of the gastrointestinal tract, such that the major problem becomes one of minimal selectivity and not a complete lack of sensitivity.

The relative sensitivity of a tumor to chemotherapeutic agents depends on many factors, including the cell proliferation kinetics, the transport of agents across membranes, the ratio of drug anabolism to catabolism, and the rate of repair of potentially lethal lesions induced by drugs. The relationship between the induction of a specific lesion by antimetabolites and cell survival in the *in vivo* situation is of particular importance, and the specific lesion induced also depends on the tumor system employed. However, a major difficulty in the evaluation of most anticancer agents, with the possible exception of acute lymphocytic leukemia, is the lack of correlation of the animal tumor models with the drug response of any specific type of human cancer (Laster, 1975). In addition, the conventional and rapidly proliferating rodent tumors used in drug screening have failed to identify new agents with marked activity in the treatment of large bowel cancer (Goldin et al., 1981; Laster, 1975). It is here that the human tumor xenograft demonstrates potential. In human xenografts, more

From the Department of Biochemical and Clinical Pharmacology, St. Jude Children's Research Hospital, Memphis, Tennessee.

Abbreviations used in this chapter

FUra, 5-fluorouracil; **FUMP,** 5-fluorouridine 5′-monophosphate; **FUDP,** 5-fluorouridine 5′-diphosphate; **FUTP,** 5-fluorouridine 5′-triphosphate; **FdUMP,** 5-fluoro 2′-deoxyuridine 5′-monophosphate; **UMP,** uridine 5′-monophosphate; **CH_2FH_4,** 5,10-methylenetetrahydrofolate; **dUMP,** 2′-deoxyurdine 5′-monophosphate; **dTMP,** thymidine 5′-monophosphate; **FUrd,** 5-fluorouridine; **FdUrd,** 5-fluoro 2′-deoxyuridine; **OPRTase,** orotate phosphoribosyltransferase; **dThd,** thymidine; **Urd,** uridine; **5-$CHOFH_4$,** 5-formyltetrahydrofolate, leucovorin, folinic acid; **10-$CHOFH_4$,** 10-formyltetrahydrofolate; **5-CH_3FH_4,** 5-methyltetrahydrofolate; **FH_2,** dihydrofolate; **FH_4,** tetrahydrofolate; **Hx,** hypoxanthine; **HPP,** allopurinol; **PRPP,** 5-phosphoribosyl-1-pyrophosphate; **R-I-P,** ribose-1-phosphate; **MTX,** methotrexate; **DHFU,** 5,6-dihydro 5-fluorouracil; **ADP,** adenosine 5′-diphosphate; **GDP,** guanosine 5′-diphosphate; **ATP,** adenosine 5′-triphosphate; **R-5-P,** ribose-5-phosphate.

specific clinical correlations and extrapolations may be made under controlled laboratory conditions.

THE MODEL

We have established a series of five human colon and one rectal adenocarcinoma xenografts, each derived from a different, untreated human primary tumor. Each line is maintained subcutaneously in thymectomized CBA/CaJ mice that have been lethally irradiated and reconstituted with syngeneic bone marrow (Houghton and Houghton, 1980a). Each line retained characteristics of the tumor of origin, including similar histology, mucin secretion, production of carcinoembryonic antigen, human isoenzyme patterns, and a human karyotype (Houghton and Taylor, 1978a; Reeves and Houghton, 1978). Rates of growth were heterogeneous between the different lines and were relatively slow in comparison to rodent tumors, with doubling times ranging from approximately 6 to 27 days after five serial transfers in mice (Houghton and Taylor, 1978b). The responses of these tumors to a series of seven clinically used agents (cyclophosphamide, 5-fluorouracil, methyl-CCNU, dactinomycin, cisdiamminedichloro platinum, pentamethylmelamine, and doxorubicin) have shown similarities to findings in the clinical disease in that each tumor exhibited an individual profile of sensitivity (Houghton et al., 1977; Houghton and Houghton, 1978, 1979). Such a model may, therefore, increase our understanding of the mechanisms that govern resistance to cytotoxic drugs in vivo and may facilitate the design of effective therapy for human adenocarcinoma of the large bowel.

SENSITIVITY OF TUMORS TO 5-FLUOROURACIL (FUra)

Of particular interest has been the use of FUra in treatment protocols for colorectal cancer. Although more than 40 single cytotoxic agents have been evaluated for therapeutic acitivity in patients with advanced disease, none has exceeded the activity of FUra, which is estimated to induce response rates in only 20% of colorectal cancer patients (Moertel, 1978).

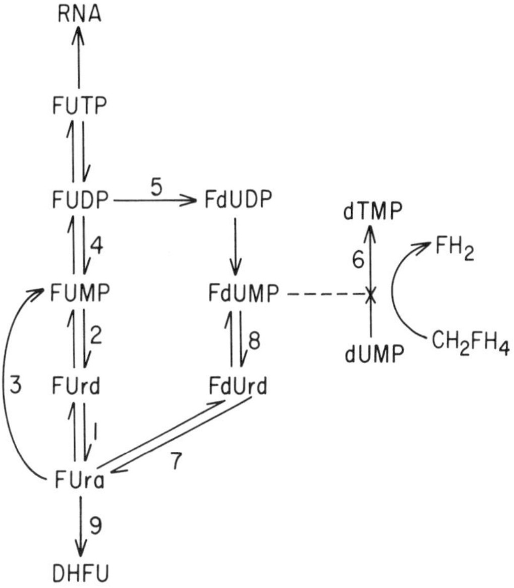

FIGURE 1. Pathways of 5-fluorouracil metabolism. The enzymes are as follows: (1) Uridine phosphorylase; (2) uridine kinase; (3) orotate phosphoribosyltransferase; (4) uridylate kinase; (5) ribonucleotide reductase; (6) thymidylate synthetase; (7) thymidine phosphorylase; (8) thymidine kinase; (9) dihydrouracil dehydrogenase.

The 2′-deoxyribonucleoside FdUrd has shown comparable activity to that of FUra (Carter and Friedman, 1974), while the FUra ribonucleoside FUrd has been less useful due to its toxicity (Currie et al., 1975). In human colorectal xenografts, these three 5-fluoropyrimidines have demonstrated some activity in two of six lines when administered intraperitoneally to mice at the maximum tolerated dose levels (Houghton and Houghton, 1980a, 1982).

METABOLISM OF 5-FLUOROURACIL

For FUra to induce cytotoxicity, it must initially be metabolized and may be cytotoxic by one of at least two known mechanisms (Figure 1). After intracellular conversion to ribonucleotides (FUMP, FUDP, FUTP), FUTP may be incorporated into RNA during transcription, with subsequent impairment of the posttranscriptional processing of rRNA (Wilkinson and Pitot, 1973; Wilkinson et al., 1975; Wilkinson and Crumley, 1976; Carrico and Glazer, 1979). Alternatively, after metabolism to FdUMP, a tight binding quasi-irreversible complex is formed with the enzyme dTMP synthetase and CH_2FH_4, the cofactor used in the conversion of dUMP to dTMP. This interaction, and the consequences of inhibition of the biosynthesis of dTMP de novo have been reviewed (Danenberg, 1977; Heidelberger, 1965, 1974; Santi, 1980). 5-Fluorouridine and FdUrd are also activated by conversion to FUTP and FdUMP by enzymes involved in pyrimidine metabolism.

The importance of nucleotide formation from FUra and OPRTase activity

TABLE 1. Concentrations of Fluorinated Ribonucleotides[a] (pmol/mg DNA)

Tumor line	Treatment		1 hr	4 hr	24 hr	Sensitivity to FUra[c] in vivo
$HxAC_4$	FUra + Hx + HPP	(A)	N.T.[b]	N.T.	N.T.	—
	FUra alone	(B)	2,231	2,414	827	
$HxELC_2$	FUra + Hx + HPP	(A)	771	539	361	
	FUra alone	(B)	867	235	322	Sensitive
	A/B		0.9	2.3	1.1	
$HxGC_3$	FUra + Hx + HPP	(A)	445	483	182	
	FUra alone	(B)	620	449	193	—
	A/B		0.7	1.1	0.9	
HxBR	FUra + Hx + HPP	(A)	340	222	58	
	FUra alone	(B)	180	111	37	—
	A/B		1.9	2.0	1.6	
$HxHC_1$	FUra + Hx + HPP	(A)	1809	1801	1074	
	FUra alone	(B)	3479	5568	2069	Sensitive
	A/B		0.5	0.3	0.5	
$HxVRC_5$	FUra + Hx + HPP	(A)	2457	1514	1194	
	FUra alone	(B)	4775	5016	4168	—
	A/B		0.5	0.3	0.3	

[a]Results represent the mean of two to six determinations.
[b]N.T. = Not tested.
[c]Data were obtained from Houghton and Houghton (1980a, 1982, 1983).
[6-^{3}H]FUra (100 mg/kg) was administered intraperitoneally to tumor-bearing mice either alone or in combination with Hx (50 mg/kg) and HPP (10 mg/kg) injected simultaneously. Concentrations of radiolabeled FUMP, FUDP, and FUTP were determined by thin-layer chromatography as previously described (Houghton and Houghton, 1980a). Hx = hypoxanthine; HPP = allopurinol.

(which is involved in this process) as determinants of intrinsic sensitivity of mammalian leukemias to FUra has been established (Kessel et al., 1966, 1973; Reyes and Hall, 1969). Acquired resistance to FUra in murine tumors is associated with decreased activities of several enzymes involved in FUra nucleotide synthesis: Urd phosphorylase (Goldberg et al., 1966; Kessel et al., 1971; Reichard et al., 1959), Urd kinase (Anderson et al., 1962; Kessel et al., 1971; Reichard et al., 1959, 1962), OPRTase (Kasbekar and Greenberg, 1963; Levinson et al., 1979, Mulkins and Heidelberger, 1982), and UMP kinase (Ardalan et al., 1980). The sensitivity of human colorectal cancer to FUra was subsequently examined in the human xenograft model by attempting to relate the concentrations of fluorinated ribonucleotides formed after administration of FUra (100 mg/kg) to the intrinsic sensitivity of tumors to this agent (Table 1). It is clear that concentrations of ribonucleotides formed from FUra varied between different tumor lines, but this did not relate to responsiveness for this agent. (Additional data in the table will be discussed subsequently.)

One factor that was considered to influence the level and duration of inhibition of dTMP synthetase in neoplastic tissues was the formation of the active metabolite, FdUMP. Consequently, studies that related the peak level (Ardalan et al., 1978; Rustum et al., 1979) and retention (Ardalan et al., 1978; Klubes et al., 1978; Rustum et al., 1979) of FdUMP to the sensitivity of rodent tumors in vivo were reported. However, in human colorectal xenografts, peak levels of FdUMP, which were observed 1 hour after FUra administration to mice, did not correlate with FUra sensitivity in these tumors; in addition, FdUMP was retained for several days at similar concentrations in both sensitive and insensitive tumors (Houghton and Houghton, 1980a). It is concluded that the metabolism of FUra, although an essential step in a complex series of interactions, is not the final determinant of tumor responsiveness in xenografts of human colorectal adenocarcinomas.

MECHANISM OF CYTOTOXICITY OF 5-FLUOROURACIL IN HUMAN COLORECTAL XENOGRAFTS

The mechanism by which FUra is cytotoxic may depend on the characteristics of the cells studied and the experimental conditions employed (Evans et al., 1980; Maybaum et al., 1980; Umeda and Heidelberger, 1968). In the xenograft model, attempts at separating the RNA and DNA targets for cytotoxicity were made by treating tumor-bearing mice intraperitoneally with FUra, FUrd, and FdUrd. The incorporation of drug into RNA, or the FdUMP concentrations, were compared with the sensitivity of $HxELC_2$ and $HxHC_1$ tumors (Houghton and Houghton, 1980a). In line $HxHC_1$, the relative efficacy as antitumor agents, as well as the relative concentrations of FdUMP between 24 and 96 hours after treatment, for equimolar doses, were in the order FUrd > FdUrd > FUra. In $HxELC_2$ tumors, however, the order for both parameters was FUrd > FUra > FdUrd. There was no relationship between ranking according to drug incorporation into RNA and relative tumor responsiveness. Evidence was subsequently presented in a series of cultured mouse cell lines, which responded to low concentrations of FUra (5 to 20 μM), that the growth-limiting event was the inhibition of dTMP synthetase (Evans et al., 1980). At higher concentrations of FUra (15 to 70 μM), incorporation of the drug into RNA appeared to become growth limiting. However, in the same study, concentrations of FUra required for growth inhibition of human cell lines were 50 to 200 μM, and cytotoxicity appeared to be produced through an RNA-mediated mechanism.

In gastrointestinal tissues of the mouse, doses of FUra, FUrd, and FdUrd that gave equivalent levels of toxicity resulted in similar levels of incorporation into RNA, but different concentrations of FdUMP (Houghton et al., 1979). These data suggest that gastrointestinal toxicity may be induced via an RNA-mediated mechanism, whereas the antitumor effects observed in human colon xenografts may be mediated by an antithymidylate effect. It is therefore possible under conditions in situ that only those tumors that are sensitive to lower concentrations of the drug will be identified as responders, and for these the antithymidylate effect may be critical. The RNA-mediated mechanism may be important at higher drug concentrations, and in most cases they may not be achievable in vivo with FUra alone due to lack of sufficient selectivity between the tumor and the tissue of origin. However, if it should be possible selectively to increase the metabolism of FUra in tumors in vivo by combining FUra with other agents, the incorporation of FUra into RNA may become a cytotoxic lesion.

NATURAL RESISTANCE OF HUMAN COLORECTAL XENOGRAFTS TO 5-FLUOROURACIL

In acquired resistance to FdUrd, an increase in the target enzyme dTMP synthetase has been reported (Baskin et al., 1975). However, in cytosols derived from human colorectal xenografts, activity of this enzyme ranged from 8.4 to 124 pmol/mg protein/hour; both the highest and lowest activities were present in FUra-insensitive tumors, while the two sensitive lines demonstrated intermediate activities (Houghton et al., 1981). One hour after treatment of tumor-bearing mice with FUra, levels of FdUMP, which were maximal at this time, exceeded by 634 to 4356 times the available FdUMP binding sites on dTMP synthetase, irrespective of 5-fluoropyrimidine sensitivity. Nevertheless, further analysis in vitro demonstrated that in nonresponsive tumors only 40 to 50% of the available binding sites were occupied by covalently bound FdUMP in the absence of exogenously administered cofactor (CH_2FH_4, see following), while in FUra-sensitive lines, all FdUMP binding sites were occupied. These data correlated with residual dTMP synthetase activity (Houghton et al., 1981; Figure 2), which has also been demonstrated in FUra-insensitive murine colon adenocarcinomas in mice treated with FUra (Spears et al., 1982).

In the inhibition of dTMP synthetase by FdUMP in the presence of CH_2FH_4, numerous association and dissociation events occur. The dissociation of the ternary complex formed is a first order, temperature-dependent, enzyme-catalyzed process, although net dissociation is slow in the presence of excess cofactor (nonphysiological levels; Santi et al., 1974), which would allow FdUMP to reassociate with the enzyme after dissociation has occurred. The rate of dissociation of the [6-^{3}H]FdUMP-labeled ternary complex in the presence of excess unlabeled FdUMP was reported to be independent of the natural substrate dUMP, and FdUMP, but was slowed by increasing the concentration of CH_2FH_4 (Lockshin and Danenberg, 1981). Dissociation of the complex in whole cells ($t\frac{1}{2}$ = 6.2 hours; Washtien and Santi, 1979) was less rapid than within cell cytosols ($t\frac{1}{2}$ = 2 hours; Washtien and Santi, 1979, $t\frac{1}{2} \approx$ 80 minutes; Spears et al., 1982), in the presence of 0.3 to 2 mM CH_2FH_4; net dissociation of the complex in the absence of a large pool of nonradioactive FdUMP was negligible in both systems (Washtien and Santi, 1979). In the absence of cofactor (which would prevent reassociation of the complex after dissociation and hence affect the net dissociation), dissociation of the complex formed from purified enzyme was rapid ($t\frac{1}{2}$ = 22 to 36 minutes; Danenberg and Danenberg, 1978; Lockshin and Danenberg, 1981), with the generation of free enzyme and FdUMP (Santi et al., 1974).

Thus, in the presence of low concentrations of CH_2FH_4 or in its absence, the rate of dissociation, the net dissociation, and hence stability of the complex may be important determinants of the inhibition of dTMP synthetase. The greater sensitivity and antithymidylate activity of FUra in S-180 in comparison with Hep-2 cells correlated with larger total pools of folates and a higher content of folate cofactors required for the biosynthesis of dTMP and purines (Yin et al., 1983). Consequently, 10-$CHOFH_4$, 5-$CHOFH_4$, FH_2, and FH_4 were higher in S-180 cells, where the principal component was FH_4. In contrast, in Hep-2 cells, 5-CH_3FH_4, required for the biosynthesis of methionine, was the major folate

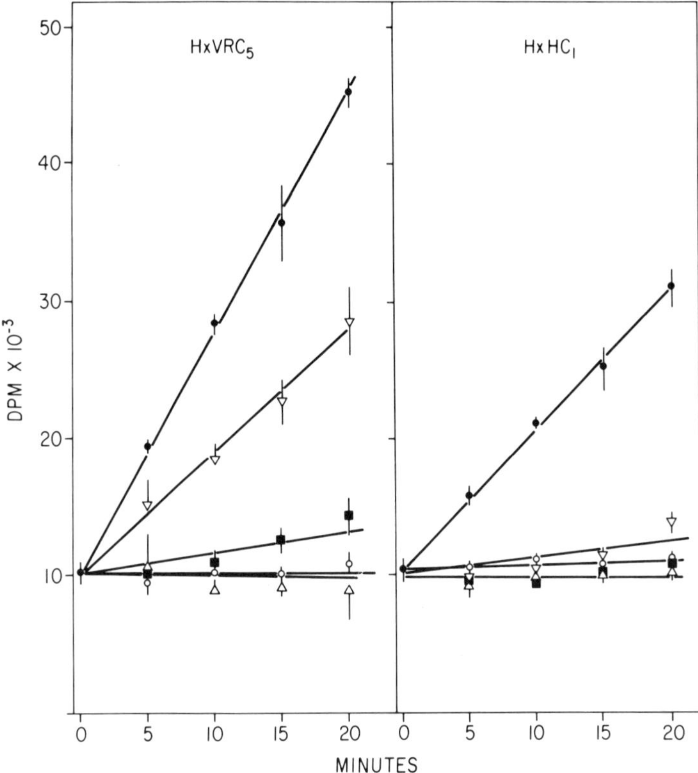

FIGURE 2. Activity of dTMP synthetase in cytosols preincubated with excess FdUMP with or without added 5,10-methylenetetrahydrofolate. Preincubation: (●) cytosol + buffer; (○) cytosol + buffer; (△) cytosol + FdUMP; (▽) cytosol + FdUMP; (■) cytosol + FdUMP + CH_2FH_4. Postincubation: [5-^{3}H]dUMP was added to each reaction mixture, and either excess CH_2FH_4 (●, ▽, ■) or buffer (○, △). Results show the mean ± SD for triplicate determinations from representative experiments using cytosols from $HxVRC_5$ and $HxHC_1$ tumors. *Source:* Houghton et al. (1981). Reproduced with permission of Cancer Research, Inc.

form, and folic acid was also present, when folate-depleted cells were grown in the presence of radiolabeled folic acid. Concentrations of CH_2FH_4 determined in human colorectal xenografts varied from 66 to 233 nM in cell water (Houghton et al., 1982a), but both the highest and lowest values were found for the two FUra-sensitive tumors. Thus, the concentration of CH_2FH_4 alone does not adequately account for sensitivity to FUra. However, all concentrations were considerably lower than the apparent Km for CH_2FH_4 (21 to 31 μM; Dolnick and Cheng, 1978; Lockshin and Danenberg, 1981) or its pentaglutamate form (2.2 μM; Dolnick and Cheng, 1978), or the cofactor concentrations reported for cultured L1210 cells (3 to 6 μM; Jackson and Harrap, 1973; Moran et al., 1976).

The data indicate that natural insensitivity to FUra relates to the inability either to form or to maintain a covalent complex due to very low levels of endogenous cofactor. However, the apparent anomaly for the FUra-sensitive xenografts (high FdUMP binding with low cofactor concentration) suggest that other factors, including the endogenous dUMP concentration, may be important. This nucleotide, which may accumulate after FUra administration, can influence the degree of inhibition of dTMP synthetase by competing for the binding site on the enzyme (Lockshin and Danenberg, 1981; Myers et al., 1975).

Although levels of dUMP have not yet been determined in human colorectal xenografts, this nucleotide could have been converted to dTMP under the experimental conditions used in the determination of ternary complex formation (Houghton et al., 1982a), thus decreasing levels of CH_2FH_4 in nonresponsive tumors. Under in situ conditions in which FdUMP concentrations rapidly decrease, high dUMP/FdUMP ratios would prevent reassociation of FdUMP with the enzyme. Endogenous concentrations of dUMP in different neoplastic cells range from approximately 5 μM (Berger et al., 1981; Jackson, 1978; Moran et al., 1979; Spears et al., 1982), to between 150 and 700 μM (Ardalan, et al., 1978; Klubes et al., 1978; Myers et al., 1975). Accumulation of dUMP in neoplastic cells after treatment with either FUra or FdUrd has also varied from 1 to 300 times control values (Ardalan et al., 1978; Berger et al., 1981; Jackson, 1978; Klubes et al., 1978; Moran et al., 1979; Myers et al., 1975; Spears et al., 1982).

A low capacity to accumulate dUMP after treatment, together with high concentrations of intracellular folic acid derivatives, has correlated with FUra sensitivity in cultured cells (Berger et al., 1981), so that the combined effects of relatively high dUMP levels and low cofactor concentration may be synergistic in their prevention of dTMP synthetase inhibition by FdUMP (Lockshin and Danenberg, 1981). Accumulation of high concentrations of dUMP has prevented dTMP synthetase inhibition from becoming critical for growth in cultured cells (Evans et al., 1980; Maybaum et al., 1980), unless excess folinic acid (10 μM) was present (Evans et al., 1981; Berger and Hakala, 1982). The ability of neoplastic cells to form polyglutamate conjugates of CH_2FH_4 may also influence their sensitivity to FUra. Polyglutamates of CH_2FH_4 containing up to seven glutamate residues have increased affinity for dTMP synthetase and are more active catalytically (Dolnick and Cheng, 1978; Kisliuk et al., 1974; Maley et al., 1979; Priest and Mangum, 1981). Thus, in S-180 cells, more than 90% of intracellular folates were in the form of polyglutamates, whereas in Hep-2 cells, only 32% of the folate cofactors were present in these forms (Yin et al., 1983). The concentration and form of CH_2FH_4 in vivo in combination with other factors such as dUMP concentration may thus be important in determining the sensitivity of colorectal tumors to FUra.

INCREASED FORMATION OF THE COVALENT TERNARY COMPLEX

As the folate requirement for optimal growth of cultured L1210 cells (100 nM) was lower than that required for maximal cytotoxicity of FdUrd (500 nM; Ullman et al., 1978), it has been suggested that administration of a reduced folate, such as folinic acid, might increase the effectiveness of dTMP synthetase inhibition by FdUMP, while folate-independent effects (for example, incorporation of FUra into RNA) would remain unchanged. Potentiation of the growth-inhibitory effects of FUra or FdUrd up to threefold by 5-$CHOFH_4$ was reported for L1210 (Ullman et al., 1978; Waxman and Bruckner, 1982), and S-180 (Evans et al., 1981) cells, while in Hep-2 cells inhibition of dTMP synthetase became growth-limiting (Evans et al., 1981; Berger and Hakala, 1982). It appeared that the extent of enzyme inhibition was not increased, but that the spontaneous recovery of enzyme acitvity was markedly slowed due to apparent stabilization of the CH_2FH_4:FdUMP:dTMP synthetase complex (Evans et al., 1981). Under these conditions, net dissociation of the complex must correlate with the recovery of dTMP synthetase activity. Folic acid (Evans et al., 1981; Ullman et al., 1978) and 5-CH_3FH_4 (Evans et al., 1981) also potentiated the growth inhibitory effects of FUra and FdUrd, presumably due to rapid incorporation into the pool of reduced folate cofactors.

Attempts were made to increase the pool of CH_2FH_4 in cytosols prepared from human colon xenografts by the addition of precursors of the cofactor. Tetrahydrofolate and, to some extent, FH_2 enhanced the covalent binding of [6-^{3}H]FdUMP to dTMP synthetase, while 5-$CHOFH_4$ and 5-CH_3FH_4 decreased covalent complex formation (Houghton et al., 1982a). In contrast, administration of FH_4 and FH_2 to tumor-bearing mice depressed subsequent formation of the covalent complex in tumor cytosols. These data indicate that FH_4 and FH_2 are not incorporated to any great extent into the pool of CH_2FH_4 in vivo. Leucovorin administered in vivo is rapidly converted to 5-CH_3FH_4 (Mehta et al., 1978), which is the principal folate component of mammalian blood and liver (Bird et al., 1965; Blakley, 1969), so that FH_4 and FH_2 are possibly also converted rapidly to this folate derivative on in vivo administration.

In the treatment of L1210 leukemia in vivo, concurrent infusion of leucovorin for up to 4 days did not increase either the therapeutic effect of a bolus dose of FUra or its toxicity to the host (Klubes et al., 1981). Data from preliminary studies with the leucovorin-FUra combination in patients suggest that toxicity of FUra to the gastrointestinal tissue may be increased by leucovorin (Bruckner et al., 1981). However, increased response rates (complete + partial, 56% and 21% in previously untreated and treated patients, respectively) using this combination have been reported clinically in colorectal adenocarcinoma (Machover et al., 1982). Thus, further studies increasing the intracellular concentration of CH_2FH_4 and the equilibrium proportion of dTMP synthetase present in the ternary complex in human colon tumors in vivo are warranted. These studies could lead to a selective and enhanced inhibition of dTMP synthetase in neoplastic cells.

SELECTIVE PROTECTION OF THE HOST DURING THERAPY WITH 5-FLUOROURACIL

Therapeutic activity of a cytotoxic agent may potentially be increased by selectively reducing conversion to the active metabolite in normal intestinal epithelium and bone marrow, but not in neoplastic cells. This may be possible where two or more pathways to the cytotoxic product exist, and where one route predominates in normal tissues while the alternative pathway is the major one in

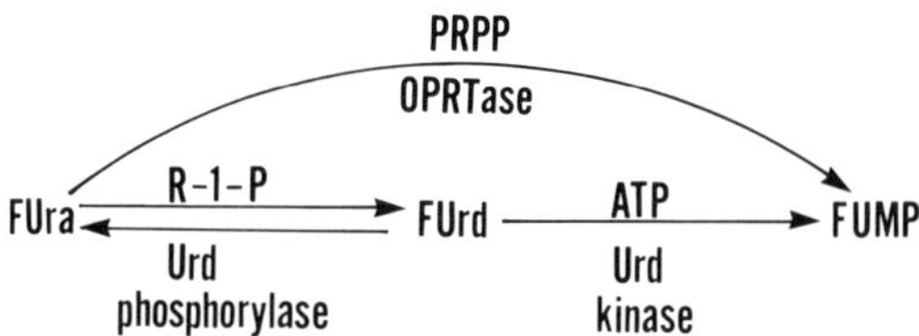

FIGURE 3. The two opposing pathways for the metabolism of FUra to ribonucleotides. Enzymes and cosubstrates required for the reactions are shown.

tumors. Thus, the opposing pathways for ribonucleotide formation from FUra (OPRTase versus the sequential acitivities of Urd phosphorylase and Urd kinase; Figure 3) were investigated.

Using cultured neoplastic cells, Hx reduced the cytotoxic effects of FUra in lines L5178Y (Yoshida et al., 1978) and S49 (Ullman and Kirsch, 1979), an effect attributed to the depletion of PRPP. The Hx analogue, HPP, antagonized the cytotoxicity of FUra in cultured S-180 and murine leukemic cells, whereas lines of Walker 256 and HeLa were unaffected by the purine (Schwartz and Handschumacher, 1979). In the latter study, accumulation of orotic acid, which can compete favorably with FUra for metabolism by OPRTase (Reyes and Guganig 1975) was postulated as the mechanism of protection. Simultaneous or prior administration of HPP protects normal tissues from the toxicity of FUra in rodents (Houghton and Houghton 1980b; Schwartz et al. 1980) and in humans (Campbell et al., 1982; Fox et al., 1979, 1981; Howell et al., 1981; Kroener et al., 1982). Such protection has been reported for both gastrointestinal tissues and bone marrow (Houghton and Houghton, 1980b; Schwartz et al., 1980). Hypoxanthine also reduces the toxicity of FUra, particularly in the bone marrow, when given by simultaneous administration either alone or in combination with HPP (Houghton and Houghton, 1980b).

These data suggested that the metabolism of FUra by OPRTase may be an important pathway in the normal tissues; the combination of Hx (50 mg/kg) and the inhibitor of its degradation, HPP (10 mg/kg), was subsequently examined further in studies using human colorectal xenografts in vivo. Five xenograft lines examined in vivo were divided into two groups (Houghton and Houghton, 1983). The first comprised those that formed relatively high levels of FUrd (21 to 74 nmol/mg DNA at 1 hour) and low concentrations of FUMP, FUDP, and FUTP (fluorinated ribonucleotides, Figure 1; 180 to 867 pmol/mg DNA at 1 hour) after the injection of FUra (100 mg/kg). These tumors showed no decrease in FUra ribonucleotide levels after the in vivo administration of Hx and HPP simultaneously with FUra (HxELC$_2$, HxGC$_3$, and HxBR tumors; Table 1). Tumors in this group possessed a high Urd phosphorylase/OPRTase ratio (7 to 24), and a high ratio of R-1-P/PRPP ($\approx$5, Table 2). These data suggest that the metabolism of FUra to ribonucleotides in these lines may proceed via the sequential activities of Urd phosphorylase and Urd kinase.

The second group was comprised of those tumors that formed lower levels of FUrd (9 to 13 nmol/mg DNA at 1 hour) and higher concentrations of fluorinated ribonucleotides (4 to 5 nmol/mg DNA at 1 hour), which were reduced by

TABLE 2. Levels of Enzymes and Cosubstrates involved in the Metabolism of 5-Fluorouracil to Ribonucleotides[a]

	Enzyme activity (pmol/min/mg protein)			Cosubstrate Concentration (pmol/mg protein)		
Tumor Line	OPRTase[b] (A)	Urd phosphorylase[b] (B)	B/A	PRPP[c] (C)	R-1-P[c] (D)	D/C
$HxELC_2$	108	2570	23.8	240	1210	5.0
$HxGC_3$	522	3860	7.4	330	1660	5.0
$HxHC_1$	2206	2600	1.2	1280	1080	0.8
$HxVRC_5$	621	1500	2.4	1180	1510	1.3

[a]These have been described by Houghton and Houghton (1983).
[b]Results represent the mean of duplicate determinations.
[c]Results represent the mean of 6 to 12 determinations.

50% during the first hour after simultaneous administration of the purine combination with FUra ($HxHC_1$ and $HxVRC_5$ tumors, Table 1). Group 2 tumors demonstrated a lower ratio of Urd phosphorylase to OPRTase (1.2 to 2.4), higher endogenous levels of PRPP, and a lower R-1-P/PRPP ratio ($\approx$1; Table 2). Data are therefore indicative of a predominant metabolism of FUra by OPRTase. Levels of PRPP were decreased by 71 to 79% in tumors from both groups ($HxELC_2$, $HxHC_1$) within 15 minutes of administration of the purine combination (Houghton and Houghton, 1983). One tumor in each group ($HxELC_2$, $HxHC_1$) was also sensitive to treatment with FUra alone (Houghton and Houghton 1980a, 1982; Table 1).

When mice were treated at seven-day intervals with FUra administered simultaneously with low dose levels of the protecting agents, no increase in therapeutic index was obtained in these two lines (Houghton and Houghton, 1982). Moreover, in $HxHC_1$ xenografts, some antagonism of the cytotoxicity of FUra was observed. These data are consistent with a report that no activity of the FUra-HPP combination could be detected clinically in patients with colon carcinoma (Kroener et al., 1982). It is apparent that FUra-sensitive tumors are heterogeneous in their pathway of metabolism of FUra to ribonucleotides. Thus, the combination of FUra with agents that can reduce its metabolism by OPRTase may reduce the overall response rate of 20% observed with the use of FUra administered alone.

SELECTIVE INCREASE IN 5-FLUOROURACIL ACTIVATION IN TUMORS

Studies in a cultured human adenocarcinoma cell line (HCT-8) indicated that the endogenous level of PRPP was elevated threefold after exposure to 10 μM MTX (Benz and Cadman, 1981); ribonucleotides of FUra and FdUMP were similarly elevated, and increased cytotoxicity resulted when FUra was added subsequent to MTX (Benz et al., 1980; Benz and Cadman, 1981). The mecha-

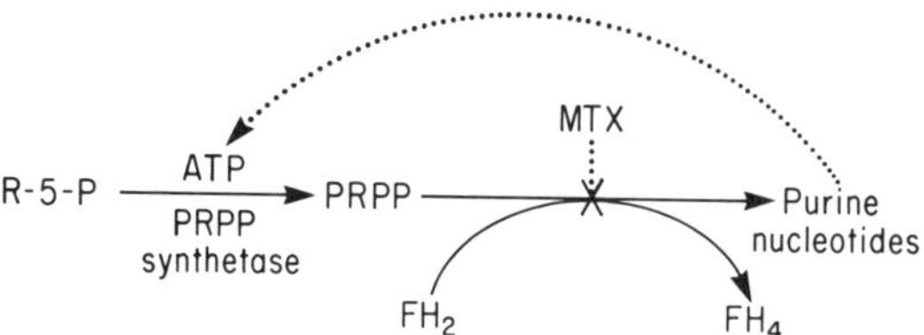

FIGURE 4. Inhibition, by MTX, of the biosynthesis of purine nucleotides, which are allosteric regulators of PRPP synthetase.

nism of elevation of PRPP by MTX has been described by Cadman and colleagues (1979, 1981) and is summarized in Figure 4. Inhibition of the conversion of FH_2 to FH_4 by MTX results in depletion of reduced folate cofactors, a reduction in the biosynthesis of purine nucleotides, and may lead to increased availability of PRPP. Purine nucleotides, of which ADP and GDP are particularly potent, also act as allosteric regulators of PRPP synthetase (Becker et al. 1979; Danks and Scholar, 1982; Fox and Kelley, 1972; Hershko et al., 1969), such that a reduction in the concentration of these nucleotides may result in disinhibition of the enzyme and increased synthesis of PRPP. Schedules in which MTX is administered 1 (Burnet et al., 1981; Cantrell et al., 1982; Tisman and Wu, 1980), 3 (Herrmann et al., 1981), 4 (Solan et al., 1980; Weinerman et al., 1982), or 7 (Drapkin et al., 1981) hours before FUra are under clinical evaluation in colorectal cancer patients. However, the ability of MTX to increase PRPP levels in vivo, the optimal scheduling for the drugs in this disease, and the feasibility of improving the therapeutic index of FUra for these patients have remained uncertain. Consequently, it was of interest to determine the feasibility of selectively increasing the metabolism of FUra in human colon xenografts in vivo by using this approach, with the prospect of inducing the RNA-mediated mechanism of cytotoxicity to become growth-limiting for the tumor.

Methotrexate, at a sublethal dose level of 100 mg/kg administered intraperitoneally increased the PRPP concentration in three of the xenograft lines to a maximum (305 to 456% of control) between 14 and 24 hours after treatment (Houghton et al., 1982b). In bone marrow of the host, concentrations of PRPP decreased progressively to 28% of control, 24 hours after MTX administration, while in ileum there was a profound increase such that by 4 hours, PRPP was 968% of control; at 14 hours, 277% of control; and at 24 hours, 494% of control. Twenty-four hours after treatment with MTX at doses of 25 to 100 mg/kg, the elevation in PRPP was greater in ileum than in tumors. The metabolism of [6-^{3}H]FUra administered 24 hours after MTX was increased in ileum, radiolabeled ribonucleotides increasing to five times control values by 6 hours after FUra treatment, but with only marginal elevation of FdUMP levels at this time (Houghton et al., 1982b). Such pretreatment with MTX also resulted in an increased rate and greater level of incorporation of [6-^{3}H]FUra into the RNA of ileum, 1 hour after the administration of [6-^{3}H]FUra, although only a slight elevation in the incorporation of drug into the RNA of one of two tumor lines studied ($HxELC_2$), was measured (Houghton et al., 1982b; Figure 5). At subsequent times, the level of incorporation of [6-^{3}H]FUra into RNA was also greater

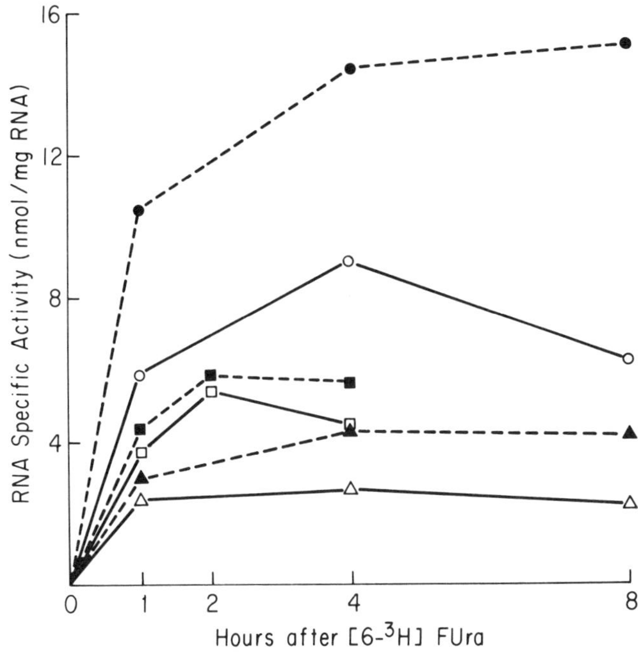

FIGURE 5. [6-^{3}H]FUra (100 mg/kg) was adminsitered intraperitoneally to mice either alone, or 24 hours after MTX (100 mg/kg). The incorporation of [6-^{3}H]FUra into RNA was examined in $HxELC_2$ and $HxVRC_5$ tumors and in ileum for up to 8 hours after treatment. Data from ileum and $HxVRC_5$ tumors represent the mean of two separate experiments. In line $HxELC_2$, results were obtained by pooling eight tumors at each time point. [6^{3}H]FUra alone: (○-○) ileum, (△-△) $HxELC_2$, (□-□) $HxVRC_5$. MTX [6-^{3}H]FUra: (●-●) ileum, (▲-▲) $HxELC_2$, (■-■) $HxVRC_5$. *Source:* Houghton et al. (1982b)

in ileum than in tumors. The scheduling of FUra at a dose level of 25 mg/kg, 24 hours after a priming dose of MTX (100 mg/kg), was at least as toxic as 100 mg of FUra per kg adminsitered alone, based on drug-induced weight loss and death. The dose-limiting toxicity was related to gastrointestinal damage, whereas bone marrow toxicity, which has been observed with high dose levels of FUra administered alone (Houghton and Houghton, 1980b), was not detected.

The pattern of toxicity is thus correlated with changes in PRPP concentrations in these tissues. In bone marrow, where data are consistent with the salvage of preformed purine bases by mammalian bone marrow (Murray 1971; Taetle et al., 1979), no enhancement of FUra incorporation into RNA of human bone marrow in vitro by MTX pretreatment has been observed (Tisman and Wu, 1980). In patients with colorectal carcinoma, the major toxicity with this combination has been gastrointestinal (Herrmann et al., 1981; Weinerman et al., 1982). Unacceptable toxicity in patients was also reported when MTX preceded FUra by 4 hours (Solan et al., 1980). The moderate increase in PRPP detected in mouse ileum at 14 hours after MTX treatment (277% of control) seems at first to suggest an increased therapeutic benefit for FUra in human colon xenografts if MTX were to precede FUra by 14 hours (Houghton et al., 1982b). However, the concentrations of PRPP in tumors at this time ranged from 289 to 456% of control, and the difference between these levels and those in ileum may not be sufficient to increase the therapeutic index. It must be concluded that the use of MTX in this system apparently does not allow a selective increase of PRPP in tumors during the first 24 hours.

CONCLUSIONS AND FUTURE DIRECTIONS

It is clear that considerable heterogeneity exists in tumors of colorectal origin and that this poses a major problem of therapy with FUra. In the xenografts of large bowel cancer that have been studied, such differences exist in their biologic and biochemical characteristics, cell proliferation kinetics, and responsiveness to chemotherapeutic agents. Derivation of a successful chemotherapeutic regimen for a high proportion of patients is complicated by heterogeneity in the pathways and extent of metabolism of FUra, levels of metabolic enzymes, and the extent to which dTMP synthetase becomes inhibited.

Under in situ conditions, the antithymidylate effect of FUra may be an important determinant of FUra responsiveness, and this appears to be only transient in sensitive tumors. Factors that may influence tumor sensitivity under conditions of low CH_2FH_4 concentration, which are present in human colon xenografts, include endogenous dUMP concentrations, the rate of dissociation, and the net dissociation of the covalent complex formed between CH_2FH_4, FdUMP, and dTMP synthetase. These must be evaluated in the xenograft model, and factors that may increase the extent and duration of covalent complex formation should be examined. The extent of polyglutamylation of CH_2FH_4, particularly under conditions of low cofactor concentration, may be an important determinant of the inhibition of dTMP synthetase in vivo, because of the enhanced affinity of the polyglutamates for the enzyme. Studies of the effect of polyglutamylation on the formation and net dissociation of the ternary complex are also needed.

Hypoxanthine and HPP, which protect normal limiting tissues from the toxicity of FUra such that a twofold higher dose of FUra may be administered in vivo, have failed to increase response rates in the treatment of colon carcinoma. Reduction in the metabolism of FUra by OPRTase in normal tissues has also occurred in human colon xenografts.

In contrast, host toxicity (gastrointestinal) was increased when MTX (which increased endogenous levels of PRPP) preceded the administration of FUra in vivo by 24 hours. Concentrations of PRPP, together with the incorporation of FUra into RNA were increased to a greater extent in ileum than in human colon xenografts, and selectivity based on the MTX-induced increase in PRPP was not apparent during the first 24 hours after MTX administration. However, the exploration of factors that may selectively increase the intratumor metabolism of FUra in tumors should be pursued. The RNA-directed mechanism of cytotoxicity, which may become operative at higher drug concentrations in vivo may be of value for increasing responsiveness in a higher percentage of tumors. The value of a colorectal xenograft model, in contrast to a cell culture model, resides in the ability to examine possible selectivity of therapy in human solid tumors under more closely defined conditions in the laboratory.

This work was supported by grants CH-172 from the American Cancer Society, CA-32613 and CA-21677 from the National Cancer Institute, and by ALSAC.

REFERENCES

Anderson EP, Ciardi JE, Brockman RW, Law LW (1962) Uridine kinase activity in fluorouridine-resistant tumor cells. Fed Proc 21:384.

Ardalan B, Buscaglia MD, Schein PS (1978) Tumor 5-fluorodeoxyuridylate concentration as a determinant of 5-fluorouracil response. Biochem Pharmacol 27:2009–2013.

Ardalan B, Cooney DA, Jayaram HN, et al. (1980) Mechanisms of sensitivity and resistance of murine tumors to 5-fluorouracil. Cancer Res 40:1431–1437.

Baskin F, Carlin SC, Kraus P, et al. (1975) Experimental chemotherapy of neuroblastoma II. Increased thymidylate synthetase activity in a 5-fluorodeoxyuridine-resistant variant of mouse neuroblastoma. Mol Pharmacol 11:105–117.

Bearden JD, Coltman CA, Moon TE, et al. (1977) Combination chemotherapy using cyclophosphamide, vincristine, methotrexate, 5-fluorouracil, and prednisone in solid tumors. Cancer 39:21–26.

Becker MA, Raivio KO, Seegmiller JE (1979) Synthesis of phosphoribosylpyrophosphate in mammalian cells. Adv Enzymol 49:281–306.

Benz C, Cadman E (1981) Modulation of 5-fluorouracil metabolism and cytotoxicity by antimetabolite pretreatment in human colorectal adenocarcinoma, HCT-8. Cancer Res 41:994–999.

Benz C, Schoenberg M, Choti M, Cadman E (1980) Schedule-dependent cytotoxicity of methotrexate and 5-fluorouracil in human colon and breast tumor cell lines. J Clin Invest 66:1162–1165.

Berger SH, Hakala MT (1982) Role of cellular dUMP and FdUMP pools and of excess folinic acid (CF) in recovery of thymidylate synthetase (dTMP-S) activity after 5-fluorouracil (FUra) treatment. Proc Am Assoc Cancer Res 23:217.

Berger SH, Yin MB, Whalen JA, Hakala MT (1981) Role of folate (FA) and dUMP pools in response to 5-fluoropyrimidines. Proc Am Assoc Cancer Res 22:215.

Bird OD, McGlohon VM, Vaitkus JW (1965) Naturally occurring folates in the blood and liver of the rat. Anal Biochem 12:18–35.

Blakley RL (1969) The biochemistry of folic acid and related pteridines. Neuberger A, Tatum EL, eds. New York: American Elsevier.

Bruckner HW, Storch JA, Holland JF (1981) Leucovorin increases the toxicity of 5-fluorouracil: Phase I clinical pharmacological trials. Proc Am Assoc Cancer Res 22:192.

Burnet R, Smith FP, Hoerni B, et al. (1981) Sequential methotrexate-5-fluorouracil in advanced measurable colorectal cancer: Lack of appreciable therapeutic synergism. Proc Am Assoc Cancer Res 22:370.

Cadman E, Heimer R, Davis L (1979) Enhanced 5-fluorouracil nucleotide formation after methotrexate administration: Explanation for drug synergism. Science 205:1135–1137.

Cadman E, Heimer R, Benz C (1981) The influence of methotrexate pretreatment on 5-fluorouracil in metabolism in L1210 cells. J Biol Chem 256:1695–1704.

Campbell TN, Howell SB, Pfeifle C, House BA (1982) High-dose allopurinol modulation of 5-FU toxicity: Phase I trial of an outpatient dose schedule. Cancer Treatm Rep 66:1723–1727.

Cantrell JE, Brunet R, Lagarde C, et al. (1982) Phase II study of sequential methotrexate–

5-FU therapy in advanced measurable colorectal cancer. Cancer Treatm Rep 66:1563–1565.

Carrico CK, Glazer RI (1979) Augmentation by thymidine of the incorporation and distribution of 5-fluorouracil in ribosomal RNA. Biochem Biophys Res Commun 87:664–670.

Carroll DS, Kemeny NE, Gralla RJ (1979) Phase II evaluation of pyrazofurin in patients with advanced colorectal carcinoma. Cancer Treatm Rep 63:139–140.

Carroll DS, Gralla RJ, Kemeny NE (1980) Phase II evaluation of N-(phosphonacetyl-L-aspartic acid (PALA) in patients with advanced colorectal carcinoma. Cancer Treatm Rep 64:349–351.

Carter SK, Friedman M (1974) Integration of chemotherapy into combined modality treatment of solid tumors. II. Large bowel carcinoma. Cancer Treatm Rev 1:111–129.

Currie VE, Burchenal JH, Sykes MP, et al. (1975) Animal and clinical studies of 5-fluorouridine (FUR). Proc Am Assoc Cancer Res 16:188.

Danenberg PV (1977) Thymidylate synthetase—a target enzyme in cancer chemotherapy. Biochim Biophys Acta 473:73–92.

Danenberg PV, Danenberg KD (1978) Effect of 5,10-methylenetetrahydrofolate on the dissociation of 5-fluoro-2′-deoxyuridylate from thymidylate synthetase. Biochemistry 17:4018–4024.

Danks MK, Scholar EM (1982) Regulation of phosphoribosylpyrophosphate synthetase by endogenous purine and pyrimidine compounds and synthetic analogs in normal and leukemic white blood cells. Biochem Pharmacol 31:1687–1691.

Dolnick BJ, Cheng Y-C (1978) Human thymidylate synthetase II. Derivatives of pteroylmono- and -polyglutamates as substrates and inhibitors. J Biol Chem 253:3563–3567.

Drapkin R, Griffiths E, McAloon E, et al. (1981) Sequential methotrexate (MTX) and 5-fluorouracil (5FU) in adenocarcinoma of the colon and rectum. Proc Am Soc Clin Oncol 22:453.

Evans RM, Laskin JD, Hakala MT (1980) Assessment of growth-limiting events by 5-fluorouracil in mouse cells and in human cells. Cancer Res 40:4113–4122.

Evans RM, Laskin JD, Hakala MT (1981) Effect of excess folates and deoxyinosine on the activity and site of action of 5-fluorouracil. Cancer Res 41:3288–3295.

Fox IH, Kelley WN (1972) Human phosphoribosylpyrophosphate synthetase: Kinetic mechanism and end product inhibition. J Biol Chem 247:2126–2131.

Fox RM, Woods RL, Tattersall MHN, Brodie GW (1979) Allopurinol modulation of high-dose fluorouracil toxicity. Cancer Treatm Rev 6(Suppl):143–147.

Fox RM, Woods RL, Tattersall MHN, et al. (1981) Allopurinol modulation of fluorouracil toxicity. Cancer Chemother Pharmacol 5:151–155.

Goldberg AR, Machledt JH, Pardee AB (1966) On the action of fluorouracil on leukemia cells. Cancer Res 26:1611–1615.

Goldin A, Venditti JM, Macdonald JS, Muggia FM, Henney JE, DeVita VT (1981) Current results of the screening program at the Division of Cancer Treatment, National Cancer Institute. Eur J Cancer 17:129–142.

Haller DG, Woolley PV, MacDonald JS, et al. (1978) Phase II trial of 5-fluorouracil, adriamycin, and mitomycin C in advanced colorectal cancer. Cancer Treatm Rep 62:563–565.

Heidelberger C (1965) Fluorinated pyrimidines. Prog Nucl Acid Res Mol Biol 4:1–50.

Heidelberger C (1974) Fluorinated pyrimidines and their nucleosides. In: Sartorelli AC, Johns DG, eds., Antineoplastic and immunosuppressive agents II. Handbook of experimental pharmacology. New York: Springer-Verlag, pp. 193–231.

Herrmann R, Manegold C, Rittinghausen R, et al. (1981) Sequential methotrexate (MTX) and 5-fluorouracil (FU) in colorectal adenocarcinoma. Results of a pilot study. Proc Am Soc Clin Oncol 22:457.

Hershko A, Razin A, Mager J (1969) Regulation of the synthesis of 5-phosphoribosyl-1-pyrophosphate in intact red blood cells and in cell-free preparations. Biochim Biophys Acta 184:64–76.

Houghton JA, Houghton PJ (1978) Evaluation of single-agent therapy in human colorectal tumour xenografts. Br J Cancer 37:833–840.

Houghton JA, Houghton PJ (1979) Evaluation of cytotoxic agents in human colonic tumor xenografts and mouse gastrointestinal tissue using 3H-thymidine fractional incorporation into DNA. Eur J Cancer 15:763–769.

Houghton JA, Houghton PJ (1980a) On the mechanism of cytotoxicity of fluorinated pyrimidines in four human colon adenocarcinoma xenografts maintained in immune-deprived mice. Cancer 45:1159–1167.

Houghton JA, Houghton PJ (1980b) 5-Fluorouracil in combination with hypoxanthine and allopurinol: Toxicity and metabolism in xenografts of human colonic carcinomas in mice. Biochem Pharmacol 29:2077–2080.

Houghton JA, Houghton PJ (1982) Combinations of 5-fluorouracil, hypoxanthine and allopurinol in the chemotherapy of human colon adenocarcinoma xenografts. Cancer Treatm Rep 66:1201–1206.

Houghton JA, Houghton PJ (1983) Elucidation of pathways of 5-fluorouracil metabolism in xenografts of human colorectal adenocarcinoma. Eur J Cancer, 19:807–815.

Houghton JA, Taylor DM (1978a) Maintenance of biological and biochemical characteristics of human colorectal tumours during serial passage in immune-deprived mice. Br J Cancer 37:199–212.

Houghton JA, Taylor DM (1978b) Growth characteristics of human colorectal tumours during serial passage in immune-deprived mice. Br J Cancer 37:213–223.

Houghton PJ, Houghton JA, Taylor DM (1977) Effects of cytotoxic agents on TdR incorporation and growth delay in human colonic tumour xenografts. Br J Cancer 36:206–214.

Houghton JA, Houghton PJ, Wooten RS (1979) Mechanism of induction of gastrointestinal toxicity in the mouse by 5-fluorouracil, 5-fluorouridine and 5-fluoro-2′-deoxyuridine. Cancer Res 39:2406–2413.

Houghton JA, Maroda SJ, Phillips JO, Houghton PJ (1981) Biochemical determinants of responsiveness to 5-fluorouracil and its derivatives in human colorectal adenocarcinoma xenografts. Cancer Res 41:144–149.

Houghton JA, Schmidt C, Houghton PJ (1982a) The effect of derivatives of folic acid on the fluorodeoxyuridylate-thymidylate synthetase covalent complex in human colon xenografts. Eur J Cancer Clin Oncol 18:347–354.

Houghton JA, Tice AJ, Houghton PJ (1982b) The selectivity of action of methotrexate in combination with 5-fluorouracil in xenografts of human colorectal adenocarcinomas. Mol Pharmacol 22:771–778.

Howell SB, Wung WE, Taetle R, et al. (1981) Modulation of 5-fluorouracil toxicity by allopurinol in man. Cancer 48:1281–1289.

Isacoff WH, Eilber F, Tabbarah H, et al. (1978) Phase II clinical trial with high-dose methotrexate therapy and citrovorum factor rescue. Cancer Treatm Rep 62:1295–1304.

Jackson RC (1978) The regulation of thymidylate biosynthesis in Novikoff hepatoma cells and the effects of amethopterin, 5-fluorodeoxyuridine, and 3-deazauridine. J Biol Chem 253:7440–7446.

Jackson RC, Harrap KR (1973) Studies with a mathematical model of folate metabolism. Arch Biochem Biophys 158:827–841.

Kasbekar DK, Greenberg DM (1963) Studies on tumor resistance to 5-fluorouracil. Cancer Res 23:818–824.

Kessel D, Hall TC, Wodinsky I (1966) Nucleotide formation as a determinant of 5-fluorouracil response in mouse leukemias. Science 154:911–913.

Kessel D, Bruns R, Hall TC (1971) Determinants of responsiveness to 5-fluorouridine in transplantable murine leukemias. Mol Pharmacol 7:117–121.

Kessel D, Dodd DC, Hall TC (1973) Some determinants of drug responsiveness in bovine leukemia cells. Biochem Pharmacol 22:1161–1164.

Kisliuk RL, Gaumont Y, Baugh CM (1974) Polyglutamyl derivatives of folate as substrates and inhibitors of thymidylate synthetase. J Biol Chem 249:4100–4103.

Klubes P, Connelly K, Cerna I, Mandel HG (1978) Effects of 5-fluorouracil on 5-fluorodeoxyuridine 5′-monophosphate and 2-deoxyuridine 5′-monophosphate pools, and DNA synthesis in solid mouse L1210 and rat Walker 256 tumors. Cancer Res 38:2325–2331.

Klubes P, Cerna I, Meldon MA (1981) Effect of concurrent calcium leucovorin infusion on 5-fluorouracil cytotoxicity against murine L1210 leukemia. Cancer Chemother Pharmacol 6:121–125.

Kroener JF, Saleh F, Howell SB (1982) 5-FU and allopurinol: Toxicity modulation and phase II results in colon cancer. Cancer Treatm Rep 66:1133–1137.

Laster WR (1975) Ridgway osteogenic sarcoma—a promising laboratory model for special therapeutic trials against an advanced staged, drug-sensitive animal tumor system. Cancer Chem Rep 5(2):151–168.

Levinson BB, Ullman B, Martin DW (1979) Pyrimidine pathway variants of cultured mouse lymphoma cells with altered levels of both orotate phosphoribosyltransferase and orotidylate decarboxylase. J Biol Chem 254:4396–4401.

Lockshin A, Danenberg PV (1981) Biochemical factors affecting the tightness of 5-fluorodeoxyuridylate binding to human thymidylate synthetase. Biochem Pharmacol 30:247–257.

Machover D, Schwarzenberg L, Goldschmidt E, Tourani JM, Michalski B, Hayat M, Dorval T, Misset JL, Jasmin C, Maral R, Mathe G (1982) Treatment of advanced colorectal and gastric adenocarcinomas with 5-FU combined with high-dose folinic acid: A pilot study. Cancer Treatm Rep 66:1803–1807.

Maley GF, Maley F, Baugh CM (1979) Differential inhibition of host and viral thymidylate synthetases by folylpolyglytamates. J Biol Chem 254:7485–7487.

Maybaum J, Ullman B, Mandel HG, et al. (1980) Regulation of RNA- and DNA-directed actions of 5-fluoropyrimidines in mouse T-lymphoma (S-49) cells. Cancer Res 40:4209–4215.

Mehta BM, Gisolfi AL, Hutchison DJ, et al. (1978) Serum distribution of citrovorum factor and 5-methyltetrahydrofolate following oral and Im administration of calcium leucovorin in normal adults. Cancer Treatm Rep 62:345–350.

Michaelson R, Kemeny N, Young C (1982) Phase II evaluation of 4′-epidoxorubicin in patients with advanced colorectal carcinoma. Cancer Treatm Rep 66:1757–1758.

Moertel CG (1978) Current concepts in cancer: Chemotherapy of gastrointestinal cancer. N Engl J Med 299:1049–1052.

Moran RG, Werkheiser WC, Zakrzewski SF (1976) Folate metabolism in mammalian cells in culture I. Partial characterization of the folate derivatives present in L1210 mouse leukemia cells. J Biol Chem 251:3569–3575.

Moran RG, Spears CP, Heidelberger C (1979) Biochemical determinants of tumor sensitivity to 5-fluorouracil: Ultrasensitive methods for the determination of 5-fluoro-2′-deoxyuridylate, 2′-deoxyuridylae and thymidylate synthetase. Proc Natl Acad Sci USA 16:1456–1460.

Mulkins MA, Heidelberger C (1982) Biochemical characterization of fluoropyrimidine-resistant murine leukemic cell lines. Cancer Res 42:965–973.

Murray AW (1971) The biological significance of purine salvage. Annu Rev Biochem 40:811–826.

Myers CE, Young RC, Chabner BA (1975) Biochemical determinants of 5-fluorouracil response *in vivo*. The role of deoxyuridylate pool expansion. J Clin Invest 56:1231–1238.

Presant CA, Ratkin G, Klahr C (1978) Phase II study of mitomycin C, cyclophosphamide, and methotrexate in drug-resistant colorectal carcinoma. Cancer Treatm Rep 62:549–550.

Priest DG, Mangum M (1981) Relative affinity of 5,10-methylenetetrahydrofolylpolyglutamates for the Lactobacillus casei thymidylate synthetase-5-fluorodeoxyuridylate binary complex. Arch Biochem Biophys 210:118–123.

Reeves BR, Houghton JA (1978) Serial cytogenetic studies of human colonic tumour xenografts. Br J Cancer 37:612–619.

Reichard P, Sköld O, Klein G (1959) Possible enzymatic mechanism for the development of resistance against fluorouracil in ascites tumours. Nature 183:939–941.

Reichard P, Sköld O, Klein G, et al. (1962) Studies on resistance against 5-fluorouracil I. Enzymes of the uracil pathway during development of resistance. Cancer Res 22:235–243.

Reyes P, Guganig ME (1975) Studies on a pyrimidine phosphoribosyltransferase from murine leukemia P1534J. J Biol Chem 250:5097–5108.

Reyes P, Hall TC (1969) Synthesis of 5-fluorouridine 5′-phosphate by a pyrimidine phosphoribosyltransferase of mammalian origin—II. Correlation between tumor levels of the enzyme and the 5-fluorouracil-promoted increase in survival of tumor bearing mice. Biochem Pharmacol 18:2587–2590.

Richards F, Pajak TL, Cooper MR, Spurr CL (1975) Comparison of 5-fluorouracil with 5-fluorouracil, cyclophosphamide, and methotrexate in metastatic colorectal carcinoma. Cancer 36:1589–1592.

Rustum YM, Danhauser L, Wang G (1979) Selectivity of action of 5-FU: biochemical basis. Bull Cancer (Paris) 66:44–47.

Saiers JH, Salvik M, McKinney DR (1982) Phase II evaluation of vindesine for patients with advanced colorectal carcinoma. Cancer Treatm Rep 66:583–584.

Santi DV (1980) Perspectives on the design and biochemical pharmacology of inhibitors of thymidylate synthetase. J Med Chem 23:103–111.

Santi DV, McHenry CS, Sommer H (1974) Mechanism of interaction of thymidylate synthetase with 5-fluorodeoxyuridylate. Biochemistry 13:471–480.

Schwartz PM, Handschumacher RE (1979) Selective antagonism of 5-fluorouracil cytotoxicity by 4-hydroxypyrazolopyrimidine (Allopurinol) in vitro. Cancer Res 39:3095–3101.

Schwartz PM, Dunigan JM, Marsh JC, Handschumacher RE (1980) Allopurinol modification of the toxicity and antitumor acitivty of 5-fluorouracil. Cancer Res 40:1885–1889.

Solan A, Vogl SE, Kaplan BH, et al. (1980) 5-Fluorouracil (FU) and methotrexate (MTX) in combination for colo-rectal cancer: Unacceptable toxicity when intermediate dose MTX precedes FU by 4 hours. Proc Am Soc Clin Oncol 21:335.

Spears CP, Shahinian AH, Moran RG, et al. (1982) In vivo kinetics of thymidylate synthetase inhibition in 5-fluorouracil-sensitive and -resistant murine colon adenocarcinomas. Cancer Res 42:450–456.

Taetle R, Mendelsohn J, Howell SB (1979) Nucleoside requirements for the protection of human marrow from methotrexate (MTX). Proc Am Soc Clin Oncol 20:399.

Taylor SG, Desai SA, DeWys WD (1978) Phase II trial of a combination of cyclophosphamide, vincristine, and methotrexate in advanced colorectal carcinoma. Cancer Treatm Rep 62:1203–1205.

Tisman G, Wu SJG (1980) Effectiveness of intermediate-dose methotrexate and high-dose 5-fluorouracil as sequential combination chemotherapy in refractory breast cancer and as primary therapy in metastatic adenocarcinoma of the colon. Cancer Treatm Rep 64:829–835.

Ullman B, Kirsch J (1979) Metabolism of 5-fluorouracil in cultured cells. Protection from 5-fluorouracil cytotoxicity by purines. Mol Pharmacol 15:357–366.

Ullman B, Lee M, Martin DW, Santi DV (1978) Cytotoxicity of 5-fluoro-2′-deoxyuridine: Requirement for reduced folate cofactors and antagonism by methotrexate. Proc Natl Acad Sci USA 75:980–983.

Umeda M, Heidelberger C (1968) Comparative studies of fluorinated pyrimidines with various cell lines. Cancer Res 28:2529–2538.

Washtien WL, Santi DV (1979) Assay of intracellular free and macromolecular-bound metabolites of 5-fluorodeoxyuridine and 5-fluorouracil. Cancer Res 39:3397–3404.

Waxman S, Bruckner H (1982) The enhancement of 5-fluorouracil antimetabolic activity by leucovorin, menadione and α-tocopherol. Eur J Cancer Clin Oncol 18:685–692.

Weinerman B, Schacter B, Schipper H, et al. (1982) Sequential methotrexate and 5-FU in the treatment of colorectal cancer. Cancer Treatm Rep 66:1553–1555.

Weiss G, Ervin TJ, Meshad MW, Kufe DW (1982) Phase II trial of combination therapy with continuous-infusion PALA and bolus-injection 5-FU. Cancer Treatm Rep 66:299–303.

White LA, Perry MC, Kardinal CG, et al. (1979) Phase II study of 5-fluorouracil, methyl-CCNU, and daunorubicin in colorectal cancer: A cancer and leukemia group B study. Cancer Treatm Rep 63:215–217.

Wilkinson DS, Crumley J (1976) The mechanism of 5-fluorouridine toxicity in Novikoff hepatoma cells. Cancer Res 36:4032–4038.

Wilkinson DS, Pitot HC (1973) Inhibition of ribosomal ribonucleic acid maturation in Novikoff hepatoma cells by 5-fluorouracil and 5-fluorouridine. J Biol Chem 248:63–68.

Wilkinson DS, Tlsty TD, Hanas RJ (1975) The inhibition of ribosomal RNA synthesis and maturation in Novikoff hepatoma cells by 5-fluorouridine. Cancer Res 35:3014–3020.

Yin M-B, Zakrzewski SF, Hakala MT (1983) Relationship of cellular folate cofactor pools to the activity of 5-fluorouracil. Mol Pharmacol 32:190–197.

Yoshida M, Hoshi A, Kuretani K (1978) Prevention of antitumor effect of 5-fluorouracil by hypoxanthine. Biochem Pharmacol 27:2979–2982.

CONTROL OF EXPERIMENTAL COLON CANCER BY SODIUM CYANATE

VINCENT G ALLFREY, PH.D.

The investigation of the antitumor effects of sodium cyanate had its origins in two independent and unrelated lines of research. Early reports that the topical administration of urea could inhibit tumor growth and cause a high incidence of regression of squamous skin carcinomas (Danopoulos and Danopoulos, 1974a) and that urea given orally prolongs the survival of patients with liver cancer (Danopoulos and Danopoulos, 1974b) led to the suggestion that cyanate present in the urea preparation may have been the actual tumor-inhibitory agent (Lea et al., 1975a,b; Allfrey et al., 1977). Analagous reasoning led to the testing of cyanate as an inhibitor of hemoglobin-S crystallization and erythrocyte sickling after prior reports of the treatment of sickle-cell anemia by the administration of urea (Cerami and Manning, 1973). Subsequent tests of cyanate in tumor-bearing animals have not only confirmed that it has a highly selective antitumor action but also indicate that this effect is mediated not by cyanate itself but by an activated form of the compound that is synthesized in the host.

The cyanate metabolite can now be prepared in vitro, and it is being used to probe the mechanism of its antitumor action. In new developments, this system is being used to monitor the expression of the malignant phenotype in transformed cells and the suppression of malignant growth characteristics by agents such as sodium butyrate.

CYANATE INHIBITION OF PROTEIN AND DNA SYNTHESIS IN TUMOR CELLS IN VIVO

The administration of cyanate to tumor-bearing animals has been shown to inhibit a number of biosynthetic reactions essential for cell growth and replication. Both DNA and protein synthesis were found to be inhibited in a diverse

From the Laboratory of Cell Biology, Rockefeller University, New York, New York.

series of Morris hepatomas of differing growth rates and degrees of differentiation and in leukemia L1210 cells (Lea et al., 1975a,b). For example, the incorporation of radioisotopically labeled amino acids into the proteins of hepatomas 7777, 9618A, and 5123C was inhibited by 80 to 90% within 1 to 2 hours after intraperitoneal injection of 250 mg/kg of sodium cyanate, but there was little or no inhibitory effect on host liver, kidney, skeletal muscle, or brain (Lea et al., 1975b). The cyanate sensitivity of the hepatomas cannot be ascribed to the higher sensitivity of dividing, as compared with nondivding, cells because cyanate had no such effect on regenerating liver (Lea et al., 1975b) or in intestinal epithelium (Allfrey et al., 1977).

Cyanate effectively blocked protein synthesis in MK3 kidney tumors with little inhibitory effect on the normal kidney (Lea et al., 1975b).

Under similar conditions, cyanate was found to inhibit protein synthesis in primary colonic adenocarcinomas [induced in rats by the repeated administration of 1,2-dimethylhydrazine (DMH)], but there was little or no effect of the drug on protein synthesis in normal epithelial cells surrounding the tumors (Allfrey et al., 1977). Autoradiographic studies (in collaboration with Dr. Eleanor E. Deschner of the Sloan-Kettering Memorial Cancer Center) confirm that cyanate inhibits protein synthesis, especially in the dividing cells in the upper luminal third of the tumors (Allfrey et al., 1981).

Cyanate has also been tested as an inhibitor of protein synthesis in transplantable colonic tumors such as T36, derived from a DMH-induced adenocarcinoma of mice (Corbett et al., 1977). In these experiments, the tumors were carried as subcutaneous transplants in BALB/c mice. Matching groups of tumor-bearing animals were given intraperitoneal injections of 250 mg/kg sodium cyanate, or NaCl, respectively. After 1 hour, each animal received a mixture of ^{3}H-amino acids and protein synthesis was allowed to proceed for one additional hour. The specific activities of the total proteins of the liver, kidneys, colonic epithelium, and T36 tumors in the cyanate-treated and NaCl-treated mice are compared in Table 1. Attention is drawn to the striking contrast in cyanate sensitivity of the normal and malignant cell populations, with more than 90% inhibition of ^{3}H-amino acid incorporation in the T36 tumors and no detectable effect on the normal tissues of the tumor-bearing animals.

TABLE 1. Selective Inhibition by Sodiuum Cyanate of Protein Synthesis in Colonic Tumor T36

		Specific ^{3}H-activities of cellular proteins in			
Experimental conditions[a]	Cyanate dosage (mg/kg)	T36 tumors (cpm/mg)	Colonic epithelium (cpm/mg)	Kidney (cpm/mg)	Liver (cpm/mg)
Control	0	5660 ± 120	4500 ± 183	5290 ± 206	6350 ± 266
Cyanate-treated	250	543 ± 145	4270 ± 150	5360 ± 136	6460 ± 295

[a]Tumor-bearing BALB/c mice were injected with Na cyanate (250 mg/kg) or NaCl. One hour later, all animals received 100 μCi of a mixture of 15 ^{3}H-amino acids. The radioactivity of the total proteins in the tumors and normal tissues was measured at 60 minutes. The specific activities of the proteins are presented in mean cpm/mg ± S.D.

Ehrlich ascites cells and Novikoff hepatomas were also found to be cyanate-sensitive in vivo (Allfrey et al., 1977). Although the mechanism of cyanate inhibition remains to be fully explained, an important aspect of cyanate treatment is its effect on the transport of metabolites into tumor cells. There is a substantial suppression of transport of amino acids, thymidine, and phosphate into hepatomas under conditions where there is no decrease (or even an increase) in their transport into the normal hepatic cells of the tumor-bearing animals (Lea et al., 1977; Lea and Koch, 1979). The resulting deprivation of these essential precursors for protein and nucleic acid synthesis represents a major causational factor in the observed restriction of protein and DNA synthesis in cyanate-treated animals, as well as in cultured tumor cells exposed to the cyanate metabolite (Boffa and Allfrey, 1982). In whole animals, the effect of cyanate is complicated by a surprising and unexplained influence of cyanate on circulation through the hepatomas (Lea and Parsons, 1981), but in cultured cells, the availability of the precursors is subject to experimental control, and the effects of the cyanate metabolite on active transport are clearly demonstrable (Boffa and Allfrey, 1982).

In any case, the empirical finding is that two biosynthetic pathways necessary for the replication of chromosomes in the malignant cell—that is, DNA and histone synthesis—are blocked almost completely in the tumors of cyanate-treated animals. The effect is dependent on the amount of cyanate administered and it persists for periods up to 24 hours after a single injection of 250 mg/kg body weight (in rats and mice) (Lea et al., 1975a,b).

In addition to these direct effects on chromosome replication, it is very likely that cyanate also induces cell cycle arrest by interfering with the phosphorylation of tumor histones. Histone phosphorylation, especially of histone H1, appears to be coupled to cell-cycle progression and agents such as sodium butyrate that inhibit histone phosphorylation (D'Anna et al., 1980; Boffa et al., 1981a) arrest cultured tumor cells in the G_1-phase (D'Anna et al., 1980; Fallon and Cox, 1979; Xue and Rao, 1981). It has been found that ^{32}P-phosphate incorporation into the histones of hepatoma 5123C is reduced to only 12% of the control value 1 to 2 hours after injection of 250 mg/kg sodium cyanate. There is virtually no effect on histone phosphorylation in the host liver under the same experimental conditions (Lea et al., 1977).

CYANATE ACTIVATION FOR SUPPRESSION OF PROTEIN SYNTHESIS IN CULTURED TUMOR CELLS

The inhibitory effects of cyanate on tumor protein and DNA synthesis in vivo and the cyanate insensitivity of normal tissues in the same animal suggested that the mechansim of cyanate inhibition could be studied more directly using cultured tumor cells under defined conditions. Surprisingly, no inhibition of amino acid uptake was detected in cells derived from a human colonic adenocarcinoma (HT-29), Novikoff rat hepatoma cells, or Ehrlich ascites tumor cells cultured in the presence of 3.85 mM Na cyanate (Allfrey et al., 1977). This negative result suggested that cyanate itself was not the active antitumor agent but that it had to be metabolized by the host to generate an inhibitory compound. This view was confirmed by comparisons of the effects of sodium cyanate on tumor cells in culture with those on the same cell lines grown and tested in the peritoneal cavity. For example, Novikoff ascites hepatoma cells and Ehrlich ascites tumor cells that were insensitive to cyanate in vitro became cyanate-sensitive when transplanted into the peritoneal cavity of rats (or mice) and tested for ^{3}H-leucine incorporation 1 hour after cyanate administration to the tumor-bearing animals. The inhibition observed—about 40% in the case of the Ehrlich ascites tumor cells—was highly selective; there was no reduction in amino acid uptake into the proteins of the liver, spleen, or kidneys of the cyanate-treated animals (Allfrey et al., 1977).

These observations established the basis for current studies of the mechanism of cyanate activation, and they have led to the development of assay systems for measuring the production and effects of cyanate metabolites on protein synthesis and active transport in cultured malignant cells.

On the premise that the cyanate effect in vivo is probably due to the activity of metabolites produced by the reaction of cyanate with the drug-metabolizing systems of the liver, attempts were made to activate cyanate in vitro, using the mixed-function oxidases of hepatic microsomes (Boffa et al., 1981b).

The assay system, diagramed in Figure 1, uses a dialysis membrane to separate the mixed-function oxidases—prepared as an S9 fraction (Garner et al., 1972; Ames et al., 1975)—in the upper reaction vessel from the tumor cell culture in the lower vessel. Metabolites produced in the reaction of cyanate with the S9 fraction diffuse through the membrane to the cellular compartment, where the uptake of isotopic amino acids into the intracellular "pools," or incorporation into protein, is measured as a function of time. These results are compared with those observed in control experiments in which sodium cyanate is replaced by an equivalent concentration of NaCl, or in which cyanate is present but the S9 fraction is omitted or inactivated.

FIGURE 1. Reaction system for generation and testing of the tumor-inhibitory metabolite of sodium cyanate. The upper vessel, which has a membrane across its base, contains the cyanate-activating enzyme system (either an S9 fraction enriched in cytochrome P_{450b} with added NADPH, or lactoperoxidase plus H_2O_2). Cyanate is added, and the products of the reaction pass through the membrane into the encircling lower vessel containing the tumor cells. After a 5-minute dialysis period facilitated by small magnetic stirrers above and below the membrane, radioactive amino acids or other metabolites are added to the cell suspension. The incorporation of isotopic precursors into intracellular macromolecules (or "pools") is measured at successive times. In control experiments, the sodium cyanate is replaced by NaCl.

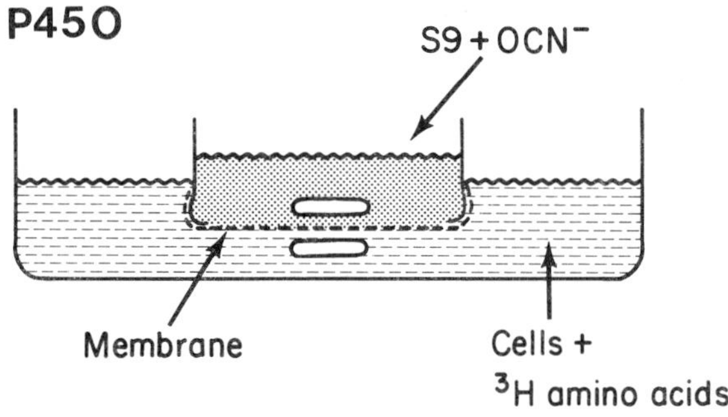

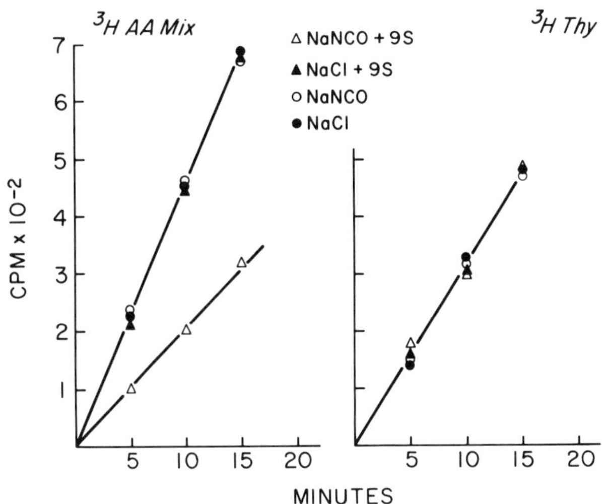

FIGURE 2. Effects of the cyanate and S9 system on the incorporation of ^{3}H-amino acids into protein and ^{3}H-thymidine into DNA of cultured T36 colonic tumor cells. The cells were treated as described in the legend to Figure 1, measuring the uptake of ^{3}H-amino acids and ^{3}H-thymidine in samples withdrawn at the indicated times. Left: kinetics of labeling of protein in cells exposed to NaCl and S9 (▲); cyanate alone (○); NaCl alone (●), and cyanate and the active S9 fraction (△).

An example of the assay, showing the selective inhibition of protein synthesis in cells of the murine colonic tumor T36, is shown in Figure 2. The incorporation of ^{3}H-amino acids into the proteins of the colonic tumor cells is inhibited very rapidly and is easily detected within 5 minutes after exposure to cyanate and the S9 fraction. Under these conditions, there is little effect on ^{3}H-thymidine incorporation into the DNA of T36 cells. It should be emphasized that cyanate alone has no effect on protein synthesis in the tumor cells and that the S9 fraction without cyanate does not produce a dialyzable inhibitor of protein synthesis. Although the reaction of sodium cyanate with the S9 fraction causes a rapid inhibition of amino acid incorporation into T36 and other malignant cells, its analogue, sodium thiocyanate, has no effect under the same conditions (Boffa et al., 1981b).

The reaction between cyanate and the hepatic S9 fraction to produce the tumor inhibitory metabolite is enzymatically catalyzed. Omission of the S9 fraction results in amino acid incorporation at control levels, as does thermal inactivation of the enzyme, or omission of the cofactor NADPH (Boffa et al., 1981b). The hepatic mixed-function oxidases comprise a complex population of drug-metabolizing enzymes, some of which can be induced selectively. Tests of a variety of inducers of cytochrome P_{450} activities show that certain inducers appreciably augment the activation of cyanate by the S9 fraction. The S9 fractions from animals treated with Arochlor 1254 were found to be more than 10 times more effective than those prepared from normal rat liver. Comparisons of other inducers show phenobarbital to be effective, whereas β-naphthoflavone is not; this result suggests that cyanate activation requires the participation of a cytochrome P_{450b} rather than a cytochrome P_{448} system (Strobel et al., 1980).

The activation of cyanate by the cytochrome P_{450} system appears to require the catalytic formation of peroxides. When catalase is added to the reaction vessel above the membrane, there is a total suppression of the cyanate effect on tumor protein synthesis. The addition of catalase to the cell suspension below the membrane does not prevent the inhibition of tumor protein synthesis by the reaction products of cyanate and the S9 fraction. Thus, the product of the reaction is not destroyed by catalase. No effect is seen when similar experiments are carried out with superoxide dismutase, further confirming that peroxide rather than superoxide radicals are likely to be involved in the reaction with cyanate (Boffa et al., 1981b).

This information provided the basis for a more direct approach, using hydrogen peroxide plus lactoperoxidase as a source of hydroxyl radicals for activation of the cyanate. This reaction is also carried out as shown in Figure 1, with the modification that catalase is always present in the cell chamber to destroy any hydrogen peroxide diffusing through the membrane. The cyanate metabolite generated by the lactoperoxidase/H_2O_2 reaction is very effective in inhibiting protein synthesis in a variety of tumor cell lines but, like the product of the cytochrome P_{450b} reaction, it has a relatively short half-life in vitro.

The stability of the cyanate metabolite was assessed in experiments in which

FIGURE 3. Studies of the stability characteristics of the cyanate metabolite produced by reaction with lactoperoxidase and H_2O_2. In these experiments HeLa cells were exposed to the cyanate metabolite without delay (□) and the uptake of ^3H-amino acids into tumor proteins was compared to that observed in the cyanate-free control (●). Delays of 5 minutes (○), 15 minutes (▲), and 30 minutes (△) were introduced before testing of the cyanate metabolite for its effects on ^3H-amino acid incorporation.

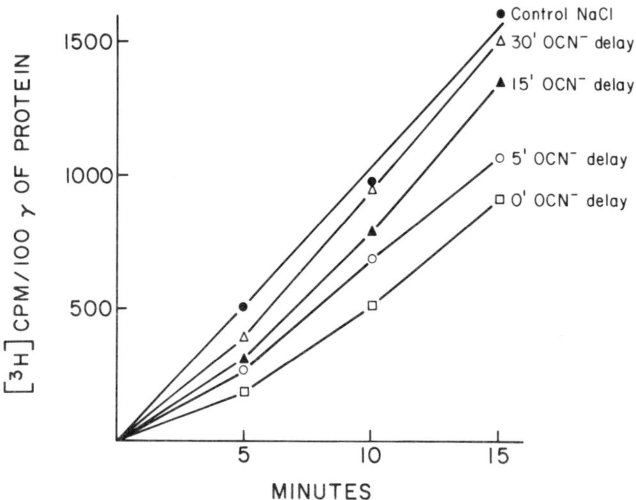

a delay was introduced between the generation of the reaction product and its introduction into the tumor cell culture. The data presented in Figure 3 compare the rates of ^{3}H-amino acid incorporation into HeLa cell proteins after delay periods ranging from 5 to 30 minutes. It is clear that even a short delay results in attentuation of the inhibitory effect on protein synthesis. After a 30-minute delay, the kinetics of amino acid incorporation approximate those seen in control experiments in which NaCl is used instead of sodium cyanate in the upper reaction vessel. Analysis of the amino acid incorporation rates following other delay periods indicate that the tumor inhibitory metabolite(s) has a half-life of only about 10 minutes under these assay conditions.

The instability of the cyanate metabolite, as generated by either lactoperoxidase/H_2O_2 or cytochrome P_{450b}, implies that the effects of cyanate in vivo (which have been detected over periods ranging from 1 to 24 hours) might depend on a continuing generation of the inhibitory factor(s) in the tissues of the tumor-bearing animals. If so, the use of cyanate in the therapy of cancer (discussed following) might be improved by combination with agents such as phenobarbital to enhance the appropriate cytochrome P_{450} activity.

It would be of greater advantage to be able to generate and employ the cyanate metabolite directly for tests of its antitumor activity in vivo. The lactoperoxidase/H_2O_2 reaction with cyanate offers considerable promise in this regard, and experiments are in progress to prepare the cyanate metabolite in a stable derivative form that will allow the slow release of the active compound in the tumor-bearing host.

MECHANISM OF CYANATE INHIBITION OF PROTEIN SYNTHESIS

The effects of sodium cyanate in vivo have generally been monitored by measuring the incorporation of radioactive amino acids into the proteins of the tumors, comparing the results with those obtained in paired tumor-bearing animals injected with NaCl in place of Na cyanate. In all cases, the uptake of isotopic amino acids into proteins is drastically curtailed in the tumors of the cyanate-treated animals (Lea et al., 1975a,b; Allfrey et al., 1977; Lea and Koch, 1979). Since there is no corresponding inhibition of protein labeling in the normal tissues of the tumor-bearing animals, it is clear that cyanate must influence selectively some essential step(s) in the protein biosynthetic pathway that is more susceptible to inhibition in malignant cells. Attempts to identify the primary site(s) of cyanate inhibition and to define the differences between normal and cancer cells in their cyanate sensitivity have converged on the phenomenon of impaired amino acid transport.

Studies of the uptake of the nonmetabolizable amino acid analogue α-aminoiso[^{3}H]butyric acid (AIB) have shown that cyanate lowers its entry into the acid-soluble fraction of hepatomas, but stimulates its uptake into the liver. The inhibition of AIB uptake into hepatoma 9618A_2 persisted for at least 18 hours after administration of 250 mg/kg sodium cyanate to the tumor-bearing rats (Lea et al., 1977). Although the inhibitions observed—greater than 80% for hepatoma 9618A_2, and more than 90% for HTC hepatomas—strongly suggest that impaired amino acid transport is largely responsible for the low rates of incorporation of other isotopic amino acids into the tumor proteins of cyanate-treated animals, it should be noted that similar studies of DMH-induced colonic tumors failed to show any significant difference in the uptake of ^{3}H-amino acids into the total acid-soluble "pool," although the incorporation of the amino acids into tumor proteins was only one-third of that observed in the tumors of control animals (Lea and Koch, 1979). Discrepancies between the specific activities of the total intracellular amino acid "pools" and the activities of newly syntehsized proteins have been noted frequently, and one cannot generally postulate a tight kinetic coupling between the entry of isotopic amino acids into the "pool" and the labeling of nascent polypeptide chains. [See Robinson (1977), Ilan and Ilan (1981), and Schneible et al. (1981) for further discussion of the problem.] However, with regard to the cyanate effect, recent evidence clearly indicates that transport systems in cultured tumor cells are rapidly damaged by exposure to the cyanate metabolite (Boffa and Allfrey, 1982).

The effects on transport can be demonstrated directly by incubating tumor cells in the presence of the cyanate metabolite—generated by the lactoperoxidase/H_2O_2 system—and isotopically labeled amino acids. Aliquots of the cell suspension are taken at periods ranging from 5 to 15 minutes and centrifuged through a density barrier (to remove free amino acids present in the medium) into a second layer containing 10% trichloroacetic acid (TCA) (to solubilize the "pools"). The isotope content of the TCA extract is measured as a function of time and compared with that observed in tumor cells incubated with the same amino acids but in the absence of cyanate.

In the case of HeLa cells tested under these conditions, there is an appreciable inhibition of amino acid uptake within 5 minutes. The effects on transport vary with the particular amino acid employed; typical figures are 66% inhibition for ^{14}C-leucine, 57% for ^{3}H-glutamic acid, and 42% for a mixture of 15 ^{3}H-amino acids. The uptake of ^{3}H-lysine is suppressed by only 24% under identical conditions. For all amino acids tested, there is good proportionality between the labeling of the "pool" and isotope incorporation into tumor cell proteins (Boffa and Allfrey, 1982). It follows that previous studies indicating that the cyanate metabolite inhibits protein synthesis in HeLa and T36 colonic tumor cells (Boffa et al., 1981b) are most likely to reflect primary damage to the transport systems of the cells.

The effect is not limited to amino acids. Similar studies of the effects of the cyanate metabolite on the uptake of nucleic acid precursors also show an inhibition of transport. For example, the entry of ^{3}H-thymidine into the acid-soluble "pool" of HeLa cells is progressively inhibited after cyanate treatment and reaches about 60% of the control value in 15 minutes. The corresponding figure for ^{3}H-uridine uptake is 30% inhibition at 15 minutes, while ^{32}P-phosphate incorporation into the "pool" is diminished by 50%. The effects on polynucleotide synthesis exceed those seen in the acid-soluble nucleotide "pool"; ^{3}H-thymidine uptake into DNA is inhibited by about 80% while ^{3}H-uridine labeling of HeLa cell RNA is reduced to 33% of that seen in control cells (Boffa and Allfrey, 1982). The results are in accord with earlier studies of cyanate inhibition of DNA synthesis in vivo (Lea et al., 1975a).

An additional point of some interest is that cyanate influences the transport of anticancer drugs; the uptake of ^{3}H-methotrexate, for example, is reduced to 24% of the control value within 15 minutes after exposure of HeLa cells to the cyanate metabolite (Boffa and Allfrey, 1982).

The damage to the transport systems of tumor cells is not limited to the entry of metabolites into the intracellular "pools"; cyanate also affects the retention of amino acids, nucleosides, and phosphate ions that are already present in the "pools." Recent studies show that HeLa cells exposed to radioactive amino acids for 10 minutes and then treated with activated cyanate lose the amino acids more rapidly than control cells do, and the ability to retain previously incorporated ^{3}H-thymidine, ^{3}H-uridine, and ^{32}P-phosphate is also impaired (Boffa and Allfrey, 1982). This is an entirely new aspect of cyanate toxicity that suggests that the reason for the differential susceptibility of malignant cells, as compared with normal cells, resides in the plasma membrane or in associated cytoskeletal systems involved in active transport. Given this rapid assay for cyanate effects on amino acid transport, and the fact that normal cells are insensitive to the cyanate metabolite, it now becomes possible to investigate those changes in cell structure and composition that are most relevant to the expression of the malignant phenotype. This approach has proven particularly useful in analyzing the suppression of the malignant phenotype by agents such as sodium butyrate (see below).

INDUCTION OF CYANATE SENSITIVITY IN CELLS TRANSFORMED BY AN ONCOGENIC VIRUS

The relationship between cyanate sensitivity and malignant growth was further investigated by comparing the responses of normal chicken fibroblasts with those of fibroblasts transformed by the Rous sarcoma virus. Both normal and transformed cells were exposed to the cyanate and S9 system, as described, and ^{3}H-amino acid incorporation was measured as a function of time. As expected, the synthesis of proteins in the normal fibroblast culture was not inhibited by the cyanate metabolite, but fibroblasts transformed by the Schmidt-Ruppin strain of the Rous sarcoma virus were cyanate-sensitive (Boffa et al., 1981b).

BUTYRATE EFFECTS ON CYANATE SENSITIVITY OF CULTURED TUMOR CELLS

Attempts have been made to extend the correlation between malignancy and cyanate sensitivity by observing the effects of sodium butyrate on the growth characteristics and response to exogenous cyanate activation systems of cultured HeLa cells. This experimental approach is based on observations that sodium butyrate in millimolar concentrations causes a loss of malignant characteristics in Syrian hamster tumor cells (Leavitt et al., 1978) and inhibits DNA synthesis in neuroblastoma cells (Schneider, 1976), hepatoma cells (Rubenstein et al., 1979) HeLa cells (Hagopian et al., 1977; Boffa et al., 1981a), and mouse kidney cells transformed by murine sarcoma virus (Altenburg and Steiner, 1979). Many tumor cell lines exposed to butyrate display a more "differentiated" phenotype, as indicated by changes in morphology, isozyme patterns, structural and secretory proteins, and hormone sensitivity (reviewed by Prasad, 1980). Human colon adenocarcinoma cells (HRT-18 and HT-29) exposed to 2 mM sodium butyrate show a marked increase in doubling time and a markedly reduced colony-forming efficiency in soft agar. In addition, there are striking changes in morphology, enzyme activities, membrane glycoproteins, and CEA production (Tsao et al., 1982; Herz et al., 1981).

The effects of butyrate on the cyanate sensitivity of HeLa cells have been examined using two different systems for cyanate activation. The first system employed cytochrome P_{450} (prepared as an S9 fraction); the dialyzable products of the reaction were tested on cells exposed to 5 mM butyrate for 15 hours. Under these conditions, there was no inhibition of amino acid incorporation into the proteins of the tumor cells (Boffa et al., 1981b). However, the cyanate sensitivity of the culture reappeared when butyrate was removed from the culture medium. A complete restoration of cyanate inhibition of amino acid uptake required 6 to 10 hours in a butyrate-free medium, but most of the sensitivity to the cyanate metabolite(s) generated by the cytochrome P_{450} reaction was restored in about 5 hours. Because the butyrate-treated cells are arrested in the G_1-phase of the cell cycle (Fallon and Cox, 1979), it became possible to analyze the cell-cycle dependency of the effect and to determine whether the reappearance of the cyanate-sensitive state requires the synthesis of DNA. Studies of ^{3}H-thymidine incorporation indicate that DNA synthesis does not begin until 6 hours after butyrate is removed from the medium. Since sensitivity to the cytochrome P_{450}/cyanate reaction products(s) is almost completely restored at that time, it was concluded that entry into the S-phase is not a prerequisite for expression of this characteristic.

This conclusion, namely, that cyanate sensitivity is not limited to the replicative phase of the cell cycle, has been confirmed using the second system for cyanate activation. The lactoperoxidase/H_2O_2/cyanate reaction differs in several respects from the cytochrome P_{450}-catalyzed reaction. The most significant difference involves DNA synthesis; this is not inhibited by the cytochrome P_{450} system but is inhibited by the product(s) of the lactoperoxidase/H_2O_2/cyanate reaction (Boffa et al., 1981b, Boffa and Allfrey, 1982). Because the chemical nature of the unstable metabolites produced in these reactions has not yet been determined, the reason for this difference remains unclear. However, the lactoperoxidase activation system is now regarded as a better model for the in vivo effects of cyanate, because cyanate administered to tumor-bearing animals does inhibit DNA synthesis in the tumors (Lea et al., 1975a).

When the lactoperoxidase/H_2O_2 reaction is used to activate cyanate, both control and butyrate-treated HeLa cells are inhibited in their capacity to transport, retain, and incorporate radioactive amino acids. Thus, unlike the findings with cytochrome P_{450} as the activating enzyme, the lactoperoxidase reaction generates a cyanate metabolite in sufficient concentration to inhibit the tumor cells whether butyrate is present or not. The reason for the difference must reside in the activation reaction systems; their chemistry is currently under investigation. However, the important point is that tumor cell sensitivity to cyanate persists in nondividing cells; this conclusion is supported by the results of experiments using both activation systems.

CYANATE INHIBITION OF GROWTH OF MURINE COLONIC TUMORS

Studies of the effects of cyanate taken orally on the growth of transplantable colonic tumors have been initiated, using the murine adenocarcinoma line T36 (Corbett et al., 1977) as a model. The tumors were transplanted subcutaneously to BALB/c mice that had been fed for 7 days on laboratory chow containing 2.6 mg/g of sodium cyanate. T36 tumors were also transplanted to equivalent numbers of paired mice fed a cyanate-free diet. Both sets of animals were maintained on the appropriate diets, and tumor size was measured at successive times, as shown in Table 2. In some experiments, complete tumor regression was observed in 28% of the cyanate-treated animals. In other trials, which employed a more malignant subline of the tumor, there were no regressions, but tumor size was greatly reduced and survivorship was prolonged (Table 2).

Recent experiments by Wattenberg (1981a) show that oral cyanate inhibits the induction of colonic tumors by 1,2-dimethylhydrazine. Three levels of the sodium cyanate were employed: 1.6, 2.4, and 3.2 mg/g of diet, and two control groups were fed a cyanate-free diet. Tumor incidence in the control groups was 72%, with an average of 4.2 tumors per mouse. In the cyanate-fed animals, the tumor incidence decreased in proportion to the cyanate content of the diet, with 50% incidence (3.4 tumors/mouse) at the lowest cyanate level, 42% incidence (2.5 tumors/mouse) at the intermediate level, and 32% incidence (2.1 tumors/ mouse) at the highest cyanate feeding level. Otherwise, the dietary intake was the same in all groups, and there was no difference in weight gain in the control and cyanate-fed animals.

Similar studies by Wattenberg (1981b) have shown that dietary cyanate inhibits the induction by benz(a)pyrene of pulmonary tumors in A/J mice, and

TABLE 2. Growth Inhibition of Murine Colonic Tumor T36 by Sodium Cyanate

Experimental conditions		Tumor characteristics			
Diet	Duration (weeks)	Incidence	Average size (mm^2)	Tumor regression (%)	Animals surviving (%)
Experiment 1[a]					
Control	7	24/27	—	—	90
	9	22/22	—	0	73
Cyanate-fed	7	25/29	—	—	97
	9	18/26	—	28	87
Experiment 2[b]					
Control	3	24/26	340	—	87
	4	22/22	550	—	74
	5	19/19	650	—	64
	6	13/13	1070	—	44
	7	2/3	1650	3	10
Cyanate-fed	3	31/31	160	—	100
	4	30/30	470	—	97
	5	27/27	550	—	87
	6	19/19	750	—	62
	7	13/13	810	—	45

[a]Animals placed on diet containing 2.6 g of Na cyanate per kg Purina chow 1 week before tumor transplantation and maintained on cyanate for 7 weeks. Normal diet thereafter.

[b]Animals placed on cyanate diet at time of tumor transplant and maintained on cyanate for duration of experiment.

reduces the incidence of mammary tumors in Sprague-Dawley rats treated with 7,12-dimethyl-benz(a)anthracene. Both the frequency of tumor induction and the number of tumors per animal were reduced by cyanate in a dose-dependent manner.

In view of all these findings, and the very low toxicity of sodium cyanate as determined in previous trials of cyanate in the treatment of sickle-cell anemia (Gillette et al., 1974), a Phase I clinical trial on colonic cancer patients is being initiated in collaboration with Dr. Arnold Mittleman of the Roswell Park Memorial Institute.

Future assessments of the clinical utility of cyanate will obviously require direct testing of the cyanate metabolite, as prepared enzymatically or by direct chemical synthesis. Its effects on the growth of animal tumors and its ability to block tumor induction by a variety of experimental carcinogens are currently under investigation. It is too early to say whether this will lead to testing in human subjects, but even if this approach does not lead to more effective chemotherapy of colon cancer, the cyanate activation reaction has already provided a useful and rapid assay for malignant transformation by carcinogens and oncogenic viruses that, in combination with studies of tumor-suppressants such as butyrate or retinoic acid, opens the way to a more incisive analysis of the differences between normal and malignant cells.

REFERENCES

Allfrey VG, Boffa LC, Vidali G (1977) Selective inhibition with sodium cyanate of protein synthesis in colon cancer cells. Cancer 40:2692–2698.

Allfrey VG, Kozak S, Boffa LC (1981) Selective inhibition of protein synthesis in colonic carcinoma. In: Malt A, Williamson CN, eds. Colonic carcinogenesis. Lancaster: MTP Press, Ltd., pp. 385–396.

Altenburg BC, Steiner S (1979) Cytochalasin B-induced multinucleation of murine sarcoma virus-transformed cells. Exptl Cell Res 118:31–37.

Ames BN, McCann J, Yamasaki E (1975) Methods for detecting carcinogens and mutagens with the salmonella/mammalian microsome mutagenicity test. Mutat Res 31:347–364.

Boffa LC, Allfrey VG (1982) Lactoperoxidase activation of cyanate for selective inhibition of metabolite transport in cultured tumor cells. (Unpublished results.)

Boffa LC, Gruss RJ, Allfrey VG (1981a) Manifold effects of sodium butyrate on nuclear function. J Biol Chem 256:9612–9621.

Boffa LC, Kozak S, Allfrey VG (1981b) Activation of sodium cyanate for selective inhibition of protein synthesis in cultured tumor cells. Cancer Res 41:60–66.

Boffa LC, Victor R, Allfrey VG (1982) Reversibility of the malignant phenotype as probed by the cyanate sensitivity of butyrate-treated tumor cells. (Unpublished experiments.)

Cerami A, Manning JM (1973) Potassium cyanate as an inhibitor of the sickling of erythrocytes in vitro. Proc Natl Acad Sci USA 68:1180–1183

Corbett TH, Griswold DP, Roberts BJ, et al. (1977) Evaluation of single agents and combinations of therapeutic agents in mouse colon carcinoma. Cancer 40:2660–2680.

D'Anna JA, Tobey RA, Gurley LR (1980) Concentration-dependent effects of sodium butyrate in Chinese Hamster Cells. Cell-cycle progression, inner-histone acetylation, histone H1 dephosphorylation and induction of an H1-like protein. Biochemistry 19:2656–2671.

Danopoulos ED, Danopoulos IE (1974a) Urea treatment of skin malignancies. Lancet 1:115–118.

Danopoulos ED, Danopoulos IE (1974b) Regression of liver cancer with oral urea. Lancet 1:132.

Fallon RJ, Cox RP (1979) Cell cycle analysis of sodium butyrate and hydroxyurea, inducers of ectopic hormone production in HeLa cells. J Cell Physiol 100:251–262.

Garner RC, Miller EC, Miller JA (1972) Liver microsomal metabolism of aflatoxin B_1 to a reactive derivative toxic to Salmonella typhimurium TA 1530. Cancer Res 32:2058–2066.

Gillette PN, Peterson CM, Yan SL, Cerami A (1974) Sodium cyanate as a potential treatment for sickle-cell disease. N Engl J Med 290:654–660.

Hagopian HK, Riggs MG, Swartz LA, Ingram VM (1977) Effect of n-butyrate on DNA synthesis in chick fibroblasts and HeLa cells. Cell 12:855–860.

Herz F, Schermer A, Halwer M, Bogart LH (1981) Alkaline phosphatase in Ht-29, a human colon cancer cell line: Influence of sodium butyrate and hyperosmolarity. Arch Biochem Biophys 210:581–591.

Ilan J, Ilan J (1981) Preferential channeling of exogenously supplied methionine into protein by sea urchin embryos. J Biol Chem 256:2830–2834.

Lea, MA, Koch MR (1979) Effects of cyanate, thiocyanate and amygdalin on uptake in normal and neoplastic tissues of the rat. J Natl Cancer Inst 63:1279–1283.

Lea MA, Parsons J (1981) Effects of cyanate on the distribution of isotope-labeled H_2O and extracellular markers in rat liver and tumors. Cancer Res 41:4988–4992.

Lea MA, Koch MR, Allfrey VG, Morris HP (1975a) Inhibition by cyanate of DNA synthesis in hepatomas. Cancer Biochem Biophys 1:129–133.

Lea MA, Koch MR, Morris HP (1975b) Tumor-selective inhibition of protein synthesis by cyanate. Cancer Res 35:2321–2326.

Lea MA, Koch MR, Beres B, Dayal V (1977) Divergent effects of cyanate on amino acid and phosphate uptake by liver and hepatoma. Biochim Biophys Acta 474:321–328.

Leavitt J, Barrett JC, Crawford BD, Ts'o POP (1978) Butyric acid suppression of the in intro neoplastic state of Syrian hamster cells. Nature 271:262–265.

Prasad KN (1980) Butyric acid: A small fatty acid with diverse biological functions. Life Sci 27:1351–1358.

Robinson JH (1977) The nature of the amino acid pool used for protein synthesis in cultured androgen-responsive tumor cells. Exptl Cell Res 106:239–246.

Rubenstein P, Sealy L, Marshall S, Chalkley R (1979) Cellular protein synthesis and inhibition of cell division are independent of butyrate-induced histone hyperacetylation. Nature 280:692–693.

Schneible PA, Airhart J, Low RB (1981) Differential compartmentation of leucine for oxidation and for protein synthesis in cultured skeletal muscle. J Biol Chem 256:4888–4894.

Schneider FH (1976) Effects of sodium butyrate on mouse neuroblastoma cells in culture. Biochem Pharmacol 25:2309–2317.

Strobel HW, Fang WF, Oshinsky RJ (1980) Role of colonic cytochrome P_{450} in large bowel carcinogenesis. Cancer 45:1060–1065.

Tsao D, Morita A, Bella A, et al. (1982) Differential effects of sodium butyrate, dimethylsulfoxide and retinoic acid on membrane-associated antigen, enzymes and glycoproteins of human rectal adenocarcinoma cells. Cancer Res 42:1052–1058.

Wattenberg L (1981a) Inhibition of carcinogen-induced neoplasia by sodium cyanate, tert-butyl isocyanate and benzyl isothiocyanate administered subsequent to carcinogen exposure. Cancer Res 41:2991–2994.

Wattenberg L (1981b) Inhibition of polycyclic caromatic hydrocarbon-induced neoplasia by sodium cyanate. Cancer Res 40:232–234.

Xue S, Rao PN (1981) Sodium butyrate blocks HeLa cells preferentially in early G_1 phase of the cell cycle. J Cell Sci 52:163–171.

HEPATIC ARTERIAL THERAPIES FOR PRIMARY AND SECONDARY HEPATIC CARCINOMAS

WILLIAM D ENSMINGER, M.D., PH.D.,
AND JOHN W GYVES, M.D.

PERSPECTIVES ON REGIONAL THERAPY FOR HEPATIC CANCERS

Liver involvement by cancer occurs frequently and is a major source of morbidity and mortality. The majority of patients with primary and metastatic tumors in the liver cannot be cured with surgical resection. However, a few patients with one or two tumor nodules in the liver are apparently cured by resection, thus indicating regional confinement in such cases (Fortner et al., 1978; Latham and Foster, 1967). Frequently in patients with hepatoma and occasionally in patients with colorectal carcinoma in the liver, the cancer may be localized to the liver, yet it will be surgically inoperable due to the anatomical location (Fortner et al., 1978; Latham and Foster, 1967; Geddes and Falkson, 1970; Lee, 1977). Effective methods for eradicating the liver of tumor cells, therefore, may cure some patients and provide effective palliation with prolonged survival in many more. Eradication of a bulk tumor within the liver might create a circumstance wherein smaller quantities or microscopic disease elsewhere could be more definitively addressed by surgery, radiotherapy, and chemotherapy. In addition, treatment modalities for liver tumors have been useful in the development of new techniques and approaches applicable to other regional therapies. Accordingly, a great deal of clinical effort has been expended in the regional therapy of hepatic cancer. To date, these regional approaches appear to generate more effective results than are achieved by systemic chemotherapy against hepatic tumors. However, although showing the value of a regional approach, these treatments usually have not been sufficiently powerful to induce complete remissions within the liver. As described herein, recent developments in drug delivery techniques make possible a new generation of clinical pharmacologic approaches aimed at improved therapeutic potency based on selective manipulation of the tumor microcirculation.

From the Departments of Internal Medicine and Pharmacology, University of Michigan, Ann Arbor.

RATIONALE FOR HEPATIC ARTERIAL CHEMOTHERAPY

The liver has a dual blood supply; under normal circumstances, approximately one-third of the blood entering the liver comes from the hepatic artery and two-thirds from the portal vein (Grindlay et al., 1941; Tygstrup et al., 1962). A number of investigations have shown that hepatic tumors derive most of their blood supply from the hepatic artery (Almersjo et al., 1966; Bierman et al., 1951; Breedis and Young, 1954; Healy, 1965; Nilsson, 1966; Blanchard et al., 1965). At an early stage, portal venous inflow to a tumor becomes occluded by the pressure of tumor growth (Bengmark and Rosengren, 1970; Ackerman et al., 1969), and tumor-evoked neovascularity (Folkman, 1975) appears to be derived from the hepatic arterial supply (Healy, 1965; Wirtanen, 1973). Recent evidence suggests that the proliferating peripheral rim of hepatic tumor nodules is often hypervascular (at the arteriolar-capillary level) compared with the normal liver (Gyves et al., 1982a; Ackerman and Hechmer, 1980). Hence, drugs infused directly into the hepatic artery should reach the important regions of intrahepatic tumors where tumor growth occurs.

According to pharmacokinetic principles, it should be possible to markedly increase the drug exposure of tumors within the hepatic arterial watershed by direct hepatic arterial infusion using drugs with high total body clearance and short plasma half-lives (Eckman et al., 1974; Chen and Gross, 1980). With agents displaying high hepatic extraction, hepatic arterial dosages can be escalated with the retention of lower, acceptable systemic drug exposure. In terms of increased hepatic drug exposure per given amount of systemic exposure, clinical pharmacologic studies using direct plasma drug level assays have demonstrated a relative advantage for hepatic arterial administration of fluorouracil (Ensminger et al., 1978a), fluorodeoxyuridine (FUDR) (Ensminger et al., 1978a), bischlorethylnitrosourea (Ensminger et al., 1978b), adriamycin (Garnick et al., 1979), dichloromethotrexate (Ensminger et al., 1981a), and mitomycin (Tseng et al., 1981). With FUDR in particular, hepatic arterial infusion can produce as much as 400-fold greater tumor exposure to the drug than is achievable with intravenous infusion (Frei, 1980).

PROBLEMS UNIQUE TO HEPATIC ARTERIAL CHEMOTHERAPY

Several difficulties unique to hepatic arterial chemotherapy are not found with systemic, intravenous drug administration. Although a drug may be pharmacologically rationale, it must be delivered directly into the tumor blood supply in a reliable and reproducible manner. With protracted (that is, greater than 3 week) hepatic arterial infusion using percutaneous angiographic catheters or surgically placed plastic catheters, progressive hepatic arterial thrombosis occurs at a high rate and gradually produces decreased blood flow and, ultimately, occlusion (Cady, 1973; Clouse et al., 1977). Any improvement in response (Patt et al., 1981) (brought about through resultant ischemia and higher drug levels generated) must be tempered by the inability to use further arterial chemotherapy (Ensminger and Gyves, 1983).

It has been shown that the pattern of distribution of agents injected into the hepatic artery is dependent on the flow rate of the infusion (Kaplan et al., 1978). Radionuclide angiography (hepatic artery perfusion scanning) using technetium-99m-macroaggregated albumin (TcMAA) appears to give the best representation of drug distribution at the low infusion rates (3 ml to 1000 ml a day) clinically used (Kaplan et al., 1980). When percutaneous angiographic catheters are used, the tip of the catheter tends to move about and lead to frequent and unpredictable flow distribution changes. When the drug is infused inadvertently into a gastric artery, severe gastric damage can result (Chuang et al., 1981; Narsete et al., 1977). Hence, a catheter system free of thrombosis and movement that reliably infuses only the liver is a prerequisite for maximum response with minimal toxicity. The more potent the cytotoxic agent for hepatic arterial use, the more important the focusing of the catheter flow so as to directly infuse only the liver.

Hepatic arterial drug infusions have been limited by the type of pumping system involved. Pumps worn externally by patients have proven to be inconvenient by their bulkiness and have been a major hindrance to normal daily activities. The pump and the external catheter connection have represented sites for the interruption of the infusion path leading to bleeding, catheter thrombosis, or infection from the introduction of pathogenic organisms (Maki et al., 1979). The fact that patients have undergone protracted outpatient treatment using external pumps is witness more to the fortitude of the cancer patient than to the ingenuity of their physicians and the biomedical engineers. The need for an extensive support system to maintain prolonged outpatient infusions and the clumsiness and unreliability of the infusion systems has limited their widespread applicability.

A totally implanted drug delivery system tested over the past several years appears to overcome many of the problems just noted (Ensminger et al., 1981b). At laparotomy, a small flexible silastic catheter is implanted so as to infuse the entire liver. Appropriate vessels are ligated to confine drug flow to the liver (Niederhuber and Ensminger, 1983). The catheter is attached to a subcutaneously placed model 400 Infusaid pump (Infusaid Corp., Norwood, MA). In the first 60 patients with colorectal cancer metastatic to the liver treated with this system at the University of Michigan, there was only one hepatic artery occlusion (immediately postoperatively) and one permanent catheter occlusion (Ensminger et al., 1982). Flow distribution to the entire liver ascertained by radionuclide angiography was maintained in the other 58 patients. Autopsies in six patients having catheters in place for up to 18 months showed no evidence of thrombosis or vessel wall damage in the catheterized artery. These patients as a group received 13,000 cumulative days of hepatic arterial infusion and 900 pump refills without a bleeding or infectious episode. More than 95% of the days of infusion were given as outpatients. Patients were able to function relatively normally since the system was totally implanted under the skin.

This system has been found to function reliably for other investigators as well (Barone et al., 1982). The model 400 Infusaid pump has a sideport allowing direct injection into the hepatic artery catheter. The 0.63 mm lumen on the hepatic arterial catheter readily allows the passage of TcMAA, starch microspheres, and other forms of microspheres (see below). The recent approval by the Food and Drug Administration of the Infusaid pump for hepatic arterial infusion with fluorodeoxyuridine (FUDR) has facilitated dissemination of the device.

Another problem associated with hepatic arterial chemotherapy is the failure to control extrahepatic tumors. Prior studies are discrepant and indicate that extrahepatic tumors in the face of hepatic metastases may (Cady et al., 1970) or may not (Mansfield et al., 1969) determine survival. Effective hepatic arterial chemotherapy may control the liver disease with little effect on extrahepatic tumors. Preliminary experience with the implanted system suggests that patients having extrahepatic disease at the time of implant have a shorter life expectancy (see below) (Ensminger et al., 1982). Drug programs in such patients need to have systemic effects as well as regional potency.

HEPATIC ARTERIAL VERSUS SYSTEMIC CHEMOTHERAPY FOR HEPATIC TUMOR

An objective response rate of approximately 60% appears to have been achieved in a variety of earlier hepatic arterial infusion studies (Ansfield et al., 1975; Petrek and Minton, 1979; Oberfield et al., 1979). In some studies, a majority of patients had failed conventional intravenous fluorouracil (FU) on a bolus schedule prior to hepatic arterial infusion and yet responded to the arterial treatment (Ansfield et al., 1975). Only one prospective, randomized study, has compared systemic FU with hepatic arterial FU (Grage et al., 1979; Shingleton and Grage, 1976). Fourteen member institutions in the Central Oncology Group (COG) entered 61 evaluable patients with hepatic metastases from colorectal cancer into the study (COG 7032) over a 5-year period. Thirty-one patients received a 3-week course of hepatic arterial FU (60% of patients had a percutaneous angiographically placed catheter, 40% had surgically placed catheters), and 30 patients received intravenous FU (on a loading course). Catheter position was checked "radiographically." After an initial 3-week hepatic arterial infusion, patients received maintenance intravenous FU. No significant differences in survival and response rate were noted. Progression and response were defined in some cases solely by changes in liver function tests.

Unfortunately, this study is not definitive due to major technical shortcomings. Most institutions entered only 1 or 2 patients in a 5-year period, certainly not enough to demonstrate technical proficiency convincingly. Drug flow distribution was not monitored, although 60% of patients had angiographic catheters, which are known to readily migrate. Most fluorouracil was administered intravenously even in patients on the hepatic arterial infusion arm, since only the initial 3 weeks of treatment was intraarterial. A major toxicity of hepatic arterial infusion can be chemical hepatitis, yet elevation in serum levels of hepatic enzymes was interpreted as progression in this study. FU was used and not FUDR, a more selective agent for hepatic arterial infusion. Staging was inadequate without the use of abdominal CT scans or laparotomy to rule out extrahepatic disease. Clearly, the probability of type II error in the study is so great as to negate its usefulness as a comparative trial. As noted previously, the implanted system recently developed makes it possible to efficiently conduct a controlled, prospective, randomized trial comparing the response rates with conventional systemic FU versus hepatic arterial FUDR in patients with colon cancer confined to the liver.

Preliminary therapeutic results have been excellent with the totally implanted system consisting of the model 400 Infusaid pump and silastic catheters implanted so as to infuse the entire liver (Ensminger et al., 1982). As noted earlier, the system has functioned reliably. The model 400 Infusaid pump holds 50 ml of solution with a typical flow rate of 2 to 3 ml/day. Pumps were refilled every 2 weeks, alternating 2 weeks of FUDR (0.3 mg/kg/day) with 2 weeks of saline in order to decrease the propensity for chemical hepatitis. Hepatic tumor response ascertained by physical examination and liver scan using standard criteria was seen in 50 of 60 (83%) of the patients. Only one patient had progressive growth of liver metastases. Response durations to initial FUDR therapy ranged from 2 to 24+ months. Hepatic arterial mitomycin (and recently starch microspheres) through the pump sideport was added to FUDR when response was no longer evident or when extrahepatic disease became manifest. Ninety-eight percent (47/48) of patients with an elevated carcinoembryonic antigen level had at least a 50% fall in levels with treatment. Median survival by life-table analysis for patients with disease confined to the liver at operation has been 24 months. For patients with disease outside the liver, median survival has been 8 to 10 months. Toxicities were all reversible and consisted of mild gastritis in 60% of patients, ulcers in 8%, and anicteric (23% of patients) and icteric (23% of patients) hepatitis. With dose-schedule modifications, all patients showing toxic effects were able to continue treatment without recurrence of toxicity.*

TUMOR MICROCIRCULATION

It has been customary to categorize tumors as being hypovascular or hypervascular relative to the normal liver on the basis of their angiographic appearance. By angiography, endocrine tumors, carcinoid tumors, and hepatobiliary carcinomas are generally considered to be hypervascular relative to the normal liver whereas most other metastatic tumors, including colorectal cancer, are hypovascular. Such a categorization masks important vascular distribution differences within the tumor nodules. Angiogenesis occurs at the periphery of tumor nodules; studies in experimental hepatic metastases, such as the Walker carcinosarcoma in rats, reveal a dense encircling arteriolar-capillary plexus at the tumor periphery and a relatively avascular core (Ackerman and Hechmer, 1980; Warren, 1979). Hepatic arterial injection of yttrium-90 microspheres in rats with the Walker tumor in the liver demonstrates that arteriolar perfusion is considerably greater in the tumor periphery than in the normal liver (Ackerman and Hechmer, 1980).

Recently, Tc99m macroaggregated albumin (TcMAA, lung-scanning agent) has been given by hepatic arterial injection to determine drug flow distribution (Kaplan et al., 1980). These albumin particles average 30 to 40 μm in diameter (range 10 to 90 μm) and thus are held in the first arteriolar-capillary bed. Assuming homogeneous mixing in the hepatic artery, relative density of TcMAA should relate directly to the relative density of the microvascularity patent at the time of microsphere injection into the hepatic artery.

When TcMAA radionuclide angiography is used, many colorectal metastases appear to have a central core that lacks vessels holding up TcMAA and a

---

**Editorial Comment:* Randomized studies of survival and response in carefully staged patients comparing intraarterial with intravenous chemotherapy are in progress in the United States. We believe these studies are essential before the intraarterial infusion pump can be regarded as a "standard" method of therapy.

peripheral rim that entraps much more TcMAA than do normal livers (with normal livers defined by Tc99m sulfur colloid scan) (Gyves et al., 1982a). This observation corresponds with pathologic findings in that the (frequently necrotic) tumor core may be hypovascular while the tumor periphery (where most cell proliferation is occurring) may be hypervascular compared with a normal liver (Breedis and Young, 1954; Healy, 1965; Ackerman and Hechmer, 1980).

The presence or absence of a hypovascular core appears to relate more to the size of the tumor nodule than to the tumor type (Gyves et al., 1982b). Nodules less than 3 cm in diameter generally are hypervascular whereas those more than 4 cm in diameter display a hypovascular core as ascertained by radionuclide tomographic angiography (Keyes et al., 1977). The density of vessels in the hypervascular regions of the tumor nodules appears to be two- to eight-fold greater than in normal livers. As noted subsequently, this provides an opportunity for selective therapy based on the relative vascularity of tumor and normal liver parenchyma.

EFFECTS OF VASOCONSTRICTORS ON LIVER AND TUMOR MICROCIRCULATION

The smooth muscle of the precapillary arterioles in the normal liver is sensitive to a variety of vasoconstrictors including epinephrine (Kaude and Wirtanen, 1970), norepinephrine (Mattson et al., 1979; Grady et al., 1980), vasopressin (Barr et al., 1975), and angiotensin (Kaplan and Bookstein, 1972). Injections or short infusions of these agents into the hepatic artery will constrict the liver arterioles at least temporarily and can markedly decrease overall blood flow through the hepatic artery (Kaude and Wirtanen, 1970; Mattson et al., 1979; Grady et al., 1980; Barr et al., 1975; Kaplan and Bookstein, 1972; Greenway and Stark, 1971). Hepatic tumor neovascularity often lacks the smooth muscle layer sensitive to these vasoconstrictors (Ackerman and Hechmer, 1980; Mattson et al., 1979; Lien and Ackerman, 1970). Thus, intraarterial epinephrine has had extensive use in angiography to constrict normal vessels and thereby to accentuate tumor vascularity ("blush") due to diminished responsiveness of tumor vessels (Kaude and Wirtanen, 1970; Abrams, 1964).

A recent study of hepatic arterial epinephrine in the Walker carcinosarcoma liver tumor model demonstrated the unique ability of this vasoconstrictor to increase blood flow to the tumor periphery as well as to open up blood flow to the relatively avascular core of tumor nodules (Ackerman and Hechmer, 1980). In this model, norepinephrine and angiotensin differed from epinephrine and had no effect on perfusion of the core tumor circulation.

There are two mechanisms whereby vasoconstrictors could be used to improve drug delivery to hepatic tumors. The first develops out of the overall reduction in hepatic arterial blood flow, which means that the drug concentration in the hepatic arterial watershed rises (at a constant heaptic arterial drug dose rate) (Chen and Gross, 1980; Ensminger and Gyves, 1983). If tumor vessels remain preferentially patent, then the tumor will be selectively exposed to this increased drug concentration. One study in the VX-2 rabbit carcinoma model showed a marked improvement in the ratio of liver tumor to normal liver uptake of mitomycin C when hepatic arterial injection of mitomycin C was preceded by a short infusion of epinephrine (Iwaki et al., 1978). However, in these rabbit studies, the total body clearance of mitomycin C must have decreased because the systemic levels of mitomycin were noted to be higher when epinephrine was given concurrently. Thus, although tumor exposure to mitomycin was increased, the major contributing factor to the improved ratio in this rabbit system was not increased tumor uptake, but a decreased liver uptake of mitomycin when epinephrine was given.

The second mechanism whereby vasoconstrictors could improve drug delivery to hepatic tumors would use the relative shunting of blood flow away from normal liver toward tumor vessels to deliver more drug with starch microspheres as described below.

MICROSPHERES TO IMPROVE SELECTIVITY BASED ON MICROCIRCULATION DIFFERENCES

Biodegradable starch microspheres, 40 μm in diameter, have recently been introduced into cancer therapy (Aronsen et al., 1979; Dakhil et al., 1981; Dakhil et al., 1982; Gyves et al., 1982c). When injected into the hepatic artery, the starch microspheres lodge in the microvasculature (precapillary arterioles/capillaries) and can block flow for 15 to 30 minutes until dissolution by serum amylase. Administration of a suspension of starch microspheres in an appropriate drug solution can result in a temporary retention of the drug solution in the microcirculation and has the potential to increase uptake of the drug into the liver and liver tumor.

Although it is not possible clinically to measure such regional uptake directly, significantly increased uptake in the liver should result in decreased potential for systemic toxicity in addition. When 9×10^7 (15 ml) microspheres were administered via the hepatic artery in a solution of bischlorethylnitrosourea (BCNU), systemic exposure to BCNU was decreased by as much as 90%, implying a potential ten-fold improvement in drug delivery to the liver (Dakhil et al., 1981; Dakhil et al., 1982). Similar studies with mitomycin demonstrated a 50% reduction in systemic mitomycin exposure when starch microspheres were coadministered with the drug (Gyves et al., 1982c). Studies aimed at determining the correct dose and schedule of microspheres to be used for maximal therapeutic effect are in progress.

Delivery of the drug solution within the tissue should be proportional to the microcirculation volume, which is in turn proportional to the number of microspheres entrapped in a given region of the tissue. The use of vasoconstrictors to decrease the normal hepatic microcirculation and to increase tumor microcirculation offers the potential for marked improvement in selective drug delivery with starch microspheres.

Yttrium-90 resin microspheres that are approximately 55 μm in diamter have been used both in model systems (Blanchard et al., 1965) and in the clinic to treat hepatic tumors with internal radiotherapy (Abel, 1965; Grady, 1979). In the Walker carcinosarcoma rat liver tumor, yttrium-90 microspheres lodge in highest concentrations in the hypervascular tumor periphery (Ackermann and Hechmer, 1980). Concurrent epinephrine administration decreases yttrium-90 microsphere concentration in normal livers and markedly increases concentrations in tumors in this rat model. In several patients who died shortly after yttrium-90 microsphere treatment, metastatic tumors were found to have three- to four-fold higher microsphere levels than normal livers (Grady, 1979; Grady et al., 1980). Yttrium-90 microspheres have a short effective kill distance of 2 to 3 mm and deliver the majority of their dose over about 3 days (Grady, 1979).

AMPLIFICATION OF THE SELECTIVE EFFECT OF YTTRIUM-90 MICROSPHERES

5-Bromo-2′deoxyuridine (BUDR) is an analogue of thymidine that is incorporated solely and specifically into the DNA of replicating cells (Djordjevic and Szybalski, 1960; Simon, 1963). BUDR undergoes debromination in the liver, and in analogy with fluorodeoxyuridine (Ensminger et al., 1978a) and thymidine (Ensminger and Frei, 1978), it can be expected to have high hepatic extraction. BUDR has other pharmacokinetic properties making it suitable to hepatic arterial infusion for selective regional effects (Schwade et al., 1981). Thus, BUDR by hepatic arterial infusion should be incorporated selectively into proliferating tumors within the liver.

For maximum incorporation of BUDR into DNA, prolonged exposure is necessary (Djordjevic and Szybalski, 1960; Sano et al., 1968; Simon, 1963; Schindler et al., 1966). Such prolonged exposure should be possible using the totally implanted system for hepatic arterial infusion described earlier. With sufficient incorporation into both strands of DNA, radiation sensitivity can be increased at least twofold.

Studies with BUDR and yttrium-90 microspheres have not been done, but the combination would be expected to have considerable selection antitumor potential. Preclinical studies with this combination are in progress. The implanted system allows continuous infusion of BUDR via the central pumping mechanism, whereas the pump sideport can be used for yttrium-90 microsphere injection. As with starch microspheres, further selectivity may be possible through the concurrent administration of vasoconstrictors to shift yttrium-90 microspheres from the normal liver into the tumor microcirculation.

PROSPECTS FOR SUCCESS WITH AN AGGRESSIVE INTEGRATED APPROACH

Successful regional treatment of hepatomas and cholangiocarcinomas is likely to cure some patients with a few isolated tumor nodules confined to the liver, which are nonetheless unresectable due to anatomic considerations. However, even in instances in which there is unrecognized or minimal extrahepatic tumor, successful eradication of the metastatic tumor within the liver may provide prolonged palliation and extension of useful life. Furthermore, as treatment of liver metastases becomes more successful, patients will be treated at earlier stages when the potential for secondary spread from the liver to other sites is less than it is in advanced disease.

The problem of extrahepatic tumors is formidable, but approachable. Hepatic arterial treatment can be sufficiently regional in its toxicity so that systemic chemotherapy can be given without fear of significant myelosuppression or other systemic toxicity from a combined approach. Effective hepatic arterial therapy can be visualized as a debulking modality for liver tumors, while combined systemic therapy can focus on microscopic, occult extrahepatic metastases. For example, hepatic arterial FUDR can be given with concurrent intravenous FU. Alternatively, with other drugs such as BCNU and mitomycin that do not display extensive first-pass hepatic extraction, hepatic arterial administration can increase hepatic tumor exposure but retain similar systemic exposure as achieved with intravenous use.

External beam radiotherapy can be combined with hepatic arterial and systemic chemotherapy to sterilize extrahepatic tumors at early stages in the pelvis and porta hepatis. Even bulky disease in these two extrahepatic sites can respond to aggressive radiotherapy (which can be given in conjunction with hepatic arterial chemotherapy).

A major site of extrahepatic tumor relapse is the peritoneal cavity. Regional chemotherapy using a "belly-bath" technique can generate much higher sustained intraperitoneal levels of drugs such as FU (Speyer et al., 1980, 1981). Intraperitoneally administered FU is removed in large part via the portal vein. The belly-bath approach can increase portal vein drug exposure by three- to four-fold and improve treatment of microscopic nests of tumor cells still fed from the portal vein (that is, prior to evoked neovascularity). Widespread application and evaluation of the belly-bath technique has recently become more feasible and convenient with the introduction of a totally implanted port that can be connected to standard peritoneal dialysis catheters (Liepman et al., 1981; Gyves et al., 1983). Patients thus need have no extracorporeal hardware between treatment courses, resulting in increased convenience and a decreased likelihood of infection.

CONCLUDING REMARKS

This chapter has attempted to delineate therapeutic approaches to more effective control of hepatic tumors. Clearly, the future is bright if an aggressive, hopeful attitude is taken. Despite all precautions, toxicity may occur. However, it is our belief that adverse effects can be controlled even as their potential severity rises with more powerful treatment modalities. Should more effective agents be developed in future years, their most efficient application is likely to benefit from the knowledge and use of the delivery principles and systems discussed in this chapter.

REFERENCES

Abel IM (1965) Treatment of inoperable primary pancreatic radioactive isotopes (Y99 radiating microspheres). Ann Surg 162:267–278.

Abrams HL (1964) Response of neoplastic renal vessels to epinephrine in man. Radiology 82:217–224.

Ackerman NB, Hechmer PA (1980) The blood supply of experimental liver metastases V. Increased tumor perfusion with epinephrine. Am J Surg 140:625–631.

Ackerman NB, Lien WM, Kondi ES, et al. (1969) The blood supply of experimental liver metastases. I. The distribution of hepatic artery and portal vein blood to "small" and "large" tumors. Surgery 66:1067.

Almersjo O, Bengmark S, Engevik L, et al. (1966) Hepatic artery ligation as pretreatment for liver resection of metastatic cancer. Rev Surg 377.

Ansfield FJ, Ramirez G, Davis G, et al. (1975) Further clinical studies with intrahepatic arterial infusion with 5-fluorouracil. Cancer 36:2413.

Aronsen KF, Hellenkant C, Holmberg J (1979) Controlled blocking of hepatic artery flow with enzymatically degradable microspheres combined with oncolytic drugs. Eur Surg Res 11:99.

Barone RM, Byfield JE, Goldfarb PB, et al. (1982) Intraarterial chemotherapy using an implantable infusion pump and liver irradiation for the treatment of hepatic metastases. Cancer 50:850–862.

Barr JW, Lakin RC, Rosch J (1975) Vasopressin and hepatic artery: Effect of selective celiac infusion of vasopressin on the hepatic artery flow. Invest Radiology 10:200–205.

Bengmark S, Rosengren K (1970) Angiographic study of the hepatic artery in man. Am J Surg 119:620.

Bierman HR, Byron RL, Kelley KH, et al. (1951) Studies of the liver by hepatic arteriography in vivo. J Natl Cancer Inst 12:107.

Blanchard RJW, Grotenhuis I, Lafare JW, Perry JF (1965) Blood supply to hepatic V2 carcinoma implants as measured by radioactive microspheres. Proc Soc Exp Biol Med 118:465–468.

Breedis C, Young G (1954) Blood supply of neoplasms in the liver. Am J Pathol 30:969.

Cady B (1973) Hepatic arterial patency and complications after catheterization for infusion chemotherapy. Ann Surg 178:156–158.

Cady B, Monson DO, Swinton NW, et al. (1970) Survival of patients after colonic resection for carcinoma with simultaneous liver metastases. Surg Gynecol Obstet 131:697–700.

Chen HSG, Gross JF (1980) Intra-arterial infusion of anticancer drugs: Theoretic aspects of drug delivery and review of responses. Cancer Treatm Rep 64:31–40.

Chuang VP, Wallace S, Stroehlein J, et al. (1981) Hepatic artery infusion chemotherapy: gastroduodenal complications. Am J Radiol 137:347–350.

Clouse ME, Ahmed R, Ryan RB, et al. (1977) Complications of long term transbrachial hepatic arterial infusion chemotherapy. Am J Roentgen 129:799–803.

Dakhil S, Ensminger WD, Cho K, et al. (1981) Improved regional selectivity of hepatic arterial bischlorethylnitrosourea plus degradable starch microspheres. Proc AACR/ASCO 22:383.

Dakhil S, Ensminger WD, Cho K, et al. (1982) Improved regional selectivity of hepatic arterial bischlorethylnitrosourea with degradable microspheres. Cancer 50:631–635.

Djordjevic B, Szybalski W (1960) Genetics of human cell lines. III. Incorporation of 5-brom- and 5-iododeoxyuridine into the deoxyribonucleic acid of human cells and its effects on radiation sensitivity. J Exp Med 112:509–531.

Eckman WW, Patlak CS, Fenstermacher JD (1974) A critical evaluation of principles governing the advantages of intraarterial infusions. J Pharmacokinet Biopharmacol 2:257–285.

Ensminger WD, Frei E, III (1978) High-dose intravenous and hepatic artery infusions of thymidine. Clin Pharmacol Ther 24:610–615.

Ensminger WD, Dakhil S, Doan K, et al. (1981a) Clinical pharmacology of dichloromethotrexate in hepatic arterial infusions. Proc AACR/ASCO 22:271.

Ensminger WD, Rosowsky A, Raso V, et al. (1978a) A clinical pharmacology evaluation of hepatic arterial infusions of 5-fluoro-2′-deoxyuridine and 5-fluorouracil. Cancer Res 38:3784–3792.

Ensminger WD, Thompson M, Come S, et al. (1978b) Hepatic arterial BCNU: A pilot clinical-pharmacologic study in patients with liver tumors. Cancer Treatm Rep 62:1509–1512.

Ensminger WD, Niederhuber J, Dakhil S, et al. (1981b) Totally implanted drug delivery system for hepatic arterial chemotherapy. Cancer Treatm Rep 65:393–400.

Ensminger WD, Niederhuber J, Gyves JW, et al. (1982) Effective control of liver metastases from colon cancer with an implanted system for hepatic arterial chemotherapy. Proc AACR/ASCO 1:94.

Ensminger WD, Gyves JW (1983) Clinical pharmacology of hepatic arterial chemotherapy. Sem Oncol 10:176–182.

Folkman J (1975) Tumor angiogenesis: A possible control point in tumor growth. Ann Intern Med 83:96.

Fortner JG, Dong KK, Maclean BJ, et al. (1978) Major hepatic resection for neoplasia. Ann Surg 188:363–371.

Frei E, III (1980) Clinical and experimental cancer chemotherapy. In: Fortner JG, Rhoads JE, eds. Accomplishments in cancer research. Philadelphia: Lippincott Co., pp. 169–179.

Garnick MB, Ensminger WD, Israel M (1979) A clinical-pharmacological evaluation of hepatic arterial infusion of adriamycin. Cancer Res 39:4105–4110.

Geddes EW, Falkson G, (1970) Malignant hepatomas in the Bantu. Cancer 25:1271–1278.

Grady E (1979) Internal radiation therapy of hepatic cancer. Dis Colon Rectum 22:371–375.

Grady ED, Auda SP, Cheek WV (1980) Vasoconstrictors to improve localization of radioactive microspheres to treat liver cancer. Presented at the 1980 Medical Association of Georgia Scientific Assembly (Georgia Chapter, American College of Surgeons) November 21, Atlanta.

Grage TB, Vassilopoulos PP, Shingleton WW, et al. (1979) Results of a prospective randomized study of hepatic artery infusion with 5-fluorouracil versus intravenous 5-fluorouracil in patients with hepatic metastases from colorectal cancer. A Central Oncology Group Study. Surgery 86:550–555.

Greenway CV, Stark RD (1971) Hepatic vascular bed. Physiol Rev 51:23–65.

Grindlay JH, Herrick JF, Mann FC (1941) Measurement of the blood flow of the liver. Am J Physiol 132:489.

Gyves JW, Ensminger WD, Yang P, et al. (1982a) Clinical utility of microspheres to assess and attack hepatic tumor microcirculation. Clin Res 30:418A.

Gyves JW, Ensminger WD, Thrall J, et al. (1982b) Dependence of hepatic tumor vascularity on tumor size. Clin Res 30:747.

Gyves JW, Ensminger WD, VanHarken D, et al. (1982c) Improved regional selectivity of hepatic arterial mitomycin by starch microspheres. Proc AACR/ASCO2 23:137.

Gyves JW, Ensminger WD, Niederhuber J, et al. (1983) A totally implanted system for intravenous chemotherapy administration in patients with cancer. Am Med 73:841–845.

Healy, JE (1965) Vascular patterns in human metastatic liver tumors. Surg Gynecol Obstet 120:1187.

Iwaki A, Nagasue N, Kobayashi M, et al. (1978) Intraarterial chemotherapy with concomitant use of vasoconstrictors for liver cancer. Cancer Treatm Rep 62:145–146.

Kaplan JH, Bookstein JJ (1972) Abdominal visceral pharmacoangiography with angiotensin. Radiology 103:79–83.

Kaplan WD, D'Orsi CJ, Ensminger WD, et al. (1978) Intraarterial radionuclide infusion: A new technique to assess chemotherapy perfusion patterns. Cancer Treatm Rep 62:699.

Kaplan WD, Ensminger WD, Come SE, et al. (1980) Radionuclide angiography to predict patient response to hepatic artery chemotherapy. Cancer Treatm Rep 64:1217–1222.

Kaude JV, Wirtanen GW (1970) Celiac epinephrine enhanced angiography. AJR 110:808–826.

Keyes JW, Orlandea N, Heetderks WJ, et al. (1977) The humongotron—A scintillation-camera transaxial tomograph. J Nucl Med 18:381–387.

Latham F, Jr, Foster JH (1967) Hepatic resection for metastatic cancer. Am J Surg 113:551–557.

Lee YT (1977) Systemic and regional treatment of primary carcinoma of the liver. Cancer Treatm Rev 4:195.

Lien WM, Ackerman NB (1970) The blood supply of experimental liver metastases. II. A microcirculatory study of the normal and tumor vessels of the liver with the use of perfused silicone rubber. Surgery 68:334–340.

Liepman M, Ensminger WD, Niederhuber JE, et al. (1981) A novel injection system for intravenous chemotherapy administration. Proc AACR/ASCO 22:527.

Maki DG, McCormick RD, Uman SJ, et al. (1979) Septic endarteritis due to intra-arterial catheters for cancer chemotherapy. I. Evaluation of an outbreak. II. Risk factors, clinical features and management. III. Guidelines for prevention. Cancer 44:1228–1240.

Mansfield CM, Kramer S, Southard ME, et al. (1969) Prognosis in patients with metastatic liver disease diagnosed by liver scan. Radiology 93:77–84.

Mattson J, Appelgren L, Hamberger B, et al. (1979) Tumor vessel innervation and influence of vasoactive drugs on tumor blood flow. In: Perterson HI, ed., Tumor blood circulation: Angiogenesis, vascular morphology and blood flow of experimental and human tumors. Boca Raton, FL: CRC Press, Inc. pp. 129–141.

Narsette T, Ansfield F, Wirtanen G, et al. (1977) Gastric ulceration in patients receiving intrahepatic infusion of 5-fluorouracil. Ann Surg 186:734–736.

Niederhuber JE, Ensminger WD (1983) Surgical considerations in the management of hepatic neoplasia. Sem Oncol 10:135–148.

Nilsson LA (1966) Therapeutic hepatic artery ligation in patients with secondary liver tumors. Rev Surg 374.

Oberfield RA, McCaffrey JA, Polio J, et al. (1979) Prolonged and continuous percutaneous intra-arterial hepatic infusion chemotherapy in advanced metastatic liver adenocarcinoma from colorectal primary. Cancer 44:414–423.

Patt YZ, Wallace S, Freireich EJ, et al. (1981) The pallative role of hepatic arterial infusion and arterial occlusion in colorectal carcinoma metastatic to the liver. Lancet 1(8216):349–350.

Petrek JA, Minton JP (1979) Treatment of hepatic metastases by percutaneous hepatic arterial infusion. Cancer 43:2182–2188.

Sano K, Hoshino T, Nagai M (1968) Radiosensitization of brain tumor cells with a thymidine analogue (bromouridine). J Neurosurg 28:530–538.

Schindler R, Ramseier L, Grieder A (1966) Increased sensitivity of mammalian cell cultures to radioimetric alkylating agents following incorporation of 5-bromodeoxyuridine into cellular DNA. Biochem Pharmacol 15:2013–2023.

Schwade JG, Myers CM, Sonnenfeld P (1981) Bromodeoxyuridine (NSC 38297) pharmacokinetics and clinical results with intravenous administration. Radiat Oncol Biol Phys 7:9.

Shingleton WW, Grage TB (1976) Final statistical report: 5-FU in the treatment of carcinoma of the colon and rectum metastatic to liver, Phase III (Central Oncology Group 7032).

Simon EH (1963) Effects of 5-bromodeoxyuridine on cell division and DNA replication in HeLa cells. Exp Cell Res (Suppl) 9:263–269.

Speyer JL, Collins JM, Dedrick RL, et al. (1980) Phase I and pharmacological studies of 5-fluorouracil administered intraperitonally. Cancer Res 40:567–572.

Speyer JL, Sugarbaker PH, Collins JM, et al. (1981) Portal levels and hepatic clearance of 5-fluorouracil after intraperitoneal administration in humans. Cancer Res 41:1916–1922.

Tseng MH, Luch J, Mittelman A, et al. (1981) Chemotherapy of advanced colorectal cancer with regional arterial mitomycin C infusion and concomittant measurement of serum drug level. Proc AACR/ASCO 22:359.

Tygstrup N, Winkler K, Mellemgaard K, et al. (1962) Determination of the hepatic arterial blood flow and oxygen supply in man by clamping the artery during surgery. J Clin Invest 41:447.

Warren BA (1979) The vascular morphology of tumors. In: Peterson HI, ed., Tumor blood circulation: Angiogenesis, vascular morphology and blood flow of experimental and human tumors. Boca Raton, FL: CRC Press, Inc. pp. 1-47.

Wirtanen GW (1973) A new angiographic technique in the diagnosis of liver tumor. Radiology 108:51-54.

DIET AND ENVIRONMENT IN THE ETIOLOGY OF GASTRIC CANCER

J V JOOSSENS, M.D., AND J GEBOERS

The importance of diet and environment in the etiology of gastric cancer has been suspected for many decades (see Wynder et al., 1963). This is confirmed by epidemiologic studies showing a marked decrease in the incidence of gastric cancer in Japanese migrants in the United States (Haenszel et al., 1972). The major problem, however, has been to select the most relevant factors from the numerous nutrients proposed (Joossens and Geboers, 1981a). The answer to this has been facilitated by the observation that gastric cancer and stroke mortality have a similar trend. This was first observed in the Miyagi prefecture of Japan by Hiraide (1959) and Fujisaku and coworkers (1960). Unaware of those findings, published only in Japanese, it was rediscovered as a chance finding in 1964 (Joossens, 1965). Since then, data from many countries have been obtained over several decades confirming the relative similarity in mortality of both diseases between and within countries, between social classes, and for both men and women (Joossens and Geboers, 1981b).

NONENVIRONMENTAL FACTORS

The difference in incidence of gastric cancer between males and females is notable. Although most nutritional factors are in general similarly distributed for both sexes when adjusted for age, height, and weight, a marked difference in gastric cancer mortality can be observed. Table 1 shows the average sex ratio of mortality for the 1970–1975 period for four gastrointestinal cancers in 33 countries and for three age ranges. The sex ratio of gastric cancer is much higher than for colon cancer, slightly higher than for rectal cancer, and smaller than for esophageal cancer.

One of the precursor lesions of gastric cancer, chronic atrophic gastritis, has

From the Division of Epidemiology, University of Leuven, Belgium.

TABLE 1. Sex Ratio of Mean Values of Gastrointestinal Cancers Obtained from 33 Countries[a] (1970–1975)

Age adjusted	Colon	Rectum	Stomach	Esophagus
45–64	1.04 (0.87–1.54)[b]	1.43 (0.92–1.83)	2.20 (1.73–2.74)	3.57 (1.57–19.21)
65–74	1.16 (0.91–1.51)	1.76 (1.05–2.36)	2.07 (1.55–2.44)	3.17 (1.33–13.90)
75+	1.05 (0.75–1.23)	1.71 (0.71–2.06)	1.62 (1.18–2.07)	2.18 (0.99–5.97)

Source: Data from WHO, Geneva; National Institute for Statistics, Brussels; National Bureau of Statistics, The Hague; the Registrar General, London; and Joossens and Geboers (1981b, 1983).

[a]For a list of countries see Table 3.

[b]Observed range.

a similar prevalence in both sexes (Correa et al., 1976), suggesting that the susceptibility to developing gastric cancer is much higher in males. This is strengthened by the observation that two environmental factors, namely cigarette smoking and alcohol drinking (which are unequally distributed between the sexes), are not important in the genesis of gastric cancer. These two factors may, however, increase the sex ratio of esophageal cancer. A higher susceptibility for gastric cancer can also be observed in persons with blood group A (Roberts, 1957) and in patients with pernicious anemia (Elsborg and Mosbeck, 1979).

DIETARY AND ENVIRONMENTAL FACTORS

Soil Factors

Certain soil factors, such as a peaty soil, the presence of certain trace elements (Stocks and Davies, 1964; Juhasz et al., 1980), nitrates in food (Hartman, 1982a) or in drinking water (Cuello et al., 1976; Zaldivar and Wetterstrand, 1978), or the use of excessive amounts of nitrate fertilizers (Armijo and Coulson, 1975; Zaldivar, 1977), have been mentioned several times as possible factors in the etiology of gastric cancer (see also Fraser et al., 1980). However, it should be noted that these factors were in general observed in a single country. They were not checked for possible confounding factors, and extrapolation to other countries was never attempted. It is difficult to reconcile the amount of trace elements in the soil with a rapidly decreasing stomach cancer mortality all over the world (Table 2).

Nitrates in fertilizer have been incriminated in the causation of gastric cancer in Chile. However, since 1968 stomach cancer rates in middle-aged persons in Chile have decreased nearly 45% over 10 years (Joossens and Geboers, 1983) (Table 2), whereas the use of nitrates as fertilizer increased markedly (Zaldivar, 1978). Similar observations can be made in most Western countries. A possible influence of nitrate fertilizers is not ruled out by these findings, since it may be confounded by increasing ascorbate intake, by local situations, and by decreasing salt intake. There are, however, no data available to ascertain this.

Nitrate and/or Nitrite Intake

Nitrate intake as a possible cause of gastric cancer is attractive because of the clear link with nitrosocarcinogens. However, the metabolism of nitrates/nitrites is very complex, as is shown in Figure 1 (Hartman, 1982a). The intragastric nitrate→nitrite→nitrosocarcinogen conversion is enhanced at a low pH by iodides and thiocyanates and at a high pH by phenols, aldehydes, alcohol, and sulfhydryls. The nitrate→nitrite conversion is slowed or blocked by ascorbate and by urea (more so at a low pH) (Hartman, 1982b). Iodides and thiocyanates compete for nitrate transport into the saliva (Hartman, 1982a).

Many epidemiologic and pathophysiologic investigations have been devoted to this subject in Colombia, Chile, Israel, Hungary, France, the United States, Japan, and other countries (references in Hartman, 1982a; National Research Council, 1981). The sources of nitrates/nitrites in the diet are cured meat, vegetables (for example, spinach and tomatoes), and drinking water. The nitrate hypothesis might explain to some extent the geographic gradient of stomach cancer, which is high in Japan and much lower in Western countries (National Research Council, 1981). The same is true for the decreasing trend in stomach cancer mortality. Cured meat consumption and the degree of nitrosation of meat are decreasing while the use of refrigeration techniques is increasing.

Nitrite intake as such does not geographically correlate with stomach cancer, but nitrates and nitrites together do (National Research Council, 1981). Vegetables are the main source (±50%) of nitrates in the United States, followed by cured meat (±25%) (Hartman, 1982b). A higher intake of vegetables may increase the nitrate intake, although this could theoretically be offset by getting vegetables from sunnier climates such as southern Europe or California; such vegetables contain less nitrate because of increased metabolism at higher temperatures (Hartman, 1982a). The data incriminating nitrates from drinking water are conflicting. In Colombia the well water of the high stomach cancer areas was higher in nitrates (Cuello et al., 1976). On the other hand, no geographical relation was found in Chile (Zaldivar and Wetterstrand, 1978) nor in Hungary (Fraser et al., 1980).

Another unsettled problem is the period in life at which nitrates become important. One opinion is that higher nitrate intake in childhood could cause atrophic gastritis (Correa et al., 1976; Hartman, 1982a). Another is that nitrates/nitrites are important in the etiology of gastric cancer in adult age when atrophic gastritis is present (Joossens and Geboers, 1981b). Due to the high pH and the concomitant bacterial invasion in the stomach, the conversion of nitrates to nitrites is enhanced, the influence of ascorbate is weakened, and the nitrosation is increased (Ruddell et al., 1976). It seems unlikely that the relatively small amounts of nitrates in the stomach are capable of inducing atrophic gastritis. This is even less evident when one takes into account that the stomach mucosa of infants is well protected by mucus and by the intact mucosa against external irritants. In fact, there is no good evidence for a mutagenic or carcinogenic effect of nitrates in normal animals (Fong et al., 1980; National Research Council, 1981). There is no evidence either that nitrates are an irritant to the normal mucosa.

Nitrates are probably only active when converted to nitrites, but this presupposes a bacterial overgrowth in the stomach. This explains the many pitfalls

TABLE 2. Gastric Cancer Mortality Trends per Thousand, Age Adjusted 45–64 Years, Average of Both Sexes

Year	United States	England and Wales	Belgium[a]	Italy	Portugal	Federal Republic of Germany	Nether-lands	Sweden	Japan	Chile
1930	0.51	0.58								
1935	0.47	0.56								
1940	0.39	0.54								
1945	0.34	0.50								
1950	0.27	0.46		0.62[b]		0.66[c]	0.55	0.46[b]	1.30	
1955	0.21	0.42	0.45	0.58	0.53	0.59	0.46	0.39	1.29	
1960	0.17	0.38	0.44	0.53	0.55	0.51	0.37	0.32	1.23	
1965	0.13	0.33	0.35	0.49	0.58	0.45	0.32	0.26	1.15	
1968	0.12	0.30	0.31	0.42	0.61	0.48	0.29	0.21	1.09	0.92
1969	0.12	0.29	0.27	0.42	0.58	0.38	0.27	0.20	1.04	0.90
1970	0.11	0.29	0.25	0.40	0.57	0.37	0.28	0.22	0.99	0.85
1971	0.11	0.28	0.25	0.39	0.57	0.35	0.25	0.20	0.96	0.86
1972	0.11	0.27	0.26	0.39	0.56	0.35	0.24	0.19	0.93	0.82
1973	0.10	0.27	0.24	0.36	0.57	0.33	0.24	0.18	0.90	0.79

1974	0.10	0.26	0.25	0.35	0.55	0.33	0.24	0.18	0.87	0.73
1975	0.10	0.24	0.23	0.35	0.52	0.33	0.23	0.18	0.83	0.71
1976	0.09	0.24	0.19	0.33	0.50	0.31	0.21	0.17	0.81	0.64
1977	0.09	0.22	0.18		0.53	0.30	0.21	0.17	0.77	0.63
1978	0.09	0.22	0.20		0.45	0.27	0.21	0.17	0.74	0.58
1979		0.22	0.18		0.46		0.19	0.16	0.71	
1980		0.20	0.17				0.19	0.15		
1981			0.17							
Percent change in 10 years since 1968[d]	−30	−33	−46	−31	−17	−35	−34	−28	−38	−45

Source: Data from WHO, Geneva; National Institute for Statistics, Brussels; National Bureau of Statistics, The Hague; the Registrar General, London; and Joossens and Geboers (1981b, 1983).

[a]In Belgium, the data are provisional from 1978 on.

[b]1951.

[c]1952.

[d]The decreases (Δ) are calculated using the formula: $\Delta = 10 \cdot 100 \cdot b/x$, in which b is the slope of the linear regression (time trend) and x the average mortality over the time period under consideration, that is, from 1968 until the last available year. Multiplying by 100 yields the number in percent. We also multiplied by 10 to obtain an estimate of the decrease over a 10-year period. Under no circumstances can we speak about extrapolation.

Nitrates and Nitrites

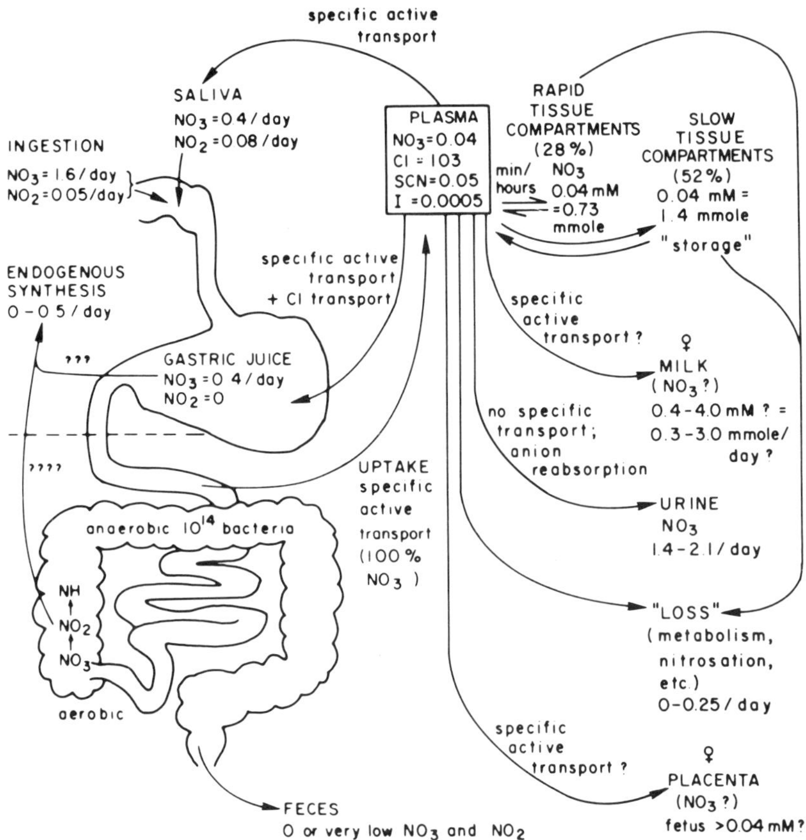

FIGURE 1. The flow of nitrates and nitrites in humans. The model is pertinent to the average U.S. adult with gastric pH below 5. All values are in mmol/day, except for plasma (mmol/L). *Source*: Courtesy of Hartman (1982a) and of Plenum Publishing Corporation.

in the epidemiology of nitrates. In Chile, Armijo and coworkers (1981) measured nitrate excretion in 700 11- to 13-year old children in low and high risk areas for stomach cancer. There was no correlation between them. The highest average urinary nitrate concentration was obtained in Antofagasta, a low risk area where more than 700 ppm NO_3 was found in the urine. The nitrate content of vegetables was significantly higher in the low risk area for lettuce, beets, and collards. There were no significant differences for three other vegetables, but the average nitrate concentration was higher in two out of three in the low risk area. The vegetable analysis was therefore consistent with the urinary results, but not with a primary mutagenic action of nitrates. Cuello and coworkers (1976) also admitted the presence of another unkown factor in order to explain the distribution of chronic gastritis and gastric cancer in Colombia.

To summarize, there is good evidence from epidemiology, biochemistry, pathophysiology, and microbiology to link nitrates, through conversion to nitrites, to stomach cancer once chronic atrophic gastritis has occurred.

Vitamin C

The production of mutagens in nitrate/nitrite food mixtures can be blocked by vitamin C (Mirvish, 1975). However, epidemiologic evidence in this field is lacking. Intake of vitamin C changed very little in the United States during the last century (Zaldivar, 1977). Potato consumption in Belgium, as in most Western countries, was three to four times higher 60 years ago than now, giving a vitamin C intake of more than 300 mg/day in 1920 from that source alone (Lederer, 1970). This was a period in which stomach cancer was the most prevalent cancer in the Western world.

In different regions of England and Wales, there is a negative correlation between stroke and average vitamin C intake (James et al., 1981). Because of the positive correlation of stroke and stomach cancer in the same regions (Joossens, 1980b), this inverse relationship must also be found between vitamin C and stomach cancer. However, the possible confounding effect of salt intake was not taken into account. There is no known influence of vitamin C on blood pressure, yet this is needed in order to explain a direct action on stroke mortality. The activity of vitamin C depends on the presence of nitrites, so it can only be active at a later stage when the stomach mucosa is abnormal.

Salt

Salt intake has been suspected as a possible factor in the etiology of gastric cancer in Japan since the late 1950s (Sato et al., 1959a, b). The very high consumption and the variability among the Japanese prefectures (much higher in the north than in the south) favored the role of salt intake (Sasaki, 1964). Further epidemiologic work in Japan gave substance to this hypothesis (Hirayama, 1967, 1979). In Hawaii, case-control studies also pointed toward salted food as an etiologic factor in gastric cancer (Haenszel et al., 1972). In the Western world, highly salted meat, fish, and vegetables were very popular 30 years ago. They still are popular in Eastern Europe, in Japan, in South Korea, in Portugal, and probably also in Colombia and Chile, which are all areas with a very high prevalence of stomach cancer. The kind of food used in those countries is generally associated with nitrates/nitrites, resulting in a high correlation between salt and nitrate intake. On the other hand, fresh vegetables may contain little salt but a high nitrate concentration.

Most food items considered to be of possible importance in the genesis of stomach cancer are salted (Joossens and Geboers, 1981a). Among such foods are cereals, salted meat, fish or vegetables, soybean sauce, miso soup, and lard. The evidence from animal studies is limited. Sato and coworkers (1959a) found that pickled, salted foods produced acute hemorrhagic gastritis. This was confirmed again by MacDonald and colleagues (1967) for pickled food. Tatematsu and coworkers (1975) found that the action of certain nitrosamides was enhanced by increasing salt intake in rats, especially when given as a concentrated solution. Experimentally, it has also been shown that, due to osmotic receptors in the duodenum, hypertonic salt solutions delay the emptying of the stomach (Hunt and Pathak, 1960).

The role of salt in stomach cancer is almost caustic, resulting in chronic atrophic gastritis when salt is used from an early age. The high acidity in the normal stomach may enhance the influence of hypertonic solutions. The deleterious nature of salt has been demonstrated in animal experiments (Sato et al., 1959a; Frenning, 1973), but it has never been tested in humans. It is, however, known that the skin of miners who extract rock salt was badly damaged by the daily contact with salt (Meyer, 1981). Skin contact with salt and brine is considered to be one of the factors in the etiology of saltwater boils and other dermatoses in lobster fishermen (Beer et al., 1968).

A high prevalence of chronic atrophic gastritis (50 to 90%) has been observed in areas with a high salt intake, such as Japan, Finland 15 years ago, and the province of Emilia-Romagna in Italy (Yoshitoshi, 1967; Siurala et al., 1968; Amadori et al., 1980). Chronic gastritis is also very common in Colombia (Correa et al., 1976). Salt intake is or was very high in Japan and Finland. It has never been measured in Colombia nor in Chile, but case control studies in Colombia have shown that the use of salted meat is more common in high risk areas (Haenszel et al., 1972). Mangoes are eaten with salt in Colombia.

The prevalence of chronic gastritis theoretically should have been higher many decades ago, when stomach cancer was very common. The only evidence we found for this is a statement of a gastroenterologist (Friedenwald, 1914) in Baltimore, Maryland, who found anacidity in 89% of 733 gastric cancer patients, but who then commented, "Yet anacidity is so frequent in other conditions that it looses much of its value!"

On the contrary, gastric cancer should be absent in populations on a no added salt diet. In one such population in Java, only one case of stomach cancer was found in 3885 autopsies studied in 1937. It was said that the native Malay population of Java who lived there used several spices but never salt (Dungal, 1958).

It is possible also to predict the average amount of salt in 24-hour urine in a given country and year based on stomach cancer mortality data (Joossens and Geboers, 1981b). The overall equation, starting from 19 observations in 10 countries was found equal to: NaCl g/24 hr $= 7.6 + 18.4 \times$ gastric cancer rate (per thousand, age adjusted 45–64 years, average of both sexes). The intercept 7.6 g NaCl is significantly different from zero, theoretically indicating that amounts of salt not producing hypertonic solutions in the stomach (taking into account the osmotic effect of other ions and molecules) will not be caustic and therefore reduce gastric cancer to near zero levels. This situation is approached in the United States (Table 2). This equation was used to calculate salt excretion in Italy. The predicted value of 13 g/24 hour and the observed one of 12.3 g were not significantly different (Mancini and Strazzullo, personal communication, 1981).

The salt hypothesis is able to explain the major epidemiologic findings.

The Geographical Gradient. As seen in Table 3, there is still a large difference in the prevalence of gastric cancer among different countries. For the

TABLE 3. Average Values of the 1970–1975 Period of Gastric Cancer, Stroke, and Noncoronary, Nonstroke Cardiovascular Mortality,[a] per Thousand, Age Adjusted 45–64 Years, Average of Both Sexes, Ranked According to Gastric Cancer

Country	Gastric cancer	Stroke	Noncoronary, nonstroke cardiovascular
United States	0.10	0.68	0.76
New Zealand	0.16	0.87	0.61
Australia	0.17	0.95	0.62
Canada	0.17	0.54	0.54
Denmark	0.18	0.46	0.51
France	0.19	0.70	0.85
Sweden	0.19	0.51	0.40
Israel	0.21	0.89	0.64
Greece	0.21	0.66	0.63
Switzerland	0.21	0.42	0.85
South Africa	0.24	1.13	1.36
Netherlands	0.25	0.49	0.51
Belgium	0.25	0.71	1.02
Norway	0.25	0.53	0.46
England and Wales	0.27	0.78	0.77
Northern Ireland	0.28	1.00	0.85
Scotland	0.30	1.12	0.76
Ireland	0.31	0.97	0.75
Finland	0.33	1.03	0.91
Federal Republic of Germany	0.34	0.68	0.97
Spain	0.36	0.77	1.24
Italy	0.37	0.79	0.99
Yugoslavia	0.37	0.95	1.49
German Democratic Republic	0.39	0.28	2.10
Austria	0.42	0.81	1.07
Czechoslovakia	0.46	1.25	0.97
Bulgaria	0.48	1.50	0.81
Venezuela	0.48	0.89	1.16
Hungary	0.50	1.06	1.47
Poland	0.55	0.51	2.02
Portugal	0.55	1.53	0.91
Chile	0.79	1.18	0.98
Japan	0.91	1.74	0.60

Source: Data from WHO, Geneva; National Institute for Statistics, Brussels; National Bureau of Statistics, The Hague; the Registrar General, London; and Joossens and Geboers (1981b, 1983).

[a]Noncoronary, nonstroke cardiovascular (arterial disease, rheumatic heart disease, hypertensive disease, other forms of heart and circulatory disease) mortality is included as a rough marker of misclassification of stroke and coronary mortality (see, for example, Poland and the German Democratic Republic).

1970–1975 period, the values (per thousand, age adjusted between 45–64 years of age, average of both sexes) are lowest in the United States and highest in Japan, a ratio of about eight. Twenty-four-hour salt excretion, corrected to a standard amount of creatinine (for example, 1.77 g*) is very high in Japan, South Korea, Bulgaria, and Portugal; high in Finland, Scotland, and Belgium (16 years ago); and medium to low in England and Wales, Belgium now, and the United States (see source of data in Joossens and Geboers, 1981b).

The Time Gradient. Gastric cancer mortality is practically decreasing in all countries where reasonable vital statistics are available (Devesa and Silverman, 1978; Joossens and Geboers, 1981b, 1983). In the United States, this decrease started before 1930. The 1977 value is five times lower than in 1930 (Table 2). In Western Europe, the decline started later, in the 1940–1950 period, whereas in Japan the decreasing mortality has only been apparent since 1957. In Belgium, mortality from gastric cancer has declined more rapidly in recent years (Table 2). There has been a slight increase in gastric cancer in Portugal after 1955, but this is most likely due to improving classification. Recently there has also been a slight decrease (Table 2).

In the salt hypothesis, salt intake must have decreased in Western countries. This has been observed in Japan, where salt consumption fell from an average of 30 g in 1937 to 18 g in 1965 (Komachi and Shimamoto, 1980) and in Belgium where it was 15 g/24 hour in 1966 and 9 g now (Joossens, 1980a). Salt intake also decreased in Finland (Pietinen and Tuomilehto, 1980), in France (Cottet, 1981), and probably also in Switzerland (Salines Suisses du Rhin Réunies, 1978). Most of this decrease was barely perceptible and has been ascribed (Joossens, 1965; Joossens and Geboers, 1981b) to the introduction and widespread use of refrigerators. Refrigerators make it possible to eliminate salt as a method for preservation of food. Meat, fish, and vegetables have been heavily salted for centuries, sometimes combined with smoking or drying. The decrease also coincided with the declining intake of cereals to which salt was frequently added, in all affluent countries.

Refrigeration techniques were introduced first in the United States, then in Western Europe, later in Eastern Europe; they are still lacking in many parts of Portugal (compare with Table 2). Of course, refrigeration of food may have other consequences that could lower the prevalence of gastric cancer. For example, it could prevent the growth of molds (Avery-Jones, 1967) and it could block the transformation of nitrates to nitrites (Weisburger and Raineri, 1975).

The Social Gradient. Stomach cancer is much more prevalent among lower socioeconomic groups. This observation could fit into the salt hypothesis, since it was shown that these groups excrete significantly more salt in 24 hours than individuals from higher groups, at least in Belgium (Joossens et al., 1980). The

*1.77 g is the average 24-hour creatinine excretion of males with mean age 40 years, weight 74 kg, and height 175 cm, as found in a large series in Belgium (Joossens et al., 1980). The standardization to creatinine is needed to correct for differences in age, weight, and height and also for eliminating the effect of over- and undercollection of 24-hour samples.

explanation for this phenomenon is that in general cheap foods, such as bread, potatoes, prepared meat products, and cheeses, are heavily salted. It was also ascertained in Belgium that the consumption of these products is higher among lower socioeconomic groups (National Institute of Statistics, 1975a, b).

The Belgian Experience. In Belgium, an intense educational campaign against salt was launched in 1968. Aid was provided by the Ministry of Health, which restricted the maximal amount of salt that could be added to bread. The campaign was also aided by all the Belgian medical faculties and by many organizations interested in hypertension and in nutrition (including the Belgian Committee Against Hypertension, the Belgian Society of Cardiology, the Belgian Cardiological Foundation, and Iban).

The campaign was widely covered by the mass media and was successful. The use of unsalted food items increased: vegetables, white cheese from skimmed milk, fresh or unprocessed deep-frozen meat and fish. Salt-free bread is now currently available, but it is not known if it is used only on medical prescription or not. In the Leuven area, the average salt content of fresh bread dropped gradually from 13.3 g/kg in 1977 to 9.8 g/kg in 1981. Low-salt hard cheese and bacon and other prepared meats are now available, although they are still relatively uncommon when compared with the available salted items.

As already mentioned, the salt excretion has decreased markedly in Belgium over the last 15 years. Whatever the mechanism, this was accompanied by a marked decrease in both stomach cancer (Table 2) and stroke mortality (Joossens, 1980b). In Europe, the rate of decrease in Belgium since 1968 ranked second only to Finland.

Fallacies About Salt. The most popular fallacy about salt is considering it as one of "the pleasures of life," implying that taking salt away from food makes it totally unpalatable, except for the newborn (Droese et al., 1973). What is forgotten, however, is that salt damages the taste buds (Bertino et al., 1982), making it necessary to adjust to the usual level of salt, either 8 to 12 g/24 hour in the United States (Luft et al., 1977; Grim et al., 1980) or 15 to 25 g/24 hour in Japan (Komachi and Shimamoto, 1980). The Japanese have nearly halved their daily intake of salt in 30 years (Komachi and Shimamoto, 1980); they still find their food enjoyable.

Experience with hundreds of families has convinced us that a gradual lowering of the amount of salt in the food is not perceived by the taste buds. They gradually and unconsciously adapt to the new level. Once used to a no added salt level, the worst thing that can happen is eating salted food. This has been confirmed in Australia (Beard et al., 1982) and in New Zealand (Thaler et al., 1982). The second fallacy is the need of increasing salt intake when sweating profusely. This is correct on a high sodium intake, but again one adapts to a low salt intake by increasing the renin-aldosterone level so that practically no sodium is lost when perspiring (Conn, 1949). This can be observed in no added salt civilizations living in the Amazon jungle (Oliver et al., 1975). The third fallacy is advocating the use of sea salt. Sea salt is slightly more toxic in rats than ordinary salt (Dahl and Heine, 1961).

THE GASTRIC CANCER-STROKE RELATIONSHIP

All the preceeding observations could be ascribed to changes in salt or nitrate intake, or both. It is probably the latter explanation that is true. Salt is considered here as the promoting agent making the stomach mucosa atrophic after many years, since atrophic gastritis is not observed before the age of 15 (Correa et al., 1976).

Nitrate, after conversion to nitrite by bacterial overgrowth in the stomach, is then combined with food amides to form nitrosocarcinogens (Sugimura and Kawachi, 1973; Tatematsu et al., 1975; Weisburger and Raineri, 1975). Nitrates therefore become important in a later stage of the natural history of the disease.

Further support for the salt hypothesis can be derived from the gastric cancer–stroke-mortality relationship (Joossens, 1965, 1980a, b). More detailed analysis can be found in Joossens and Geboers (1981a, b; 1983). The major points will be summarized here.

Geographic Correlation

There is a good geographic correlation ($P < .0001$) between gastric cancer and stroke mortality (Table 3). Certain manifest aberrant observations such as those in Poland and in the German Democratic Republic can be explained by errors of classification. This is confirmed by the abnormally high nonstroke and noncoronary cardiovascular mortality (Table 3). This mortality (arterial disease, rheumatic heart disease, hypertensive disease, other forms of heart and circulatory diseases) is also somewhat high in Belgium, but the error can be traced to the underclassified coronary mortality.

Time Relationship

Both types of mortalities have decreased in many countries, and the slope within a particular country (time relationship) is not significantly different from the slope between countries (geographic relationship) (Joossens and Geboers, 1981b). The slope between stomach cancer and stroke is independent of lung, colon, rectum, esophageal, and genital cancer and infectious diseases (Joossens and Geboers, 1981b).

The last observations are most important because both the geographic correlation and the time relationship may be spurious. However, the spurious origin of relationships that are quantitatively similar under a variety of conditions (for example, in England and Wales and in Japan) is improbable.

Socioeconomic Status

As with gastric cancer, there is also a social gradient for stroke. Stroke is more common among the lower socioeconomic groups.

Correlation with Stroke Mortality

It is possible to estimate gastric cancer from observed stroke rates over many years in Japan, Hungary, Israel, and New Zealand using a regression equation obtained in England and Wales (Joossens and Geboers, 1983).

The stroke-gastric cancer relationship emphasizes the role of salt because nitrate intake as far as is known does not increase blood pressure. On the contrary, it has a tendency to lower it. Many researchers have become convinced of the role of salt in the genesis of essential hypertension, although there is still some controversy. This is exemplified by recent recommendations of WHO (1982) and by the recommendations of the FDA about salt intake in relation to hypertension.

SUMMARY

Evidence is given for the environmental, mostly nutritional, factors important in the etiology of gastric cancer: namely salt added to food, nitrate/nitrite in combination with salt (cured meat), or from the soil (drinking water, vegetables) and vitamin C. The last-named may be protective. The majority of food factors thought to be related to the etiology of gastric cancer contain added salt, some also contain nitrates/nitrites. It is difficult to make a choice between all these factors, but the striking relationship between gastric cancer and stroke mortality makes it possible to look for a linking factor common to both diseases.

The consistency of the stomach cancer-stroke data within countries as different as England and Wales, Italy, Western Germany, Switzerland, and Japan, the similarity of the relationships between countries and between social classes, the prediction of salt consumption at the population level from mortality data, the estimation of gastric cancer from stroke mortality data, and the strength of the association are all in favor of salt being the linking factor.

Salt would then influence stroke mortality by its effect on blood pressure and stomach cancer mortality by its irritant properties as a hypertonic solution in the stomach. High salt intake goes together with chronic atrophic gastritis in Japan, in Finland, and in certain parts of Italy and Colombia.

Chronic atrophic gastritis favors bacterial overgrowth, making it possible to convert nitrates to nitrites, hence the formation of potent nitrosocarcinogens. The possible beneficial influence of vitamin C comes from blocking the nitrate-nitrite conversion. A deliberate attempt to decrease salt intake at the population level was made in Belgium in 1968, with subsequent decreases in gastric cancer and stroke mortality.

Although the salt hypothesis is not 100% proved, we believe some recommendations can already be made to the general public. A gradual decrease in the amount of salt added to food can be obtained through health education. The availability of refrigerators and deep freezers will facilitate this process. If less salted food is eaten, this will automatically result in a lower nitrate-nitrite intake. In conformity with recent WHO recommendations, a salt level of 5 g/day or less is advised as a goal for the future.

We are grateful to Dr. P.E. Hartman, Department of Biology, the Johns Hopkins University, Baltimore, Maryland, for numerous data on nitrate/nitrite related problems. He also provided us with pertinent old U.S. literature on gastric cancer. We are indebted to the National Institute of Statistics, Brussels, for recent mortality data in Belgium. We thank J. Smisdom-Rongy and A. Menten-Mellaerts for the typing of the manuscript and especially of the references. L. Cooreman and G. De Vadder of the faculty Campus Library were of great help in the bibliographic research. FWGO, Brussels, aided us with important grants. We reiterate to all of them our most sincere thanks and appreciation.

REFERENCES

Amadori D, Ravaioli A, Gardini A, et al. (1980) N-nitroso compound precursors and gastric cancer: Preliminary data of a study on a group of farm workers. Tumori 66:145-152.

Armijo R, Coulson AH (1975) Epidemiology of stomach cancer in Chile—The role of nitrogen fertilizers. Int J Epidemiol 4:301-309.

Armijo R, Gonzalez A, Orellana M, et al. (1981) Epidemiology of gastric cancer in Chile: II. Nitrate exposures and stomach cancer frequency. Int J Epidemiol 10:57-62.

Avery-Jones F (1967) The epidemiology of gastric cancer with special reference to causation. In: Proceedings of the 3rd world congress of gastroenterology, Tokyo, 1966. Tokyo: Nankodo, pp. 93-98.

Beard TC, Cooke HM, Gray WR, Barge R (1982) Randomised controlled trial of a no-added-sodium diet for mild hypertension. Lancet 2:455-458.

Beer WE, Jones M, Eifion Jones W (1968) Dermatoses in lobster fishermen. Br Med J 1:807-809.

Bertino M, Beauchamp GK, Engelman K (1982) Long-term reduction in dietary sodium alters the taste of salt. Am J Clin Nutr 36:1134-1144.

Conn JW (1949) The mechanism of acclimatization to heat. Adv Intern Med 3:373-393.

Correa P, Cuello C, Duque E, et al. (1976) Gastric cancer in Colombia. III. Natural history of precursor lesions. J Natl Cancer Inst 57:1027-1035.

Cottet J (1981) Evolution de la consommation du sel en France. Bull Acad Roy Méd Belg 136:556-565.

Cuello C, Correa P, Haenszel W, et al. (1976) Gastric cancer in Colombia. I. Cancer risk and suspect environmental agents. J Natl Cancer Inst 57:1015-1020.

Dahl LK, Heine M (1961) The enhanced hypertensogenic effect of sea salt over sodium chloride. Am J Cardiol 8:726-731.

Devesa SS, Silverman DT (1978) Cancer incidence and mortality trends in the United States: 1935-74. J Natl Cancer Inst 60:545-571.

Droese W, Stolley H, Schlage C, Wortberg B (1973) Significance of the salt level in food for infants and children. Bibl Nutr Diet 18:215-223.

Dungal N (1958) Stomach cancer in Iceland. In: Raven RW, ed., Cancer. London: Butterworth, pp. 262-271.

Elsborg L, Mosbeck J (1979) Pernicious anemia as a risk factor in gastric cancer. Acta Med Scand 206:315-318.

Fong LYY, Wong FWT, Chan WC (1980) Do chronic urinary tract infections induce cancer in the rat fed nitrate and aminopyrine? IARC Sci Publ 31:693-704.

Fraser P, Chilvers C, Beral V, Hill MJ (1980) Nitrate and human cancer: A review of the evidence. Int J Epidemiol 9:3-11.

Frenning B (1973) The effects of large osmolality variations on the gastric mucosa surface ultrastructure. Scand J Gastroent 8:185-192.

Friedenwald J (1914) A clinical study of one thousand cases of cancer of the stomach. Am J Med Sci 148:660–680.

Fujisaku S, Ito T, Kamoi M, Hiraide H (1960) Age-adjusted death rates for cerebral apoplexy by cities, towns and villages in Miyagi prefecture in 1955–58. Tohoku Igaku Zasshi 61:628–634.

Grim CE, Luft FC, Miller JZ, et al. (1980) Racial differences in blood pressure in Evans County, Georgia: Relationship to sodium and potassium intake and plasma renin activity. J Chronic Dis 33:87–94.

Haenszel W, Kurihara M, Segi M, Lee RKC (1972) Stomach cancer among Japanese in Hawaii. J Natl Cancer Inst 49:969–988.

Hartman PE (1982a) Nitrates and nitrites: Ingestion, pharmacodynamics, and toxicology. Chem Mutagens 7:211–294.

Hartman PE (1982b) Overview: Nitrite load in the upper gastrointestinal tract: Past, present and future. In: Magee PN, et al., eds., Banbury report: The possible role of nitrosamines in human cancer. Cold Spring Harbor: Cold Spring Harbor Laboratory.

Hiraide H (1959) Age adjusted death rates for stomach cancer by cities, towns and villages in Miyagi prefecture (1948–1957). Tohoku Igaku Zasshi 59:286–293.

Hirayama T (1967) The epidemiology of cancer of the stomach in Japan with special reference to the role of diet. In: Harris RJC, ed., Proceedings of the 9th International Cancer Congress, Tokyo, 1966, UICC Monograph Series 10. Berlin: Springer-Verlag, pp. 37–49.

Hirayama T (1979) Cancer epidemiology in Japan. Environ Health Perspect 32:11–15.

Hunt JN, Pathak JD (1960) The osmotic effects of some simple molecules and ions on gastric emptying. J Physiol 154:254–269.

James WPT, Powles J, Williams DRR (1981) The prevalence of diet-related diseases in Britain. In: Turner MR, ed., Preventive nutrition and society. New York: Academic Press, pp. 1–54.

Joossens JV (1965) The problem of cancer mortality (Dutch). Verh Kon Vlaam Akad Geneesk Belg 27:489–545.

Joossens JV (1980a) Dietary salt restriction. The case in favor. In: Robertson JIS, Pickering GW, Caldwell ADS, eds., The therapeutics of hypertension. London: Academic Press and Royal Society of Medicine, pp. 243–250.

Joossens JV (1980b) Recent mortality trends. Acta Clin Belg 35:65–70.

Joossens JV, Geboers J (1981a) Nutrition and gastric cancer. Proc Nutr Soc 40:37–46.

Joossens JV, Geboers J (1981b) Nutrition and gastric cancer. Nutr Cancer 2:250–261.

Joossens JV, Geboers J (1983) Epidemiology of gastric cancer: A clue to etiology. In: Sherlock P, Morson BC, Barbara L, Veronesi U, eds., Precancerous lesions of the gastrointestinal tract. New York: Raven Press, pp. 97–113.

Joossens JV, Claessens J, Geboers J, Claes J (1980) Electrolytes and creatinine in multiple 24-hour urine collections (1970–1974). In: Kesteloot H, Joossens JV, eds., Epidemiology of arterial blood pressure. The Hague: Martinus Nijhoff Medical Division, pp. 45–63.

Juhasz L, Hill MJ, Nagy G (1980) Possible relationship between nitrate in drinking water and incidence of stomach cancer. IARC Sci Publ 31:619–623.

Komachi Y, Shimamoto T (1980) Salt intake and its relationship to blood pressure in Japan. Present and past. In: Kesteloot H, Joossens JV, eds., Epidemiology of arterial blood pressure. The Hague: Martinus Nijhoff Medical Division, pp. 395–400.

Lederer J (1970) Evolution de la consommation du pain et santé publique. In: Lederer J, ed., Pain et santé. Louvain: Nauwelaerts, pp. 17–39.

Luft FC, Grim CE, Higgins JT Jr., Weinberger MH (1977) Differences in response to sodium administration in normotensive white and black subjects. J Lab Clin Med 90:555–562.

MacDonald WC, Anderson FH, Hashimoto S (1967) Histological effect of certain pickles on the human gastric mucosa: A preliminary report. Can Med Assoc J 96:1521–1525.

Meyer P (1981) L'homme et le sel: Réflexions sur l'histoire humaine et l'évolution de la médecine. Paris: Editions Fayard.

Mirvish SS (1975) Blocking the formation of N-nitroso compounds with ascorbic acid in vivo and in vitro. Ann NY Acad Sci 258:175–180.

National Institute of Statistics (1975a) Family budget enquiry 1973–1974. Statistische Studiën 38: Brussels.

National Institute of Statistics (1975b) Family budget enquiry 1973–1974. Statistische Studiën 41: Brussels.

National Research Council (1981) The health effects of nitrate, nitrite and N-nitroso compounds. Washington, D.C.: National Academy Press.

Oliver WJ, Cohen EL, Neel JV (1975) Blood pressure, sodium intake and sodium related hormones in the Yanomano Indians, a "no-salt" culture. Circulation 52:146–151.

Pietinen P, Tuomilehto J (1980) Estimating sodium intake in epidemiological studies. In: Kesteloot H, Joossens JV, eds., Epidemiology of arterial blood pressure. The Hague: Martinus Nijhoff Medical Division, pp. 29–44.

Roberts JAF (1957) Blood groups and susceptibility in disease. A review. Br J Prev Soc Med 11:107–125.

Ruddell WS, Bone ES, Hill MJ, et al. (1976) Gastric-juice nitrite. A risk factor for cancer in the hypochlorhydric stomach. Lancet 2:1037–1039.

Salines Suisses du Rhin Réunies (1978) La Situation du Sel Iodé en Suisse. Schweizerhalle, Switzerland, pp. 1–18.

Sasaki N (1964) The relationship of salt intake to hypertension in the Japanese. Geriatrics 19:735–744.

Sato T, Fukuyama T, Urata G, Suzuki T (1959a) Studies of the causation of gastric cancer. 1. Bleeding in the glandular stomach of mice by feeding with highly salted foods, and a comment on salted foods in Japan. Bull Inst Publ Health 8:10–13.

Sato T, Fukuyama T, Suzuki T, et al. (1959b) Studies of the causation of gastric cancer. 2. The relation between gastric cancer mortality rate and salted food intake in several places in Japan. Bull Inst Publ Health 8:187–198.

Siurala M, Isokoski K, Varis K, Kekki M (1968) Prevalence of gastritis in a rural population. Bioptic study of subjects selected at random. Scand J Gastroent 3:211–223.

Stocks P, Davies RI (1964) Zinc and copper content of soils associated with the incidence of cancer of the stomach and other organs. Br J Cancer 18:14–24.

Sugimura T, Kawachi T (1973) Experimental stomach cancer. In: Bush H, ed., Methods in cancer research. New York: Academic Press, pp. 245–308.

Tatematsu M, Takahashi M, Fukushima S, et al. (1975) Effects in rats of sodium chloride on experimental gastric cancers induced by N-methyl-N'-nitro-N-nitrosoguanidine or 4-nitroquinoline 1-oxyde. J Natl Cancer Inst 55:101–106.

Thaler BI, Paulin JM, Phelan EL, Simpson FO (1982) A pilot study to test the feasibility of salt reduction in a community. NZ Med J 95:939–942.

Weisburger JD, Raineri R (1975) Dietary factors and the etiololgy of gastric cancer. Cancer Res 35:3469–3474.

WHO Expert Committee Report (1982) Prevention of coronary heart disease. Geneva: World Health Organization.

Wynder EL, Kmet J, Dungal N, Segi M (1963) An epidemiological investigation of gastric cancer. Cancer 16:1461–1496.

Yoshitoshi Y (1967) Gastritis: Incidence and pathogenesis of gastritis. In: Proceedings of the 3rd World Congress of Gastroenterology, Tokyo, 1966. Tokyo: Nankodo, pp. 179–185.

Zaldivar R (1977) Epidemiology of gastric and colo-rectal cancer in the United States and Chile with particular reference to the role of dietary and nutritional variables, nitrate fertilizer pollution and N-nitroso compounds. Zbl Bakt Hyg I Alt Orig B 164:193–217.

Zaldivar R (1978) The agricultural use of nitrate fertilizers (tons of N) in provinces of Chile with high- and low-risk populations for gastric carcinoma. Bull Cancer 65:3.

Zaldivar R, Wetterstrand WH (1978) Nitrate nitrogen levels in drinking water of urban areas with high- and low-risk populations for stomach cancer: An environmental epidemiology study. Z Krebsforsch 92:227–234.

THE SIGNIFICANCE OF CHROMOSOMAL CHANGES IN HUMAN LARGE BOWEL TUMORS

AMELIA REICHMANN, M.D., AND BERNARD LEVIN, M.D.

In this review we will summarize earlier cytogenetic studies in human large bowel tumors and provide a detailed examination of the current state in this area of investigation. To date, most of the data correlating cytogenetic findings in large bowel tumors with clinical and histopathologic features have been derived from this laboratory.

The significance of chromosomal abnormalities in neoplasia has been the subject of investigation and speculation for many years (Boveri, 1914), and this topic has been extensively reviewed (German, 1974; Atkin, 1976; Sandberg, 1980). In spite of numerous investigations, the possible relationship of chromosomal abnormalities to malignant transformation remains obscure. A crucial point may be the inability to monitor by cytogenetic means the early stages of evolution of human cancer, particularly solid tumors. The human large bowel offers an exceptional opportunity to understand aspects of neoplastic growth disorders by studying cytogenetic patterns of benign and malignant tumors.

CHROMOSOMAL ABNORMALITIES IN HUMAN LARGE BOWEL TUMORS

Deviations from the normal chromosome complement in large bowel cancers can be classified into those involving an abnormal number of chromosomes and those involving structural changes (Sonta et al., 1977; Sonta and Sandberg, 1978; Kovacs, 1978a,b; Martin et al., 1979; Reichmann et al., 1981, 1982a, unpublished data). Homogeneously staining regions (HSRs) and double minutes (DMs) are cytogenetic abnormalities of considerable interest (Schimke, 1982). These ele-

From the Melamid Cytogenetics Laboratory, Section of Gastroenterology, Department of Medicine, University of Chicago (AR); and the Gastrointestinal Oncology Service, University of Chicago Hospitals and Clinics (BL).

ments (HSRs and DMs) differ from each other. They cannot be explained by the classic mechanisms of numerical or structural chromosomal change. Much more study is required to explain their origin (Schimke, 1982).

Numerical Abnormalities

Most colorectal cancers show *aneuploidy*, with only 8% of patients having an apparently normal karyotype in the tumor cells (Reichmann et al., 1981, 1982a). The *hypodiploid* state, which refers to the presence of less than 46 chromosomes usually combined with structural aberrations, is observed in 11% of patients (Reichmann et al., 1981). Chromosomal gains are commonly observed as single, double, or triple *trisomies*. Sometimes gains are combined with losses of chromosomes and more frequently as gains and losses of whole chromosomes combined with structural abnormalities (Reichmann et al., 1981, 1982a).

Single or double trisomies are unusual in large bowel cancers, but they are more frequently present in large bowel adenomas (Reichmann et al., 1982b, 1983a). In cancers, triple trisomies or multiple gains of chromosomes are more common. *Polyploidy* in large bowel cancer is not generally present as an exact multiple of 23 (*triploidy* = 69 chromosomes, or 92 chromosomes = *tetraploidy*) probably because of numerous chromosome losses. *Hypotriploidy* or *hypotetraploidy* are observed in approximately 50% of patients.

Polyploidy can be produced when a nuclear division occurs without simultaneous division of the cytoplasm or by fusion of cells (Reichmann and Levin, 1981). Elias and Hyde (1982) have described multiple fragmentation of nuclei into "nucleotesimals" and postulate that these fragments facilitate rapid growth of some colon cancer cells in spite of a low mitotic index.

In primary large bowel tumors, chromosomal number ranges from approximately 44 *(hypodiploidy)* to 91 *(hypotetraploidy)*. A karyotype of more than 92 chromosomes has never been observed in primary colonic cancer (Sonta and Sandberg, 1978; Kovacs, 1978a, b; Martin et al., 1979; Reichmann et al., 1981).

Structural Abnormalities

A prominent characteristic of large bowel cancer is the presence of marker chromosomes: only 16% of tumors lack markers (Reichmann et al., 1981). The origin of the markers can be identified in some instances. *Deletions, duplications, isochromosomes*, and *translocations* have been recognized (Reichmann et al., 1981). Unknown markers with variations in number and complexity are sometimes present with areas of indistinguishable bands that seem to be similar to HSRs (Reichmann et al., 1981). One or more breakages may be involved in the formation of a marker chromosome.

Double Minutes and Homogeneously Staining Regions

Double minutes are small paired chromatin bodies whose number and size vary from cell to cell; most of them are seen in malignant tumors. Their origin and function are uncertain (Figure 1a). The homogeneously staining regions are regions of metaphase chromosome that lack the cross-striational patterns

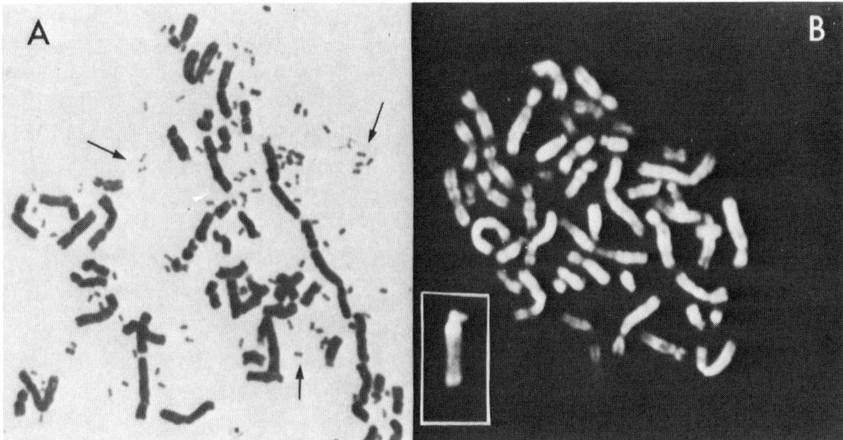

FIGURE 1. (**a**) Part of a metaphase in a primary rectal adenocarcinoma showing numerous double minutes (arrows). (Giemsa stained). (**b**) An apparently "normal"metaphase in a colon transverse adenocarcinoma. Quinacrine-banding technique. The inset shows a chromosome with abnormal banding regions.

revealed by chromosome banding (Figure 1b). These phenomena (DMs and HSRs) seem to be related to the acquisition of resistance to various drugs employed in cancer chemotherapy. Schimke (1982) reported that resistance to methotrexate was associated with amplification of the dihydrofolate reductase gene.

Double minutes are present in many large bowel cancer cells, particularly in advanced cancers, but they can also be seen infrequently in adenomas (Reichmann et al., 1980, unpublished data). Homogeneously staining regions have only been observed in a few instances in primary solid tumors (Kovacs, 1979). We have observed markers with areas of indistinguishable bands in direct preparations of colorectal cancer that seem to be similar to HSRs (Figure 1b). They are recognized also as abnormal banded regions (ABRs). In our study on marker chromosomes on colorectal cancers, we have observed that the ABRs are seen as repeated sequences of bands, nonrepeated but distinct band regions, nonfluorescent regions, and unrecognizable patterns of E or F chromosomes (Reichmann et al., 1983b).

It is too early to speculate about the importance of these phenomena (DMs, HSRs, or ABRs). It will be very useful to determine what genes are amplified and to understand the relationship of these to the development of neoplasia.

Nonrandom Patterns of Chromosomal Aberrations

It is probably not by chance that the most prevalent autosomal trisomic conditions in large bowel tumors involve one of the pair of chromosomes 7, 8, 13, 19, 20, 21, loss of one of the chromosome 17, or structural aberrations of chromosomes 1 and 5. Changes in chromosome 1 were observed in 39% of colorectal cancers (Reichmann et al., 1984); in addition, sex chromosome aberrations are present in 42% of cases (Reichmann et al., 1981). However, there are many different types of chromosomal changes that do not fall into the nonrandom pattern, and tumors exhibit marked karyotypic diversity. This variability is present prominently in left-sided colorectal tumors and in metastatic cancer (Reichmann et al., 1981). It may be the expression of marked tumor heterogeneity.

KARYOTYPIC PATTERNS AND THE CORRELATION WITH ANATOMIC DISTRIBUTION IN LARGE BOWEL TUMORS

Chromosomes were studied in 49 cancers (Martin et al., 1979; Reichmann et al., 1981, unpublished data) from different anatomic areas of the large bowel: cecum, ascending colon, hepatic flexure, transverse colon, splenic flexure, descending colon, sigmoid and rectum (Figure 2). The changes ranged from "normal karyotypes" with no apparent (or submicroscopic abnormalities) to tetraploidy. The karyotypic patterns represented by different symbols are displayed in Figure 2: cases with normal karyotypes or cases with few chromosomal abnormalities predominated on the right side of the colon; those with marked variability and chromosomal instability were more common on the left side (Reichmann et al., 1982a).

Chromosomal abnormalities were also correlated with Dukes' staging. Of 49 patients, 25 (52%) showed polyploidy: 1 was an in situ carcinoma; 12 cases were B_1 and B_2 (11 on the left and 1 on the right); 9 were stage C (6 on the left and 3 on the right side of the colon), and 3 cases were metastatic. Only one polyploid tumor occurred in a patient who had a Dukes' B_2 lesion in the cecum (Figure 2). These findings suggest that left-sided lesions may exhibit polyploidy as an early event in neoplastic transformation (Reichmann et al., 1982a). The remaining 24 cases were in the diploid range, with no more than 52 chromosomes and Dukes' staging was randomly distributed.

THE RELATIONSHIP BETWEEN CHROMOSOMAL ABNORMALITIES AND EMBRYOLOGIC AND PHYSIOLOGIC CHARACTERISTICS

Embryologically and functionally, the colon is divisible into two parts. The portion proximal to the middle of the transverse colon, adjacent to the small intestine, arises from the embryonal midgut and receives its blood supply from the superior mesenteric artery. It, too, has important absorptive functions. In this area, the chromosomal findings in cancer are very close to the normal karyotype. Tumors contain 46 chromosomes, or they are in a near-diploid range with few aberrations.

The distal half of the colon is derived from the embryonal hindgut and receives its blood supply from the inferior mesenteric artery and its branches. In the left half of the colon, we have found that the karyotypes of malignant tumors are very abnormal with a large degree of karyotypic variation; hypotriploidy or hypotetraploidy predominate (Reichmann et al., 1982a). It has been suggested (Reichmann et al., 1982a) that variation in karyotypic abnormalities may be related to the differences in function of the proximal and distal portions of the colon.

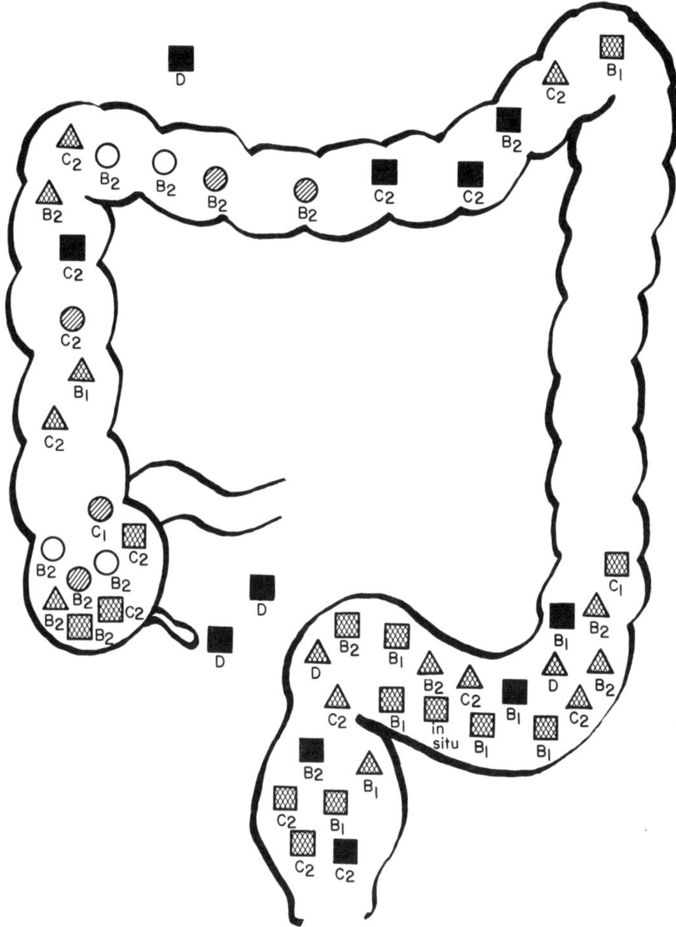

FIGURE 2. Karyotypic patterns and anatomic distribution of 49 large bowel cancers. ○ "normal karyotypes" (46 chromosomes). ⊘ near-diploid karyotype with simple gains (49 and 50 chromsomes). ▲ near-diploid karyotypes with gains, losses, and rearragnements (44–52 chromosomes). ▩ hypotriploid-hypotetraploid karyotypes (60–91 chromosomes). ■ hypotriploid-hypotetraploid cells with marked karyotypic variation. Subscripts indicate Dukes' stages. Symbols outside the large bowel represent metastases in liver and pelvis. Polyploidy, a feature that may have a significant role in the evolution of malignancy is present predominantly in left-sided Dukes' B cancers.

BENIGN COLONIC ADENOMAS AND THEIR PREMALIGNANT POTENTIAL

Studies of the cytogenetics of tubular adenomas and tubulovillous and villous adenomas are scanty (Baker and Atkin, 1970; Atkin 1976; Mark et al., 1973; Mitelman et al., 1974; Reichmann et al., 1982b). Benign tumors have a low mitotic index and rarely provide metaphases for chromosomal studies. Our experience shows that karyotypes in tubular and tubulovillous adenomas are predominantly in the diploid range with simple trisomy (47 chromosomes) or double trisomy (48 chromosomes) in C or D chromosomal groups (Reichmann et al., 1983a). Karyotypic analysis of a villous adenoma of the ascending colon showed more than 48 chromosomes (Reichmann et al., 1982b). Because villous adenomas have a higher malignant potential than do tubular adenomas, the karyotypic evolution in that patient may be an important element in the development of the neoplasm. This karyotypic evidence tends to confirm that tubular adenoma, villous adenoma, and adenocarcinoma may be interrelated steps of a disordered growth.

A patient with familial polyposis coli offered an unusual opportunity to analyze both benign and malignant lesions in the same colon (Reichmann et al., 1982c). The adenocarcinoma arose in the sigmoid area with structural abnormalities in chromosomes 1 and 13. Abnormalities in chromosome 13 were observed in the adenomas of the same patient. Although it is not possible to recognize if a chromosome change was connected with transformation, it is possible that the change permitted gene deletion, transposition, duplication, or amplification, which may have favored tumor invasion. On the other hand, chromosomal changes can precede invasion and support the clinical concept that adenomas are the precursors of large bowel adenocarcinomas.

SIGNIFICANCE OF CHROMOSOMAL CHANGES IN HUMAN LARGE BOWEL TUMORS

It is too early to draw any firm conclusions about the significance of chromosome studies in large bowel tumors. It is evident that embryologic, anatomic, histopathologic, and pathologic characteristics of the large bowel may be important in understanding the nature of the different chromosomal abnormalities observed. For example, there may be a difference between right- and left-sided colorectal tumors due to regional variations in structure, function, and microenvironment. The interaction of hereditary influences is a matter of speculation, but it may be critical in the process of malignant transformation. Clinically, different chromosomal patterns in large bowel cancers may indicate prognostic differences that may ultimately guide the use of various types of adjuvant therapy.

GLOSSARY OF CYTOGENETIC TERMS

Aneuploidy Deviation of the chromosome number from that characteristic for the species; for example, in humans, a chromosome complement that is not an exact multiple of the haploid (n) number (23 chromosomes).

Autosome A chromosome other than a sex chromosome.

Chromosome band Areas of light or dark cross-striational patterns produced by a number of techniques. C(Constitutive Heterochromatin)-bands; G(Giemsa)-bands; Q(Quinacrine)-bands; R(Reverse)-bands. Bands are so designated because of the technique used.

Deletion The loss of a segment of the genetic material from a chromosome. The size of the deletion can vary from a single nucleotide to sections containing a number of genes. If the lost part is at the end of a chromosome, it is called a *terminal deletion*. Otherwise it is called an *intercalary deletion*.

Diploid The chromosome state in which each type of chromosome (except the sex chromosomes) is represented twice (2n).

Double minutes (DMs) Small, paired DNA-containing structures that replicate themselves.

Duplication A term used when a chromosomal segment is present twice, often in tandem.

Homogeneously staining regions (HSRs). Unbanded regions within a chromosome.

Hypodiploid Less than the diploid number of chromosomes; for example, less than 46 in humans.

Hypotetraploid Less than the tetraploid number of chromosomes; for example, less than 92 in man.

Hypotriploid Less than the triploid number of chromosomes; for example, less than 69 in humans.

Isochromosome A chromosome with two identical arms. Isochromosomes have arms that are mutually homologous.

Marker chromosome An abnormal chromosome easily identified by its peculiar morphology. (Marker chromosomes are always abnormal.)

Nondisjunction Failure of sister chromatids to separate at anaphase, one daughter nucleus receiving both (resulting in hyper- and hypoploid products of mitosis).

Polyploid Designating an individual having more than two sets of chromosomes.

Tetraploidy (4n) Cell containing twice (4n) the number of chromosomes in diploid cells; for example, in the human, 92 chromosomes.

Translocation Breakage followed by transfer of chromosome material between chromosomes.

Triploidy (3n) In humans, the presence of 69 (3n) chromosomes.

Trisomy The presency of an extra (third) chromosome in addition to a normal homologous pair.

The authors appreciate the cytogenetic collaboration of Paulette Martin.

REFERENCES

Atkin NB (1976) Cytogenetic aspects of malignant transformation. Experimental biology and medicine, vol. 6, Basel: S. Karger.

Baker MC, Atkin NB (1970) Chromosome abnormalities in polyps and carcinomas of the large bowel. Proc R Soc Med 63(suppl):9–10.

Boveri T (1914). Zur frage der entstehung maligner tumoren. Jena: Gustav Fisher, S.

Elias H, Hyde DM (1982) Separation and spread of nuclear fragments ("nucleotesimals") in colonic neoplasms. Hum Pathol 13:635–639.

German J (1974) Chromosomes and cancer. New York: John Wiley and Sons.

Kovacs G (1978a) Banding analysis of three primary cancers. Acta Cytol 22:538–541.

Kovacs G. (1978b) Abnormalities of chromosome number in human solid malignant tumours. Int J Cancer 21:688–694.

Kovacs G (1979) Homogeneously staining regions on marker chromosomes in malignancy. Int J Cancer 23:299–301.

Mark J, Mitelman F, Dencker H, et al. (1973). The specificity of the chromosomal abnormalities in human colonic polyps. Acta Pathol Microbiol Scand 81:85–90.

Martin P, Levin B, Golomb HM, Riddell RH (1979) Chromosome analysis of primary large bowel tumors: A new method for improving the yield of analyzable metaphases. Cancer 44:1656–1662.

Mitelman G, Mark J, Nilsson PG, et al. (1974). Chromosome banding pattern in human colonic polyps. Hereditas 78:63–68.

Reichmann A, Levin B (1981) Premature chromosome condensation in human large bowel cancer. Cancer Genet Cytogenet 3:223–225.

Reichmann A, Riddell RH, Martin P, Levin B (1980). Double minutes in human large bowel cancer. Gastroenterology 79:334–339.

Reichmann A, Martin P, Levin B (1981). Chromosomal banding patterns in human large bowel cancer. Int J Cancer 28:431–440.

Reichmann A, Levin B, Martin P (1982a) Human large-bowel cancer: Correlation of clinical and histopathological features with banded chromosomes. Int J Cancer 29:625–629.

Reichmann A, Martin P, Levin B (1982b) Karyotypic findings in a colonic villous adenoma. Cancer Genet Cytogenet 7:51–57.

Reichmann A, Martin P, Levin B (1982c) Chromosomal banding patterns in familial polyposis coli associated with adenocarcinoma. Am J Hum Genet 139A (Abstract).

Reichmann A, Martin P, Levin B (1983a) Chromosomes in human large bowel adenomas: Significance of karyotypic changes. Gastroenterology 84:1283 (Abstract).

Reichmann A, Martin P, Levin B (1983b) Are marker chromosomes in human large bowel cancer related to stage of invasion and location of tumor? Am J Hum Genet 35:69A (Abstract).

Reichmann A, Martin P, Levin B (1983c) Chromosomes in human large bowel tumors. I: A study of chromosome no. 1. Cancer Genet Cytogenet (In press).

Reichmann A, Martin P, Levin B. Chromosomes in human large bowel tumors. Banding studies in 12 cases (unpublished data).

Sandberg AA (1980) The chromosomes in human cancer and leukemia. New York: Elsevier North Holland.

Schimke RT (1982) Gene amplication. Cold Spring Harbor, NY: Cold Spring Harbor Laboratory.

Sonta S, Sandberg AA (1978) Chromosomes and causation of human cancer and leukemia. XXX. Banding patterns of primary intestinal tumors. Cancer 41:164–173.

Sonta S, Oshimura M, Evans JT, Sandberg AA (1977). Chromosomes and causation of human cancer and leukemia. XX. Banding patterns of primary tumors. J Natl Cancer Inst 58:49–53.

CELL CLONING TECHNIQUES IN THE SELECTION OF CHEMOTHERAPEUTIC AGENTS FOR GASTROINTESTINAL TUMORS

DAVID M LOESCH, M.D.,* GARY M. CLARK, PH.D., AND DANIEL D VON HOFF, M.D.

In 1955, established tumor cell lines were first cloned in soft agar by Puck and associates (1955). Evolution of this soft agar cloning technique continued through the work of Park and coworkers (1971) with the successful growth of mouse and human myeloma in 1971. From this early research, Hamburger and Salmon (1977a, b) were able to demonstrate consistent cloning of human multiple myeloma in a two-layer soft agar system. After this initial success, other tumors were found to clone in the assay, including neuroblastoma (Von Hoff et al., 1980), cancer of the lung (Pollard et al., 1980), breast carcinoma (Sandbach et al., 1980), melanoma (Meyskens and Salmon, 1980), ovarian carcinoma (Hamburger et al., 1978), and colon carcinoma (Buick et al., 1980). This human tumor cloning assay used in retrospective studies has demonstrated a 70% accuracy for positive prediction (sensitivity) and a 94% accuracy for negative prediction (specificity) between in vitro responses and chemotherapeutic responses in patients (Von Hoff, 1981a). This chapter describes the growth of gastrointestinal carcinoma in the two-layer soft agar system in our laboratory. Alternative applications of the cloning assay will be discussed in the area of drug screening and new drug development.

MATERIALS AND METHODS

Two-hundred-seventeen adenocarcinomas of the large bowel, 88 pancreatic carcinomas, 44 gastric adenocarcinomas, 41 hepatic carcinomas, and 7 esophageal adenocarcinomas were submitted for routine cloning. All specimens were obtained during routine diagnostic and therapeutic procedures from mul-

From the Department of Medicine, Division of Oncology, University of Texas Health Science Center at San Antonio.

*Present address: Wright-Patterson Air Force Base, Dayton OH.

tiple hospitals across the United States. The specimens were obtained by surgical excision, thoracentesis, paracentesis, or bone marrow aspiration and were handled with aseptic technique.

Solid tumors or suspected solid metastases were obtained at surgery, placed in McCoy's 5A media supplemented with 10% fetal calf serum for transport to the cloning laboratory, and on arrival were mechanically dissociated under aseptic conditions. These solid tumors were minced with a tissue scissors, passed through 0.3-mm stainless steel mesh, and subsequently passed through 25-gauge needles until a single cell suspension was achieved. The resulting cell suspension was then washed by centrifugation as previously described (Hamburger and Salmon, 1977a, b; Von Hoff et al., 1980).

Bone marrows and ascitic, pleural, and pericardial fluids were obtained at surgery or by standard techniques. Each fluid was placed in a sterile container with 100 units of preservative-free heparin per milliliter of body fluid. After centrifugation at 150 $\times$ g for 10 minutes, the cells were harvested and washed twice with McCoy's 5A media with 10% heat-inactivated fetal calf serum. Effusions contaminated with red blood cells were treated with an ammonium chloride lysing buffer and then washed in McCoy's 5A media plus 10% heat inactivated fetal calf serum.

Culture Technique for Tumor Colony-Forming Cells

Cells were cultured as described by Hamburger and Salmon (1977a, b). Cells to be tested were suspended in 0.3% agar in enriched CMRL 1066 medium supplemented with 15% heat-inactivated horse serum, penicillin (100 units/ml), streptomycin (2 mg/ml), glutamine (2 mM), $CaCl_2$ (4 mM), and insulin (3 units/ml). Prior to plating, asparagine (0.6 mg/ml), DEAE-dextran (0.5 mg/ml), and freshly prepared 2-mercaptoethanol (final concentration, 50 mM) were added to the cells. One milliliter of the resultant mixture was pipetted onto 1-ml feeder layers in 35-mm plastic petri dishes. The final concentration of cells in each culture was 5×10^5 cells in 1 ml of agar medium. The feeder layers used in this study consisted of McCoy's 5A media plus 15% heat-inactivated calf serum and a variety of nutrients as described by Pike and Robinson (1970). Immediately before use, 10 ml of 3% tryptic soy broth, 0.6 ml of asparagine, and 0.3 ml of DEAE-dextran were added to 40 ml of the enriched medium and underlayers were poured in 35-mm petri dishes (Von Hoff et al., 1980).

After preparation of both bottom and top layers, the plates were examined the next day under an inverted microscope to assure the presence of a good single cell suspension. Day zero background counts were performed using a Bausch and Lomb FAS II image analysis system. Day zero counts had to be $\leq$ 4 features ($\geq$ 60 μm) in order for the specimen to be considered evaluable.

All plates for drug sensitivity studies were done by incubating the cells with the drug of interest for 1 hour at 37°C. The drug was used in a concentration equal to one-tenth of the peak plasma level achievable in humans. The cells were then washed and plated as previously noted. All studies including control plates were done in triplicate. The cells were left in culture at 37°C with a 7.5% carbon dioxide 100% humidified atmosphere. After 14 to 28 days, cultures were examined and counted using an inverted phase microscope. The percent

TABLE 1. Growth Characteristics of Colon Carcinoma

Total number of specimens	217
Number of contaminated specimens	40 (18%)
Number of specimens without tumor by pathologic or cytologic review	10 (4.6%)
Number of specimens that grew (defined as > 5 colonies per 5 × 10^5 cells plated)	136 (81%)
Number of specimens that gave evaluable growth (defined as ≥ 30 colonies per 5 × 10^5 cells plated)	96 (58%)
Number of specimens that gave evaluable growth with sufficient cells to test drugs	86 (51%)
Median number of colonies formed for all growing specimens	87
Mean number of colonies formed for all growing specimens	169
Median number of drugs tested against evaluable specimens	4.0
Mean number of drugs tested against evaluable specimens	4.9

decrease in colony-forming units was calculated. A colony was defined as a spherical aggregate of 20 more cells.

To document that the colonies were indeed carcinoma cells and not granulocyte-macrophage or fibroblast colonies, slides were made from some of the tumors according to the method of Salmon and Buick (1979) and subjected to pathologic review.

RESULTS

Colorectal Carcinoma

Two-hundred-seventeen specimens were submitted for evaluation in the assay with diagnoses of adenocarcinoma of the colon and rectum. Forty (18%) specimens were contaminated, and 10 (4.6%) specimens had no tumor seen on cytologic or pathologic analysis. All 10 of the pathologically negative specimens failed to grow tumor in the cloning assay. The remaining 167 tumor-positive uncontaminated specimens were composed of 18 body fluids and 149 solid tumor lesions (see Tables 1 and 2 for growth characteristics).

TABLE 2. Percent of Colon Cancers that Grew in the Clonogenic System Detailed by Specimen Source

Source	> 5 Colonies	≥ 30 Colonies
Primary lesions	66/77 (85.7%)	53/77 (68.8%)
Lymph nodes	10/13 (76.9%)	8/13 (61.5%)
Liver metastases	16/18 (88.8%)	9/18 (50%)
Malignant effusions	13/18 (72.2%)	8/18 (44.4%)

TABLE 3. Percentage of Colon Cancer that Grew in the Clonogenic System Detailed by Previous Chemotherapy

Therapy status	> 5 Colonies	≥ 30 Colonies
No prior chemotherapy	110/131 (83.9%)	77/131 (58.7%)
Prior chemotherapy	14/20 (70%)	10/20 (50%)

Eighty-six of the specimens had sufficient growth and sufficient numbers of cells to allow for drug testing. The median number of drugs tested against these 86 specimens was 4.0, with a range of 1 to 22 drugs.

Table 3 details the growth of adenocarcinoma of the colon or rectum according to prior treatment status. Prior chemotherapy did not appear to influence the growth of colorectal carcinoma in soft agar.

Table 4 details results of drug sensitivity testing on the 86 specimens that had enough growth for drug sensitivity testing. The criteria for in vitro sensitivity are currently being examined to determine what will be the most useful criteria for calling a tumor sensitive to a particular agent in vitro. For our analysis we have used both a < 50% and a < 30% survival of tumor colony forming units.

Overall, a single drug with a < 50% survival of tumor colony-forming units (TCFUs) was found in 24 specimens (28%) giving evaluable growth with sufficient cells for drug testing. If a ≤ 30% survival of TCFUs was used to define a sensitive agent, then only nine (10.4%) specimens met this latter criteria. Conventional agents demonstrating some antitumor activity (≤ 50% survival of TCFUs in vitro) against at least one tumor specimen were 5-FU, 6/78; BCNU, 7/63; mitomycin C, 3/51; methylglyoxal bis(guanylhydrazone)(MGBG), 6/32; bisantrene, 2/20, vincristine, 3/7; 6 thioguanine (6-TG), 3/7; tamoxifen, 1/2, and Adriamycin, 1/11 (see Table 4). If a < 30% survival of TCFUs is used as a criterion for in vitro sensitivity, the activity of all these agents is minimal.

TABLE 4. Results of Drug Sensitivity Testing for Colorectal Carcinoma

Drug	Concentration (μg/ml)	Evaluable tests (No.)	≤ 50% Survival[a]	≤ 30% Survival[a]
5-FU	6.00	78	6	2
BCNU	0.10	63	7	3
Mitomycin C	0.10	51	3	1
MGBG	10.00	32	6	2
Bisantrene	0.50	20	2	0
Mitoxantrone	0.05	16	1	0
Adriamycin	0.04	11	1	0
Vincristine	0.01	7	3	0
6-Thioguanine	20.00	7	3	1
Tamoxifen	0.20	2	1	1

[a]Survival of tumor colony-forming units—drug versus control.

TABLE 5. Growth Characteristics of Gastric Carcinoma

Total number of specimens	44 (all pathologically positive)
Number of specimens that grew (> 5 colonies)	20 (45%)
Number of specimens that gave evaluable growth (≥ 30 colonies)	10 (23%)
Number of specimens available for drug testing	10 (23%)
Median number of colonies formed	30
Mean number of colonies formed	58
Median number of drugs tested	5.0
Mean number of drugs tested	5.7

Gastric Carcinoma

Forty-four pathologically proven specimens were received and plated in soft agar. These consisted of 35 solids and 9 fluids. The solid tumor specimens consisted of 26 primary tumors, 6 lymph nodes, and 3 liver metastases. The fluid specimens consisted of 8 ascitic fluids and 1 pleural effusion.

Of the 44 pathologically positive specimens received, 20 (45%) formed at least five colonies in control plates. However, only 10 (25%) formed enough colonies in control plates for drug sensitivity testing. The median number of colonies formed by all specimens was 30 (mean = 58). The median number of drugs tested in specimens that formed ≥ 30 colonies in control plates was five (mean 5.7)(see Table 5).

Table 6 details growth by source of tumor specimens. Because the numbers are small in most categories, no source appears particularly good for cloning in soft agar. Table 7 demonstrates that prior treatment with chemotherapy probably does effect the ability of tumors to form ≥ 30 colonies in soft agar ($P = .049$).

Of the conventional agents tested against the 10 evaluable specimens, only mitomycin C, bisantrene, mitoxantrone, MGBG, and vinblastine gave a ≤ 50% survival of tumor colony-forming units for at least one specimen. Only mitoxantrone gave a ≤ 30% survival in a single patients tumor (Table 8). Of note, Adriamycin demonstrated no activity against these patients' tumors in vitro (four of the patients had received and failed prior therapy with Adriamycin).

TABLE 6. Percent of Gastric Cancers that Grew in the Clonogenic System Detailed by Specimen Source

Source	> 5 Colonies	≥ 30 Colonies
Primary lesions	9/26 (35%)	6/26 (23%)
Lymph node	3/6 (50%)	1/6 (16%)
Liver metastases	3/3 (100%)	1/3 (33%)
Malignant effusions	5/9 (55%)	2/9 (22%)

TABLE 7. Percent Gastric Cancers that Grew in the Clonogenic System Detailed by Previous Chemotherapy

Therapy status	> 5 Colonies	≥ 30 Colonies
No prior chemotherapy	11/29 (38%)	4/29 (14%)
Prior chemotherapy	9/15 (60%)	6/15 (40%)

Pancreatic Tumors

Eighty-eight specimens were submitted for routine cloning in patients with diagnoses of adenocarcinoma of the pancreas (82) and islet cell tumors (6). Of these specimens, 59 (67%) specimens grew (≥ 5 colonies in control plates) and 35 (40%) gave evaluable growth (> 30 colonies in control plates). The median number of colonies formed per evaluable specimen was 85. The median number of drugs tested per evaluable specimen was 5.0. Those agents demonstrating a ≤ 30% survival of TCFUs in the assay for at least one specimen included 5-FU, Adriamycin, mitoxantrone, MGBG, bisantrene, and vinblastine (see Table 9).

Hepatocellular Carcinoma

Forty-one specimens with diagnoses of primary hepatocellular carcinoma were submitted for routine cloning and drug testing. Twenty-two (54%) grew, and 10 (24%) specimens gave evaluable growth (≥ 30 colonies in control plates) in the cloning assay. The median number of colonies formed per evaluable specimen was 50. The median number of drugs tested was 3.5. The drug screening results are detailed in Table 10. Only five agents gave a ≤50% survival of TCFUs.

TABLE 8. Drug Sensitivity Results for Gastric Carcinoma (Fraction of Tumors Showing Reponse to Individual Drugs by Reduction in Tumor Colony-Forming Units—T-CFUs)

Drug	Concentration (μg/ml)	Evaluable tests (No.)	≤50% Survival	≤30% Survival
Adriamycin	0.04	10	0	0
5-FU	6.00	7	0	0
Mitomycin C	0.10	8	2	0
BCNU	0.10	9	0	0
Bisantrene	0.50	6	2	0
Mitoxantrone	0.05	6	2	1
MGBG	10.00	2	1	0
Methotrexate	0.30	1	0	0
Vinblastine	0.05	2	1	0
Vincristine	0.01	1	0	0
m-AMSA	0.50	1	0	0

TABLE 9. Results of Drug Sensitivity Testing for Pancreatic Tumors

Agent	Concentration (μg/ml)	Evaluable tests (No.)	≤ 50% Survival	≤ 30% Survival
5-FU	6.00	26	7	2
BCNU	0.10	21	1	0
Adriamycin	0.04	14	7	1
Mitomycin C	0.10	21	3	0
Mitroxantrone	0.05	15	4	2
MGBG	10.00	12	3	3
Bisantrene	0.50	12	5	2
m-AMSA	0.50	5	0	0
Vincristine	0.01	5	1	1
Vinblastine	0.05	10	3	3
Bleomycin	0.20	5	1	0
Chlorambucil	0.10	5	0	0
Methotrexate	0.30	4	2	0
Cisplatinum	0.20	4	0	0
Streptozotocin	0.10	4	0	0
Melphalan	4.00	1	0	0
Melphalan	40.00	1	0	0

Esophageal Adenocarcinoma

Seven specimens were submitted from patients with diagnoses of adenocarcinoma of the esophagus. Three specimens formed ≥ 5 colonies in control plates (43%), and only one specimen gave evaluable growth (≥ 30 colonies in control plates). The results of drug sensitivity testing with a variety of agents is detailed in Table 11.

TABLE 10. Results of Drug Sensitivity Testing for Hepatic Tumors

Agent	Concentration (μg/ml)	Evaluable tests (No.)	≤ 50% Survival	≤ 30% Survival
5-FU	6.00	8	0	0
Adriamycin	0.04	7	0	0
Mitoxantrone	0.05	2	0	0
Bisantrene	0.50	4	1	0
BCNU	0.10	2	1	0
Vinblastine	10.00	2	0	0
MGBG	10.00	2	1	0
Mitomycin C	0.10	1	0	0
Chlorambucil	0.10	1	1	0
Methotrexate	0.30	1	1	0
Cisplatinum	0.20	1	0	0
Vinblastine	0.05	2	0	0

TABLE 11. Results of Drug Sensitivity Testing for Esophageal Adenocarcinomas

Agent	Concentration (μg/ml)	Evaluable tests (No.)	≤ 50% Survival	≤ 70% Survival
Vinblastine	0.05	2	2	2
Adriamycin	0.04	1	0	0
Mitoxantrone	0.05	1	0	0
Cisplatinum	0.20	1	0	0
Vincristine	0.01	1	1	0
VP-16-213	3.00	1	1	1

DISCUSSION

Although we have cloned more than over four times the number of colorectal cancer specimens since the report published in an earlier gastrointestinal malignancy symposium (Perkins and Von Hoff, 1980), the current results are almost identical to our earlier results. Previously published results by other investigators attempting to clone adenocarcinoma of the colon are quite variable. In an early attempt by Buick and colleagues (1980), using mechanical disaggregation, all solid tumors failed to grow. A more recent attempt by Agrez and associates (1982) at the Mayo Clinic showed a 26% growth rate using both mechanical and enzymatic means of dispersing cells.

Our studies have employed only mechanical dispersion of the tumor tissue, and we have demonstrated an evaluable growth rate of 58% for colorectal carcinoma. The reason for the growth disparity may well be due to our processing specimens the day of arrival, whereas the Mayo Clinic experience allows such tumors to sit overnight with enzymes or after mechanical mincing followed by plating the next morning (Agrez et al., 1982). However, this 50% evaluable growth rate is still disappointing. Our ability to grow gastric carcinoma (23%), pancreatic carcinoma (40%), hepatoma (21%), and esophageal adenocarcinoma (14%) is still less than optimal.

The future of the human tumor cloning assay in growing gastrointestinal tumors will be aided by at least two important factors: (1) A modification of the assay for each tumor type such that a greater percentage of tumors will grow; (2) a better mechanism for making single cell suspensions without affecting drug sensitivity.

All the tumors featured relatively few specimens, demonstrating in vitro sensitivity. One might immediately remark on the relative insensitivity of the Hamburger-Salmon assay to demonstrate drug sensitivity for such tumors. The plausible explanation for insensitivity of adenocarcinoma of the colon, pancreas, liver, stomach, and esophagus is that our present day chemotherapeutic armamentarium lacks sufficient agents to yield adequate responses both in vitro and in vivo. Thus, the assay may only reflect the current state of chemotherapy for patients with gastrointestinal malignancies.

Even in its present form, the assay demonstrates promise in screening for new agents with activity in gastrointestinal malignancy. For example, both MGBG and mitoxantrone demonstrated rather low in vitro activity against colo-

TABLE 12. In Vitro Cloning Drug Sensitivities for MGBG and Mitoxantrone for Gastrointestinal Tumors

Tumors	Concentration (μg/ml)	Evaluable tests (No.)	≥ 50% Kill	≥ 70% Kill
For MGBG				
Colon	10.00	32	6	2
Gastric	10.00	2	1	0
Hepatoma	10.00	2	1	0
Pancreatic	10.00	12	3	3
For mitoxantrone				
Colon	0.05	16	1	1
Gastric	0.05	6	2	1
Esophageal	0.05	1	0	0
Hepatic	0.05	2	0	0
Pancreatic	0.05	15	4	2

rectal tumors (Table 12). Subsequent prospective testing of both MGBG and mitoxantrone against colorectal carcinoma in Southwest Oncology Group trials and other trials have shown no substantial antitumor activity of these agents (Von Hoff et al., 1981b, c; Myers et al., 1981; Knight et al., 1979; Cowan et al., 1982; Bonnem et al., 1982; Bedikian et al., 1982).

The true test will come when an agent is found to have in vitro activity and is carried into trials to ascertain its in vivo response rate. Should such a trial demonstrate a good correlation of in vitro and in vivo results, it may then be feasible to consider using the cloning assay for directing initial phase II trials. Phase II trials planned in this manner may have a greater chance of successfully demonstrating activity, expedite anticancer agents into trials where first-line treatment is poor, and save patients from treatment with an agent for which the chance of response is remote.

This research supported in part by National Cancer Institute grants CM-07327 and CA KGAHM-30-312-416, NCI training grant KGAHM-30-460-1-16, and American Cancer Society grant CH 162

REFERENCES

Agrez MV, Kovach JS, Beart RW, et al. (1982) Human colorectal carcinoma: Patterns of sensitivity to chemotherapeutic agents in human tumor stem cell assay. J Surg Oncol 20:187–191.

Bedikian AY, Stroehlein JR, Korinek J, et al. (1982) Phase II evaluation of dihydroxyanthracenedione (DHAD) in patients with metastatic colorectal cancer. Am Soc Clin Oncol 1:95.

Bonnem E, Mitchell E, Smith R, et al. (1982) A Phase II trial of dihydroxyanthracenedione (DHAD) in advanced colon cancer. Am Soc Clin Oncol 1:97.

Buick RN, Fry SE, Salmon SE (1980) Application of *in vitro* soft agar techniques for growth of tumor cells to the study of colon cancer. Cancer 45:1238–1242.

Callahan SK, Falcon E JR., Von Hoff DD (1983) Growth of human gastric carcionoma in a human tumor cloning system. Cancer Treatm Symp 1:7–10.

Cowan J, Von Hoff DD, MacDonald B, et al. (1982) Phase II evaluation of mitoxantrone in previously untreated patients with colorectal cancer. Am Soc Clin Oncol 1:99.

Hamburger AW, Salmon SE (1977a) Primary bioassay of human stem cells. Science 197:461–463.

Hamburger AW, Salmon SE (1977b) Primary bioassay of human myeloma stem cells. J Clin Invest 60:846–854.

Hamburger AW, Salmon SE, Kim MB, et al. (1978) Direct cloning of human ovarian carcinoma cells in agar. Cancer Res 38:3438–3443.

Knight WA III, Livingston RB, Fabian C, Costanzi J (1979) Phase I-II trial of methyl-GAG: A Southwest Oncology Group pilot study. Cancer Treatm Rep 63:90–94.

Knight WA III, Loesch DM, Leichman LH, et al. (1982) Methyl-glyoxal bisguanylhydrazone (MGBG, Methyl-GAG) in advanced colon cancer. A Phase II trial of the Southwest Oncology Group. Cancer Treatm Rep 66:2099–2100.

Meyskens FL Jr, Salmon SE (1980) Regulation of human melanoma clonagenic cell expression in soft agar by follicle stimulating hormone, nerve growth factor, and melatonin (Abstract). Proc Am Assoc Cancer Res and ASCO 21:199.

Myers JW, Knight WA III, Livingston RB, et al. (1981) Phase I-II trial of methyl-GAG in advanced colon cancer. A Southwest Oncology Group pilot study. Cancer Clin Trials 4:277–279.

Park CH, Bergsagel DE, McCulloch EA (1971) Mouse myeloma tumor stem cells. A primary cell culture assay. J Natl Cancer Inst 46:411–422.

Perkins M, Von Hoff DD (1980) Experience with a two-layer soft agar system for growing gastrointestinal tumors. In: Stroehlein JR, Romsdahl MM, eds., Gastrointestinal cancer. New York: Raven Press, pp. 381–390.

Pike B, Robinson W (1970) Human bone marrow colony growth *in vitro.* J Cell Physiol 76:77–81.

Pollard EB, Tio F, Whitecar JP, et al. (1980) Utilization of a soft agar system monitor for marrow involvement with small cell carcinoma of the lung. Proc Am Assoc Cancer Res and ASCO 21:192.

Puck TT, Marcus PI (1955) A rapid method of viable cell titration and clone production with HeLa cells in tissue culture. Use of x-irradiated cells to supply conditioning factors. Proc Natl Acad Sci USA 41:432–437.

Salmon SE, Buick RM (1979) Preparation of permanent slides of intact soft agar colony cultures of hematopoeitic and tumor stem cells. Cancer Res 39:1133–1136.

Sandbach JM, O'Brien D, Welch D, et al. (1980) Assay for clonogenic cells in human breast cancer. (Abstract) Proc Am Assoc Cancer Res and ASCO 21:139.

Von Hoff DD, Casper J, Bradley E, et al. (1980) Direct cloning of human neuroblastoma cells in agar: A potential assay for diagnosis, response and prognosis. Cancer Res 40:3591–3597.

Von Hoff DD, Casper J, Bradley E, et al. (1981a) Clinical correlations of drug sensitivity in tumor stem cell assay. Association between human tumor colony-forming assay results and response of an individual patient's tumor to chemotherapy. Am J Med 70:1027–1032.

Von Hoff DD, Coltman CA JR, Foreseth B (1981b) Activity of mitoxantrone in a human tumor cloning system. Cancer Res 41:1853–1855.

Von Hoff DD, Cowan J, Harris G, Reisdorf G (1981c) Human tumor cloning: Feasibility and clinical correlations. Cancer Chemother Pharmacol 6:265–271.

COST-EFFECTIVENESS OF COLORECTAL CANCER SCREENING

DAVID M EDDY, M.D., Ph.D.

Before a practicing physician or health planner can recommend screening for colorectal cancer, he or she must address the question: Is screening worth the effort? More specifically, what proportion of invasive cancers can be prevented by finding and removing adenomatous polyps? How much will screening change long-term survival, and how much will mortality be decreased? How long will screening prolong a patient's expected lifetime? How much will it cost, and what are the risks? In terms of the use of time and resources, how does screening for colorectal cancer compare with other medical activites we might do? If the decision is made to screen, another set of questions must be answered. What tests should be used? At what age? at what frequency?

METHODS

To help answer these questions, the Third International Symposium on Colorectal Cancer conducted a cost-effectiveness analysis using a computer model of colorectal cancer screening.

Computer Model

The basic structure of the model has been described elsewhere (Eddy, 1980). For this particular exercise, the structure was modified to include both random and biological false-negative rates and to incorporate some special aspects of the natural history of colorectal cancer (for example, adenomatous polyps and the staging of invasive disease). In brief, the model consists of a set of mathematical equations that describe the relationships between the important factors

From the Center for Health Policy Research and Education, Duke University, Durham, North Carolina.

that affect the outcomes of a colorectal cancer screening program. These factors include

Age- and sex-specific incidence rates

Risk factors

Natural history of colorectal cancer, including
- proportion of cancers that arise from adenomatous polyps
- time for a precancerous polyp to develop into invasive cancer[1]
- time for an invasive cancer to progress through local, regional, and distant stages (or Dukes' A, B, C, and D)
- proportion of adenomatous polyps and cancers that develop in various regions of the colon and rectum

Clinical progression
- time from invasion to clinical signs and symptoms
- patient delay after onset of signs and symptoms

Effectiveness of fecal occult blood test (FOBT)[2]
- proportion of precancerous adenomatous polyps that bleed prior to invasion
- time from first detectable bleeding to invasion
- random false-negative rate[3]

Effectiveness of sigmoidoscopy (rigid and flexible)
- time adenomatous polyps are detectable by sigmoidoscopy prior to invasion
- proportion of adenomatous polyps and cancers that develop within range of various sigmoidoscopic instruments
- random false-negative rates of various instruments

Effectiveness of therapy (relative case-survival rates, by stage)

False-positive rates of fecal occult blood tests

Risk of sigmoidoscopy (perforation)

Financial costs, including
- screening examinations

---

[1]Not all adenomatous polyps develop into invasive cancer. The term "precancerous polyp" will designate an adenomatous polyp that would eventually become invasive cancer if not detected or treated.

[2]The term "fecal occult blood test" will designate the Hemoccult test (a registered trademark of SmithKline Diagnostics, Inc.) applied in a 3-day sequence with two samples a day. There are other brands of fecal occult blood tests that have different characteristics; the estimates of parameters and results in this analysis are based on the Hemoccult.

[3]There are two main types of false-negative rates. One, which might be called a biological false-negative rate, depends on certain biological or anatomical features such as location, size, appearance, or presence of bleeding. This false-negative rate is not constant but depends on the state of development of the lesion and the results of previous applications of the test. Information about this biological false-negative rate is contained in estimates of the time from first detectability to invasion. The second false-negative rate depends on nonbiological factors such as sampling technique, preparation of the test, and accuracy of interpretation and can be considered random.

workups of patients with positive test results
initial treatment, by stage
terminal treatment

Data on some of these factors, such as age- and sex-specific incidence rates; relative case-survival rates of patients with local, regional, and distant invasive disease; proportion of patients with cancer detected in various stages in the absence of screening; and average financial costs of initial therapy for invasive cancer (by stage) can be obtained from published sources (Anderson, 1974; Axtell et al., 1976; Evans et al., 1978; Falterman et al., 1974; Godwin and Brown, 1975; Mettlin et al., 1982; Polissar et al., 1981; Reilly et al., 1982; SEER Report, 1981; Third National Cancer Survey, 1976).

Data on some other factors, however, including many aspects of the natural history of colorectal cancer and the effectiveness of various screening tests, are not as readily available in the published literature. Estimates for these factors were obtained by surveying the attendees of the Third International Symposium.

Prior to the meeting on March 23–26, 1983, a questionnaire was sent to each invited member to request his or her best estimate of the critical numbers. Members were also invited to state ranges for their answers, indicate their degrees of confidence, and provide comments, which could include supporting data or references. The answers were compiled and then presented to the respondents at the time of the meeting. Where there was a wide divergence of opinion about a particular factor, and where the range of disagreement had an important impact on the estimated outcomes of screening, a panel of three to five persons was asked to discuss the issues before the entire Symposium audience, and audience members were invited to question the panelists and add comments. Following these panel discussions, the questionnaire was recirculated and filled out a second time by each of the respondents. The answers to this second questionnaire were then compiled, and the average values and distributions of the answers were calculated.

The invitees consisted of about 100 people from about a dozen countries, chosen for their experience and interest in colorectal cancer screening. Altogether, the expertise of the Symposium members covered a wide range of topics including genetics, epidemiology, pathology, biochemistry, gastroenterology, endoscopy, radiology, surgery, the day-to-day management of screening programs, economics, statistics, and health planning. Different people were knowledgeable about different aspects of colorectal cancer screening, and for each question there were about 40 responses. From their comments, it was clear that respondents tended to answer the questions that fell in their area of expertise.

The average values of the respondents for some of the most important variables are as follows.

1. Ninety percent of colorectal cancers arise from adenomatous polyps.
2. A precancerous adenoma is potentially detectable by sigmoidoscopy for 7 years before it becomes invasive (range, 0 to 14 years).
3. Forty-four percent of precancerous adenomas bleed prior to invasion (and are potentially detectable by an FOBT).

4. For adenomas that do bleed prior to invasion, bleeding begins an average of 2½ years prior to invasion (range, 0 to 6 years).
5. Thirty percent of precancerous adenomas and cancers arise within practical reach of the rigid sigmoidoscope.
6. Fifty percent of precancerous adenomas and cancers arise within practical reach of the flexible sigmoidoscope.
7. The random false-negative rate of the FOBT is 45%.
8. The random false-negative rate of the sigmoidoscope is 20%.
9. The false-positive rate of the FOBT is 1.5%.
10. In the absence of screening, it takes an average of 2 years for an invasive cancer to progress through local to regional disease and 1 year to progress through regional to distant disease.
11. An FOBT costs $5. A rigid sigmoidoscopy costs $40. A flexible sigmoidoscopy costs $65. A workup of a patient with a positive FOBT costs $820. (All financial costs are in U.S. dollars.)

These average values were used for the "base case" of the cost-effectiveness analysis, and the distributions of the estimates were used to define a set of optimistic and pessimistic assumptions.

The use of subjective judgments to estimate the consequences of different medical activities is not unusual; virtually all medical policies and decisions are based on subjective impressions. This exercise differs from the usual application of clinical judgment and consensus in that it employed a formal and explicit process for structuring the problem, estimating parameters, synthesizing the information, estimating results, and exploring the consequences of uncertainty and changes in assumptions.

RESULTS

The published data coupled with the estimates provided by the Symposium members imply the following results.

No Screening

The impact of colorectal cancer on a 40-year-old average-risk man or woman who is not screened is shown in Table 1. In the absence of screening, the chance that a man or woman over 40 will be diagnosed as having colorectal cancer in the coming year is about 1 in 750. The chance that an average-risk 40-year-old man will develop clinical colorectal cancer over the rest of his life is about 5.9%. For a 40-year-old average-risk woman, the lifetime chance of developing the disease is about 6.1%. (The age-specific incidence rates for women are slightly lower than for men, but women tend to live longer, giving them a higher overall probability of developing the disease.) The probability that a 40-year-old man or woman will die of colorectal cancer is 3.3 and 3.4%, respectively. Colorectal cancer reduces the life expectancy of a 40-year-old average-risk man by about 143 days, and of the 40-year-old average-risk woman by about 165 days. (For reference, the reduction in life expectancy caused by all cancers is about 2⅝ years for a man and 2¾ years for a woman.)

TABLE 1. Effect of Colorectal Cancer on 40-Year-Old Average-Risk Person if No Screening

Effect	Male	Female
Lifetime probability, get colorectal cancer	5.9%	6.1%
Lifetime probability, die of colorectal cancer	3.3%	3.4%
Probability "cured," if get colorectal cancer	44%	44%
Effect of colorectal cancer on life expectancy	143 days	165 days
Effect of colorectal cancer on life expectancy, if get colorectal cancer	6.4 years	7.4 years
Expected cost of treatment	$456	$453
Expected lost earnings due to premature death	$895	$635

For those who have the misfortune to develop symptomatic invasive colorectal cancer, the chances it will be diagnosed in local, regional, and distant stages are 40%, 30%, and 30%, repectively. With treatment, there is about a 44% chance such a patient will be "cured," in the sense that he or she will not die of colorectal cancer. The loss in life expectancy for a person diagnosed as having the disease is about 7 years (6.4 years for a man, 7.4 years for a woman), the actual loss of life varying from less than 1 year to more than 20 years, depending on the patient's age at diagnosis and how early in its natural history the cancer is detected.

Taking into account the fact that a 40-year-old person has about a 6% chance of developing colorectal cancer in the rest of his or her life, the expected financial cost of treating colorectal cancer is about $455 (present value at age 40). The expected lost earnings due to the possibility of premature death from colorectal cancer is about $895 for a man and about $635 for a woman.

Annual Fecal Occult Blood Test

The effectiveness of screening for colorectal cancer depends on the configuration of the screening program. Consider first the effect of screening a man from age 50 to age 75 with an annual fecal occult blood test.

The impact of screening with an annual FOBT on some of the more important clinical and economic outcomes is shown in the second column of Table 2. So that comparisons can be made with the no-screening case (Table 1), all the outcomes are calculated for a 40-year-old man—in this case screening is conducted from age 50 to 75, but the outcomes are computed for every year from age 40 until death. Table 2 shows a significant reduction (by about 14%) in the probability that the person will ever be diagnosed as having colorectal cancer, due to the fact that annual fecal occult blood tests can detect some potentially malignant neoplasms while they are still adenomatous polyps. Screening with an annual FOBT can also be expected to reduce significantly (by about 28%) the probability that a person will die of the disease. The probability that a patient who was otherwise destined to get colorectal cancer will

TABLE 2 Effect of Annual Screening with a Fecal Occult Test, Average-Risk Male

	Age screening begun				
Effect	53	50	47	44	41
Decrease in probability get colorectal cancer	13.7%	14.3%	14.8%	15.1%	15.3%
Decrease in probability die of colorectal cancer	26.6%	28.1%	29.2%	29.9%	30.7%
Increase in probability "cured," if get colorectal cancer or precancerous polyp	33.9%	35.7%	36.9%	37.8%	38.2%
Increase in life expectancy	37 days	41 days	44 days	46 days	48 days
Increase in life expectancy, if get colorectal cancer or precancerous polyp	1.72 years	1.90 years	2.04 year	2.14 years	2.23 years
Cost of screening and workups	$106	$131	$159	$190	$224
Decrease in cost of treatment	$48	$54	$58	$62	$65
Net financial cost	$58	$77	$101	$128	$159
Decrease in lost earnings	$120	$169	$214	$259	$298

not die of the disease (the probability of a "cure") is increased from about 44% to about 60% (an increase of about 35%).

Annual screening with an FOBT will increase the life expectancy of an asymptomatic 40-year-old average-risk male who complies with the program by about 41 days. This number appears to be low because the great majority of people (about 94%) do not have and never will get colorectal cancer, and the 41 days takes this small probability that a man will get the disease into account. The increase in life expectancy for a 40-year-old man who is destined to get the disease is about 1.9 years, ranging from less than 1 to more than 20 years, depending on his age at diagnosis and how early the cancer is detected. Thus, if in the absence of screening the loss of life expectancy was about 6.4 years, an annual FOBT from age 50 to 75 recovers about 30% of the loss of life attributable to colorectal cancer.

For these benefits, there are some risks and costs. The main risk is from false-positive test results. The expected number of false-positive test results per person over the 25-year period is about 25%. Roughly translated, this means that about one out of four people who are screened from age 50 to 75 will have a false-positive test result sometime during the 25-year period of screening. If colonoscopy is included in the workup of a positive test result, about one out of 8000 people who enter a screening program with an annual FOBT will suffer a perforated colon (assuming a perforation rate of one per 2000 examinations). Concerning costs, at $5 for a 3-day series of fecal occult blood tests, the present value of the financial costs of annual tests from age 50 to 75 is $52.[4] The workup for such a false-positive test result may include a sigmoidoscopy, barium enema, or colonoscopy, and can cost from a few hundred dollars to more than $1000. Taking these probabilities and costs into account, the present value of the expected financial costs of false-positive test results is about $79 (giving a total cost for screening examinations and workups of $131). Some treatment costs are saved because of the reduction in the chance the person will be diagnosed as having colorectal cancer and because the invasive cancers that do occur tend to be found in earlier stages when treatment is less expensive; these savings amount to about $54. Taking all the financial costs and savings into account, the net financial cost of a lifetime screening program is $77 (calculated as the present value at age 40 using a discount rate of 3%). The decrease in earnings lost to premature death from colorectal cancer is about $169.

Concerning cost-effectiveness, an increase in life expectancy of about 41 days for a total financial cost of about $77 translates on a population-wide basis into a person-year of life expectancy for about $685. Compared with other medical practices, this is a very good use of resources; for its financial costs, screening for colorectal cancer appears to deliver a very high yield in terms of decreasing the chance a patient will get or die of colorectal cancer and in prolonging a patient's expected life. It is also notable that the savings in lost earnings exceed the costs of screening.

The effect of starting annual fecal occult blood testing at ages 41, 44, 47, and 53, instead of age 50, is shown in the other columns of Table 2. The effect of biennial testing (every two years) starting at age 50 is shown in Table 3, column 5.

Annual FOBT and Sigmoidoscopy

If a 25-cm rigid sigmoidoscope is added to this screening protocol at 1-, 3-, or 5-year intervals, from age 50 to 75, then one obtains the outcomes shown in the first three columns of Table 3, which for comparison also includes data on the FOBT alone (column 4) and a biennial FOBT alone (column 5). The addition of rigid sigmoidoscopy decreases both the incidence of invasive disease (by detecting more precancerous polyps) and mortality; adding annual sigmoidoscopy is about one-third more effective than annual FOBT alone. But there is also an increase in financial cost, as well as a small risk of a perforation (about one in 40,000 examinations).

[4]Calculating the present value is a way to condense a sequence of future costs (or benefits) into a single number. It can be thought of as the amount of money that would have to be paid at age 40 so that, after interest and inflation are taken into account, it will generate the precise amount needed to pay each of the future expected costs at the exact time they are due.

TABLE 3 Effect of Screening with a Fecal Occult Blood Test and Rigid Sigmoidoscopy on 50-Year-Old Average-Risk Male Screened from Age 50 to 75

Effect	Screening strategies				
	1-yr FOBT 1-yr scope	1-yr FOBT 3-yr scope	1-yr FOBT 5-yr scope	1-yr FOBT no scope	2-yr FOBT no scope
Decrease in probability get colorectal cancer	30.6%	24.7%	23.1%	14.3%	9.5%
Decrease in probability die of colorectal cancer	39.4%	36.4%	33.3%	28.1%	18.2%
Increase in probability "cured," if get colorectal cancer of precancerous polyp	53.2%	47.7%	46.4%	35.7%	24.4%
Increase in life expectancy	56 days	50 days	48 days	41 days	28 days
Increase in life expectancy, if get colorectal cancer or precancerous polyp	2.60 years	2.32 years	2.23 years	1.90 years	1.30 years
Cost of screening and workups	$562	$285	$231	$131	$67
Decrease in cost of treatment	$89	$75	$70	$54	$37
Net financial cost	$473	$210	$161	$77	$30
Decrease in lost earnings	$200	$177	$175	$169	$118

Choice of Tests and Frequencies

To compare the value of screening with different tests at different frequencies, it is convenient to examine some measures of effectiveness and financial costs of different screening strategies. Figure 1 compares the net financial costs with three measures of effectiveness: the increase in life expectancy for an asymptomatic average-risk male who may or may not get colorectal cancer, the increase in life expectancy for an average-risk male who is destined to get colorectal cancer, and the proportion of loss of life prevented by the screening program. The results for an average-risk female are slightly more favorable.

By any of these measures, an annual fecal occult blood test alone delivers about two-thirds of the effectiveness achievable by annual fecal occult blood tests and annual rigid sigmoidoscopic examinations. If sigmoidoscopy is to be performed, then sigmoidoscopic examinations can be conducted at 3- or 5-year intervals. A biennial fecal occult blood test delivers about 68% of the effectiveness of an annual fecal occult blood test, at less than 40% of the cost.

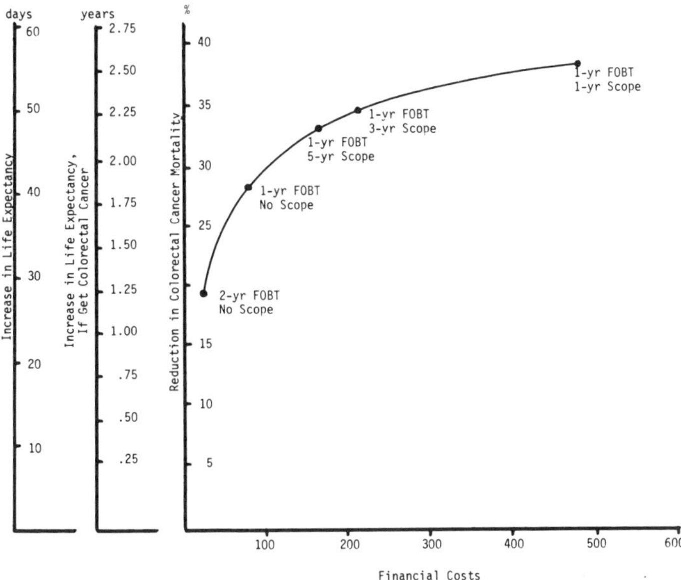

FIGURE 1

Flexible Sigmoidoscopy

Some of the costs and effectiveness of screening with 25-cm rigid sigmoidoscopes, and 60-cm flexible sigmoidoscopes are compared in Table 4 and Fig. 2. The main assumptions are that about 30% of colorectal cancers and adenomatous polyps are within the practical range of a rigid 25-cm sigmoidoscope, whereas approximately 50% of adenomatous polyps and invasive cancers are within practical range of a 60-cm flexible sigmoidoscope, and that an examination with a 60-cm flexible sigmoidoscope costs more than the rigid sigmoidoscope (about \$65 compared to \$40). If sigmoidoscopies are performed every 3 years (center two columns of Table 4), using a rigid sigmoidoscope is about 18% less effective, and 24% less expensive, than using a flexible 60-cm sigmoidoscope.

Age to Begin Screening

The question of the age to begin screening is addressed in Table 2 and Figure 3, which show the increase in life expectancy and the net financial cost of screening starting at various ages (41, 44, 47, 50, and 53) for two cases: a screening program consisting of an annual fecal occult blood test alone, and a screening program consisting of an annual fecal occult blood test combined with a 3-year rigid sigmoidoscopic examination. Beginning examinations at age 44 instead of age 50 increases the benefits of screening (as measured by the three indices in the figure) by about 15% if both FOBT and sigmoidoscopy are used, and about 17% with only fecal occult blood tesing. The costs are about doubled if screening begins at age 41 instead of age 50. Because the annual incidence

TABLE 4. Comparison of Rigid versus Flexible Sigmoidoscopy on 50-Year-Old Average-Risk Male Screened from Age 50 to 75

	Screening strategy					
	1-yr FOBT 1-yr scope		1-yr FOBT 3-yr scope		1-yr FOBT 5-yr scope	
Effect	Rigid	Flexible	Rigid	Flexible	Rigid	Flexible
Decrease in probability get colorectal cancer	30.6%	42.4%	24.7%	34.5%	23.1%	31.9%
Decrease in probability die of colorectal cancer	39.4%	48.5%	36.4%	45.5%	33.3%	42.4%
Increase in probability "cured," if get colorectal cancer or precancerous polyp	53.2%	65.8%	47.7%	58.4%	46.4%	56.3%
Increase in life expectancy	56 days	68 days	50 days	61 days	48 days	58 days
Increase in life expectancy, if get colorectal cancer or precancerous polyp	2.60 years	3.16 years	2.32 years	2.83 years	2.23 years	2.69 years
Cost of screening and workups	$562	$823	$285	$377	$231	$292
Decrease in cost of treatment	$89	$118	$75	$98	$70	$90
Net financial cost	$473	$705	$210	$279	$161	$202
Decrease in lost earnings	$200	$242	$177	$212	$175	$206

rate of invasive colorectal cancer in people 40 to 50 years old is quite small (on the order of one case per 6000 people per year), most of the benefit of screening in this age group is achieved from removing precancerous polyps.

VARIATIONS

It is important to examine how these results are affected by different assumptions. There are two main categories of assumptions: those concerning costs and those concerning effectiveness.

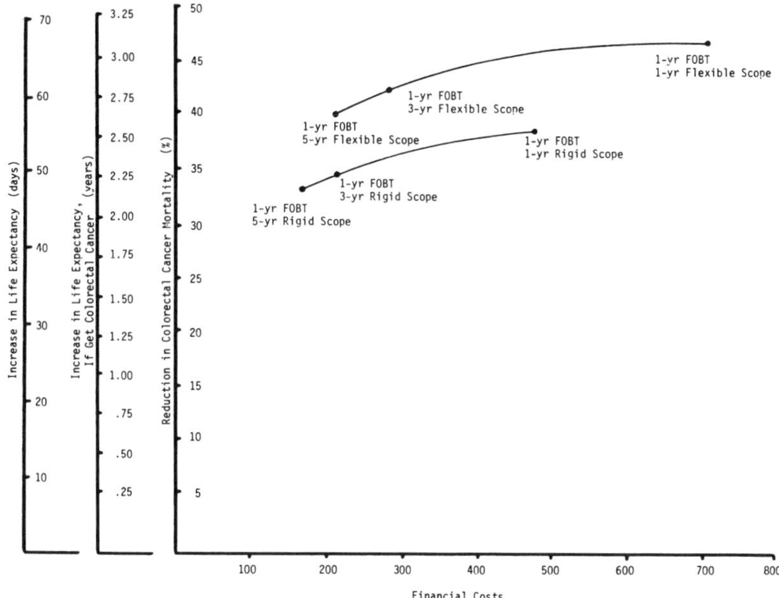

FIGURE 2

FIGURE 3

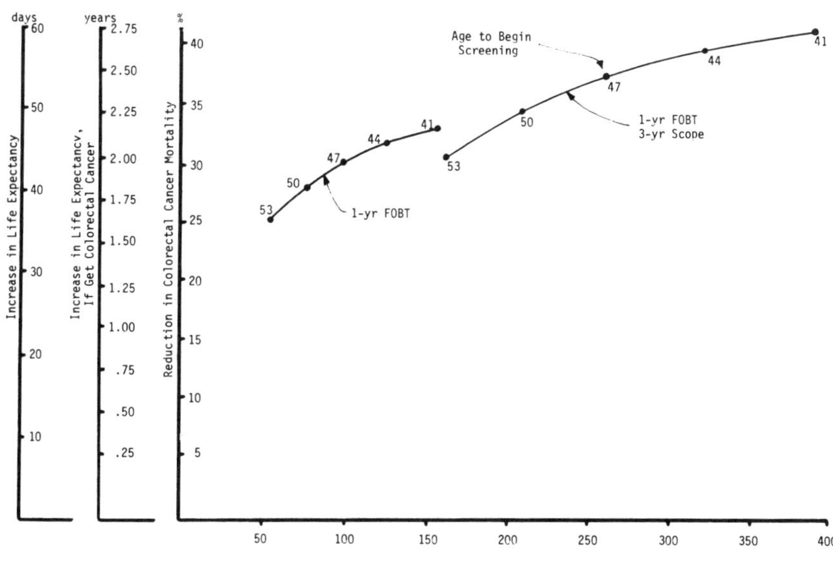

Costs

Cost vary widely from region to region and from physician to physician. In general, they are easily measured, and it is fairly simple to recalculate the financial costs of a particular screening strategy for different costs based on local conditions. The main effect of using different assumptions about costs is to shift or stretch the curves in Figures 1 through 3 horizontally. For example,

1. These analyses assumed that a 3-day set of tests with an FOBT costs $5. If the cost of the 3-day set of tests is doubled to $10, the net cost of screening from age 50 to 75 with any regimen that included an annual FOBT will be increased by about $52 (from about $77 to about $129). A $15 test would add about $104. If testing is begun at age 40, these numbers are almost doubled. If testing is done every 2 years, they are about halved.
2. Just as important as the cost of the FOBT itself is the financial cost of a false-positive FOBT result. Assuming a false-positive rate of 1.5% per examination and a workup cost for a false-positive test result of $500, the present value of the cost of workups for false-positive FOBTs, with annual FOBT from age 50 to 75, is about $79 (compared with a $52 cost for the tests themselves). If the false-positive rate is twice as high as assumed (3% versus 1.5%), the net costs are increased by $79. If the false-positive rate is 1.5% but a workup costs $1000 instead of $500, the net financial effect would be the same, an increase of about $79. Increasing both the false-positive rate (to 3%) and the cost of a false-positive workup (to $1000) will add about $237 to the bill. If screening is begun at age 40 instead of 50, these numbers are almost doubled. If fecal occult blood testing is done every 2 years, the numbers are about halved.
3. Annual rigid sigmoidoscopy (at $40 per examination) adds about $418 to the net costs of screening from age 50 to age 75. Including sigmoidoscopy, however, also increases the effectiveness of the program, which in turn decreases treatment costs by about $24, delivering a net increase in total costs of about $396. If the examination costs $80, the net costs are increased another $418. If examinations are begun at age 40, instead of 50, doubling the cost of rigid sigmoidoscopy to $80 increases the net cost of an annual program by about $750. Reducing the cost of rigid sigmoidoscopy by 50% to $20 per examination saves about $214 if examinations are begun at age 50, and about $375, if they are begun at age 40.
4. Doubling the cost of flexible sigmoidoscopy (from $65 to $130) adds about $680 to an annual program that begins at age 50.
5. The results in Tables 2 through 4 and Figures 1 through 3 do not include any indirect financial costs or nonfinancial costs that occur with screening or the workup of false-positive test results. In addition to the direct financial cost of the tests and workups, a person may incur indirect financial costs because of lost time from work, transportation, or similar expenses. In addition, many people find the act of being tested or examined unpleasant. Although it is impossible to put a precise financial value on these subjective feelings, it is possible to obtain a rough measure of these intangible costs by asking how much people would be willing to pay to avoid them. For example, some may be willing to pay several hundred

dollars to avoid an examination with a rigid sigmoidoscope or colonoscope.

These indirect financial and nonfinancial costs can be included in this analysis as follows. For a program consisting of annual examinations from age 50 to 75, one can take one's estimate of the indirect financial or nonfinancial costs of a fecal occult blood test, and/or sigmoidoscopy, and multiply that estimate by 10 to get a measure of the increase in net cost due to the indirect or nonfinancial costs of either of these tests. To examine the indirect or nonfinancial costs of a workup for a false-positive FOBT, one can take one's estimate of the cost of the events associated with a workup (for example, visit to doctor's office, barium enema, colonoscopy), and multiply it by 15% to get a measure of the increase in net costs attributable to false-positive fecal occult blood tests. For example, if one is willing to pay $1000 to avoid an unnecessary workup, one should add $150 to the net cost of screening.

Effectiveness

Changes in assumptions about how early a screening test can detect an adenomatous polyp or early invasive cancer will affect the estimate of the effectiveness of screening.

Fecal Occult Blood Test. To explore the impact of different assumptions about the value of the FOBT, two additional cases were defined. A "pessimistic" case was constructed from values at the pessimistic ends of the spectra of the important variables estimated by Symposium members. Similarly an "optimistic" case was constructed with values from the optimistic ends of the spectra of estimates. Specifically, the pessimistic case assumed the following:

1. Thirty percent (instead of 40% in the base case) of precancerous adenomatous polyps bleed before invasion.
2. Those that bleed are detectable an average of only 1.5 years (base case, average of 2 years) prior to invasion (maximum, 4 years).
3. The random false-negative rate of the FOBT is 55% (base case, 45%).

The optimistic case assumed that

1. Sixty percent of precancerous adenomatous polyps bleed before becoming invasive.
2. These polyps bleed an average of 3 years (maximum, 6 years) prior to invasion.
3. The random false-negative rate of the FOBT is 35%.

Both these cases simultaneously incorporate changes in three important variables, and it is unlikely that all three variables would take these extreme values. Thus, based on the judgments of the members of the Symposium, these two cases should be considered quite unlikely.

The results of these two cases are compared with the base case in Tables 5 and 6, Table 5 showing the effect of screening a man from age 50 to 75 with an annual FOBT only, and Table 6 showing the effect of screening a man from age

TABLE 5. Impact of Changes in Assumptions about the Effectiveness of FOBT on 50-Year-Old Average-Risk Male Screened from Age 50 to 75 with Annual FOBT

Effect	Optimistic case	Base case	Pessimistic case
Decrease in probability get colorectal cancer	21.7%	14.3%	5.8%
Decrease in probability die of colorectal cancer	36.4%	28.1%	18.2%
Increase in probability "cured," if get colorectal cancer or precancerous polyp	46.4%	35.7%	21.9%
Increase in life expectancy	53 days	41 days	25 days
Increase in life expectancy, if get colorectal cancer or precancerous polyp	2.46 years	1.90 years	1.21 years
Cost of screening and workups	$131	$131	$131
Decrease in cost of treatment	$76	$54	$28
Net financial cost	$55	$77	$103
Decrease in lost earnings	$220	$169	$106

50 to 75 with an annual FOBT and a rigid sigmoidoscopic examination every 3 years.

Table 5 shows that if the FOBT is used alone, in the pessimistic case the reduction in incidence of invasive cancer is about 6%, the decrease in probability a person dies of the disease is about 20% and the increase in proportion "cured" is also about 20%. In Table 6, adding sigmoidoscopy every 3 years to

TABLE 6. Effect of Screening with Annual FOBT and 3-Year Sigmoidoscopy on 50-Year-Old Average-Risk Male Screened from Age 50 to 75

Effect	Optimistic case	Base case	Pessimistic case
Decrease in probability get colorectal cancer	31.6%	24.7%	16.1%
Decrease in probability die of colorectal cancer	42.4%	36.4%	27.3%
Increase in probability "cured," if get colorectal cancer or precancerous polyp	57.2%	47.7%	35.1%
Increase in life expectancy	62 days	50 days	35 days
Increase in life expectancy, if get colorectal cancer or precancerous polyp	2.88 years	2.32 years	1.63 years
Cost of screening and workups	$284	$285	$285
Decrease in cost of treatment	$96	$75	$47
Net financial cost	$188	$210	$238
Decrease in lost earnings	$231	$177	$105

the "pessimistic" FOBT has a greater impact on the effectiveness of the screening program, because the FOBT is not as powerful as in the base case (Table 3). The optimistic assumptions yield higher estimates of the effectiveness of the FOBT, as shown in the tables. While the base case represents the best estimates of the Symposium members, there is uncertainty about the actual values of the important outcomes; Symposium members can be fairly certain that the actual values lie somewhere between the optimistic and pessimistic cases.

Sigmoidoscopy. The effectiveness of sigmoidoscopy is controlled primarily by the proportion of invasive cancers that arise from adenomatous polyps (assumed to be 90% in the base case), the time it takes a polyp to progress from first detectability by sigmoidoscopy to invasion (assumed to take an average of 7 years), and the random false-negative rate of the instrument (assumed to be 20%). The range in estimates provided by Symposium members was quite narrow for each of these factors, and changing assumptions about them within a reasonable range did not appreciably affect the estimated impact of screening strategies that employ sigmoidoscopy.

SUMMARY AND CONCLUSIONS

The estimates generated by this study can be used to help answer the questions posed in the introduction.

1. What proportion of invasive cancers can be prevented by finding and removing adenomatous polyps?

   With an annual FOBT, about 15%; with an annual FOBT and a rigid sigmoidoscopy every 3 years, about 25%

2. How much will screening change long-term survival?

   Screening will increase the chance a colorectal cancer patient will be cured (not die of the disease) by about 30 to 50%, depending on the screening strategy.

3. How much will mortality be decreased?

   By about one-third (20 to 40% depending on the strategy).

4. How long will screening prolong a patient's expected lifetime?

   With screening, the life expectancy of a colorectal cancer patient is increased by about 2 to 2.5 years, depending on the strategy.

5. How much will it cost and what are the risks?

   The lifetime costs vary from less than $100 to about $700, depending on the strategy. The main risk is from the workup of false-positive FOBT results. If a person is screened annually with an FOBT from age 50 to 75, he or she will have about a one in four chance of eventually needing a workup.

6. In terms of costs and resources, how does screening for colorectal cancer compare with other medical activities?

Considering the increase in life expectancy and the financial costs, screening adults for colorectal cancer appears to be a quite effective and efficient use of resources compared with other medical activities, delivering a person-year of life in a large population for about $1000.

7. What tests should be used?

Compared to annual tests with both FOBT and rigid sigmoidoscopy, an annual FOBT alone delivers about two-thirds of the effectiveness at about one-sixth the cost. Using a flexible sigmoidoscope rather than a rigid sigmoidoscope increases the benefit by about 25%, at an increase in cost of about 50%.

8. At what age?

Compared with screening with an annual FOBT from age 50 to 75, beginning screening at age 41 increases the benefit by about 17%, at about twice the cost.

9. At what frequency?

Compared with an annual FOBT, a biennial FOBT delivers about two-thirds of the benefit at about 40% the cost. Compared with an annual FOBT and an annual sigmoidoscopy, changing the frequency of sigmoidoscopies to every 3 years decreases the benefit by about 10%, while decreasing the cost by about 50%.

10. Is screening worth the effort?

These estimates do not directly answer the question as to whether screening for colorectal cancer is worthwhile, nor do they identify the "optimum" strategy or tell which screening age or frequency or choice of tests is the "best." In the end, these are value judgments requiring comparison of the potential benefits of different strategies with the costs and risks. The purpose of this analysis is to provide practicing physicians and health planners with some of the information needed to make those comparisons.

It should be stressed that the results of this analysis are estimates, estimates based on the judgments of a particular group of experts in colorectal cancer screening. The members of the Third International Symposium on Colorectal Cancer based their judgments on the most current information available from clinical trials and other research, but the data are incomplete and their judgments are subject to uncertainty. The estimates produced in this analysis must continually be reevaluated as new and better information becomes available. These results are offered on the rationale that today's decisions must necessarily be based on today's information and our best judgments about what it implies.

The author would like to thank Josephine Mauskopf, Ph.D for her valuable assistance. The preparation of this paper was supported by a grant from SmithKline Diagnostics.

REFERENCES

Anderson WAD (1974) Stage classification and end results reporting for carcinoma of the colon and rectum. Cancer 34:909–911.

Axtell LM, Asire AJ, Meyers MH, eds (1976) Cancer patient survival, Report Number 5, DHEW Publication No. (NIH)77–992. Bethesda, MD: National Cancer Institute.

Eddy DM (1980) Screening for cancer: Theory, analysis and design. Englewood Cliffs, NJ: Prentice-Hall, Inc.

Evans JT, Vana J, Aronoff BL, et al. (1978) Management and survival of carcinoma of the colon: Results of a national survey by the American College of Surgeons. Am Surg 188:716–720.

Falterman KW, Hill CB, Markey JC, et al. (1974) Cancer of the colon, rectum and anus: A review of 2313 cases. Cancer 34:951–959.

Godwin JD II, Brown CC (1975) Some prognostic factors in survival of patients with cancer of the colon and rectum. J Chron Dis 28:441–454.

Mettlin C, Natarajan N, Mittleman A, et al. (1982) Management and survival of adenocarcinoma of the rectum in the United States: Results of a national survey by the American College of Surgeons. Oncology 39:265–273.

Polissar L, Sim D, Francis A (1981) Survival of colorectal cancer patients in relation to duration of symptoms and other prognostic factors. Dis Colon Rectum 24:364–369.

Reilly JC, Rusia LC, Theuerkauf FJ (1982) Colonoscopy: Its role in cancer of the colon and rectum. Dis Colon Rectum 25:532–538.

Surveillance, Epidemiology, End Results (1981) Incidence and Mortality Data. 1973–77, NCI Monograph 57, USDHHS, PHS, NIH, NIH Publication No. 81–2330.

Third National Cancer Survey (1976) Hospitalizations and Payments to Hospitals. USDHEW, PHS, NIH, NCI.

RADIOLABELED ANTIBODIES IN THE TREATMENT OF PRIMARY LIVER MALIGNANCIES

STANLEY E ORDER, M.D., Sc.D., JERRY L KLEIN, Ph.D., PETER K LEICHNER, Ph.D., MOODY D WHARAM, M.D., JEANNIE CHAMBERS, R.N., KEN KOPHER, B.S., DAVID S ETTINGER, M.D., AND STANLEY S SIEGELMAN, M.D.

Several new concepts have emerged from our laboratory during the past decade, during which time modes of therapy using radiolabeled antibody have been developed and have reached phase I–II clinical trials. The laboratory research and clinical investigations have resulted in the following observations:

1. Specific antiserum against tumor-associated antigens may induce macrophage cytotoxicity as demonstrated in experimental ovarian cancer. This approach is now undergoing evaluation in a randomized prospective clinical trial (Order et al., 1973, 1974, 1981; Pino y Torres et al., 1982).
2. Specific antiserum in experimental ovarian cancer was additive to chemotherapeutic cytotoxicity (Davies and O'Neill, 1973; Ghose and Blair, 1957; Wright et al., 1979), and is now being clinically evaluated in a randomized prospective study (Pino y Torres et al., 1982).
3. Tumor antigens need not be "tumor specific," that is, totally unique, in order to allow preferential targeting by immunospecific radiolabeled antibodies as demonstrated in clinical scans in Hodgkin's disease and hepatoma (Order et al., 1980, 1981a) and, more recently, quantitated in an experimental hepatoma model (Rostock et al., 1983).
4. Polyclonal immunospecific antibody may be administered for tumor therapy, and the patients treated initially demonstrated hematopoietic toxicity that was dose related (Ettinger et al., 1979).
5. Tumor saturation with radiolabeled antibody may be achieved with modest doses of radiolabeled polyclonal antibody (30–20 mCi) (Leichner et al., 1981).
6. Cyclic administration of radiolabeled antibody may be achieved by altering the species of derivation of the immunoglobulin (presently rabbit, pig, chicken, and goat) (Order, 1982).

From the Departments of Radiation Oncology (SEO, JLK, PKL, MDW, JC, KK), Medical Oncology (DSE), and Diagnostic Radiology (SSS), The John Hopkins Hospital, Baltimore, Maryland.

7. Quantitation of tumor dose could be determined with radiolabeled antibody; at the present time this can best be evaluated in primary hepatic malignancies (Leichner et al., 1981).
8. The administration of polyclonal radiolabeled antibody in nonsensitized patients (skin and eye test negative) does not cause acute symptoms (Order et al., 1981b; Order, 1982).
9. Radiolabeled antibody may be administered concomitantly with chemotherapy, which may potentiate the dose rate effects of radiation (currently under study).

ANTIGENS

Ferritin

The antigen with which we have had the most experience has been ferritin, which has now been shown to be synthesized and secreted by T-lymphocytes in Hodgkin's disease (Sarcione et al., 1977), hepatoma cells (Beck and Bollack, 1974), the blast cell of acute myelogenous leukemia (White et al., 1974), some myeloma cells (Humphrey et al., 1982), and neuroblastoma (Hann et al, 1979). Ferritin is also a normal tissue component in the bone marrow, heart, and spleen, yet radioactive antiferritin IgG preferentially localizes in ferritin-bearing tumors. We have coined the term "biologic window" to describe the preferential effect of tumor localization by radiolabeled antibody (Order, 1982). This phenomenon will be described later in this review.

Carcinoembryonic Antigen

Carcinoembryonic antigen (CEA) occurs in a wide variety of malignancies and is of most practical value when a patient's tumor produces the antigen allowing monitoring of the serum level as a prognostic indicator. Controversy exists as to the value of radiolabeled antiCEA in the diagnosis of tumors bearing CEA (Mach et al., 1980). This will not be addressed by our review. In our experience, ^{131}I antiCEA is concentrated in intrahepatic biliary cancer in sufficient concentrations to warrant therapeutic investigation, whereas its reduced concentration in metastatic colon carcinoma requires investigation of other antigens before further therapeutic trials.

Alpha-Fetoprotein

The value of alpha-fetoprotein (AFP)-detecting hepatoma has been described (Matsumoto et al., 1982). To date, our own experience indicates that 20/61 hepatomas have had AFP elevations whereas >60% of the American hepatomas have not had elevated AFP titers. Clinical experience to date in our trial has indicated a poorer prognosis and the greater virulence of AFP positive hepatoma then in patients whose hepatoma lacks this biomarker.

INITIAL PILOT STUDIES OF PRIMARY LIVER TUMORS

Patients with primary liver malignancies were accepted into our initial program regardless of failure in previous therapeutic trials, metastatic disease, jaundice, and ascites. However, all patients were required to be capable of self-care to receive radiolabeled antibody. Realizing that the dosimetry of radiolabeled ^{131}I antiferritin or ^{131}I antiCEA was unknown, the treatment regimen began with external irradiation. Previous experience in the external irradiation of liver metastasis had indicated the relative efficacy of 2100 rad (Sherman et al., 1978; Order and Leibel, 1982) and the lack of significant toxicity of 2100 rad integrated with 15-mg doxorubicin (Adriamycin) and 500-mg 5-fluorouracil on alternate treatment days (Friedman et al., 1979). Remission of liver metastasis by external irradiation was known to be complete by the third week (>80%) and by the fourth week in all patients that remitted (Order and Leibel, 1982). Therefore, 1 month later, two cycles of Adriamycin 50 mg/M^2 and 600 mg/M^2 5-fluorouracil were given and followed 1 month later by single doses of ^{131}I antiferritin IgG (rabbit). New data was obtained that indicated the effective half-life whole body was 3 days or more and the tumor effective half-life was 3–7 days (effective half life = biological plus physical half-life). The administered dose was not related to tumor dose, but tumor volume and tumor dose were proportional in 11/12 patients studied (Order, 1982). Therefore, after having administered 50, 100, and 150 mCi to a series of patients, the administered dose was reduced to 50 mCi and the specific activity was altered from 1 mCi/2.5 mg IgG to 8 to 10 mCi/mg of IgG.

Initially, the effective half-life was reduced. However, we soon recognized that 50 mCi of ^{131}I incubated for 24 hours with 5 to 6 mg of IgG would lead to significant irradiation of the Fab end of the molecule. This might reduce the binding capacity of the Fab end by ionizing damage not sufficient to allow determination of damage in vitro but to alter in vivo binding. Therefore, we initiated studies to dilute the ^{131}I antiferritin IgG with immunospecific nonlabeled antiferritin, and later with normal rabbit IgG. Finally, human serum albumin was used, raising the concentration to 250 mg total protein as in our original preparations. The dilution with human serum albumin seemed to correct the adherence of antibody to the tumor by reducing radiolysis as reflected by the tumor effective half-life of 3 to 5 days. The use of human serum albumin dilution was not associated with acute reactions and was less costly than either immunospecific IgG or normal IgG as dilutents.

Based on physical data generated by transmission scans, daily probe readings over the tumor-bearing region, and computerized three-dimensional tumor volume reconstruction from CAT scans, tumor saturation was determined. Then a dose schedule of 30 mCi on day 0, and 20 mCi on day 5, was initiated and has become our standard regime with the present ^{131}I-labeled antiferritin IgG.

TOXICITY

To date, using Eastern Cooperative Oncology Group toxicity criteria, hematologic toxicity of leukopenia and thrombocytopenia were described (Ettinger et al., 1982). The hematologic depression occured 4 to 6 weeks after administration, with recovery most often evident by 8 weeks. Toxicity was dose dependent, and it was established that over 100 mCi led to significant depression. One patient who had received 150 mCi developed a minor cerebrovascular accident, recovered, and remains alive and in remission at 38 months. With the reduction in administered dose of ^{131}I antiferritin, there has been a reduction in hematopoietic toxicity. There was no acute toxicity in patients whose skin and eye sensitivity tests were negative before administration of radiolabeled antibody.

RESPONSE

In the initial studies of patients, remissions were noted. Remission was determined by physical examination, CAT scans, and planar and later volumetric tumor to normal tissue reconstruction in conjunction with laboratory tests and functional status.

As the studies have progressed, the use of cyclic radiolabeled antibody from different species, that is, rabbit, pig, chicken, and goat, every 2 months was introduced. This became the new approach in the phase I–II trial in hepatoma.

To date, the first 61 patients treated with the variety (different labeling ratios and diluents) of ^{131}I antiferritins preparations have been analyzed. The sepa-

FIGURE 1. The cumulative survival of alpha-feto protein positive hepatoma patients treated with radiation plus chemotherapy and not attaining self-care status (dashed line) and receiving ^{131}I radiolabeled antiferritin (solid line). Two of 13 patients receiving radiolabeled antiferritin were considered to demonstrate significant tumor remission.

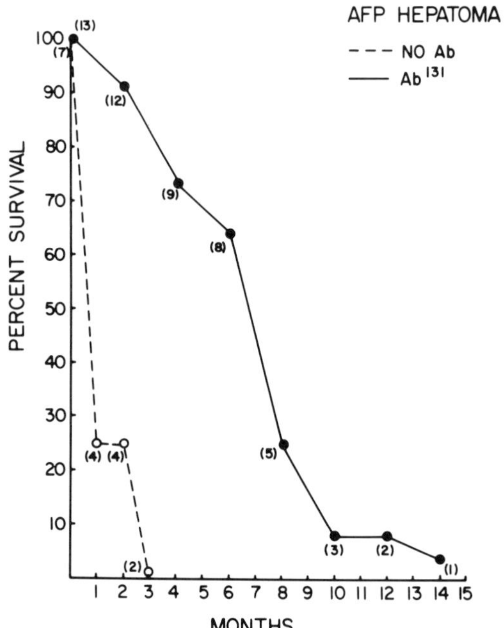

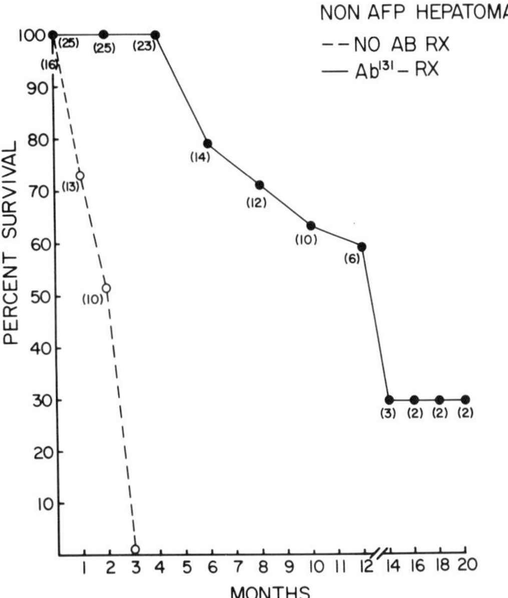

FIGURE 2. Patients with non-AFP hepatomas treated with radiation and chemotherapy and not attaining self-care for ^{131}I antiferritin administration (dashed line) and receiving ^{131}I antiferritin (solid line). Of 25 patients treated with radiolabeled antibody, 11 (44%) were considered to demonstrate tumor remission to radiolabeled antiferritin.

ration of hepatomas into those positive or negative for alpha-fetoprotein hepatomas appears to be valid based on these results. Of the 20 AFP positive patients, 7 patients received radiation and chemotherapy with a median survival of 1 month. The 13 patients who were capable of self-care and received radiolabeled antibody had a median survival of 6 months. However, we considered only 2 of 13 patients with AFP positive hepatomas that received radiolabeled antibody to have shown signficant tumor remission following radiolabled antiferritin (Figure 1).

In contrast, 41 patients with non-AFP hepatomas were treated with radiation, and chemotherapy. Of the 41 non-AFP hepatoma patients, 16 were not capable of self-care at the end of their treatment course (therefore, they did not receive radiolabeled antibody) and had a median survival of more than 2 months. Twenty-five patients were administered radiolabeled antiferritin and had a median survival of greater than 12 months (Figure 2). Eleven of 25 patients (44%) have had objective remissions and represent an advance in the treatment of this malignancy (Figure 3).

INTRAHEPATIC BILIARY CARCINOMA

Of seven patients treated with the same protocol design as in the pilot hepatoma studies except for the use of ^{131}I antiCEA, six patients received radiolabeled antiCEA. One patient did not remit with initial therapy (external beam and

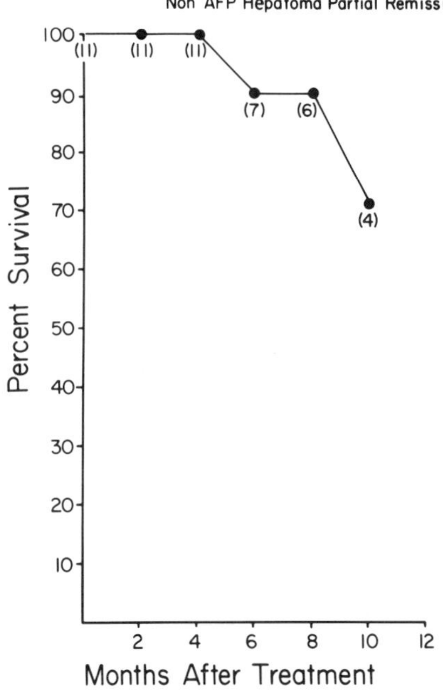

FIGURE 3. (**A**) cumulative survival of non-AFP hepatoma patients treated with ^{131}I antiferritin that demonstrated tumor remission.

(**B**) Volumetric reconstruction from serial CAT scans of a patient that had failed chemotherapy and autologous bone marrow transplant and responded to radiolabeled antiferritin. The patient remains in remission.

chemotherapy) and could not receive radiolabeled antibody. Of the six remaining patients that received ^{131}I antiCEA, one patient had such severe ascites as to not target the tumor, but instead lost the antibody into the peritoneal space. Of the five remaining patients, one was AFP positive and had no response and four responded for 5, 11, 15, and 27 months. None of the patients were treated at the time of the present protocol with cyclic radiolabeled antibody, although one patient achieved two cycles and a 15-month remission (Figure 4). However, we have been able to establish that 20 mCi ^{131}I antiCEA saturates the tumor volume in intrahepatic biliary cancer and may be followed by 10 mCi during the second administration day 4–5 for resaturation of the tumor.

PRESENT CONCLUSIONS

It has been established that radiolabeled antibody to tumor-associated antigens was capable of targeting hepatic malignancies for therapeutic purposes without significant acute toxicity. The major toxicity was hematopoietic depression, and it was related to the administered dose. Primary liver malignancies were ideal, since they allowed for quantitation of tumor dose due to present technologic approaches with CAT scan–tumor volume reconstruction and clearly definable masses. Remission rates in nonAFP hepatomas suggest the usefulness of further protocol development toward a phase III randomized prospective trial. However, a new investigative approach is needed for those with AFP-positive hepatoma and we are presently investigating ^{131}I antiAFP.

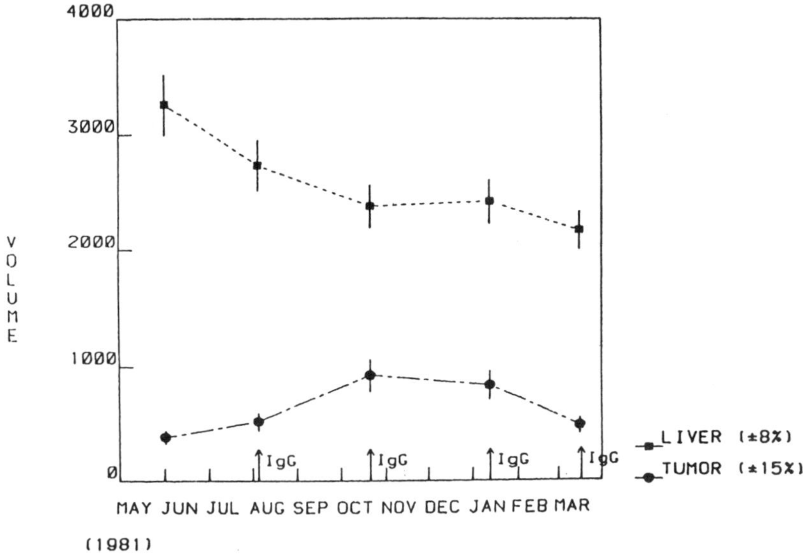

FIGURE 3.B

FIGURE 4. Tumor volume and normal tissue volume reconstruction of a patient's serial CAT scans demonstrating remission following ^{131}I antiCEA IgG. The duration of remission was 15 months prior to intraperitoneal dissemination.

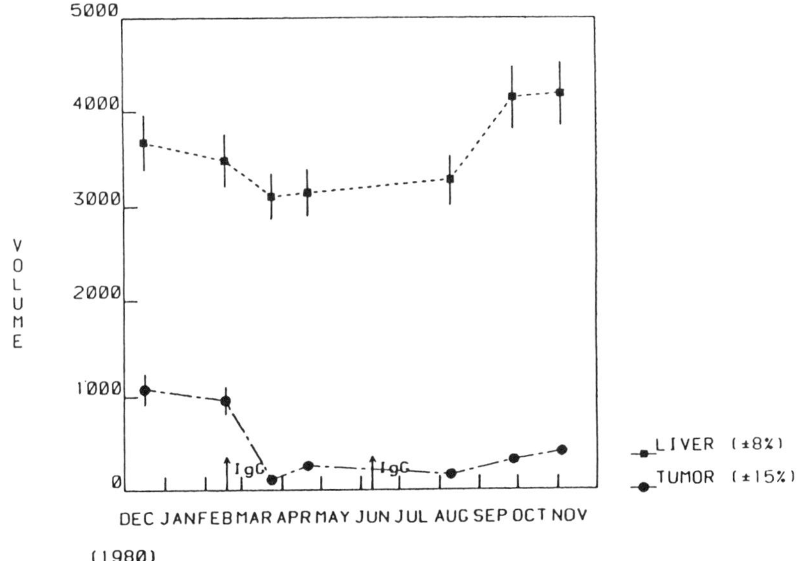

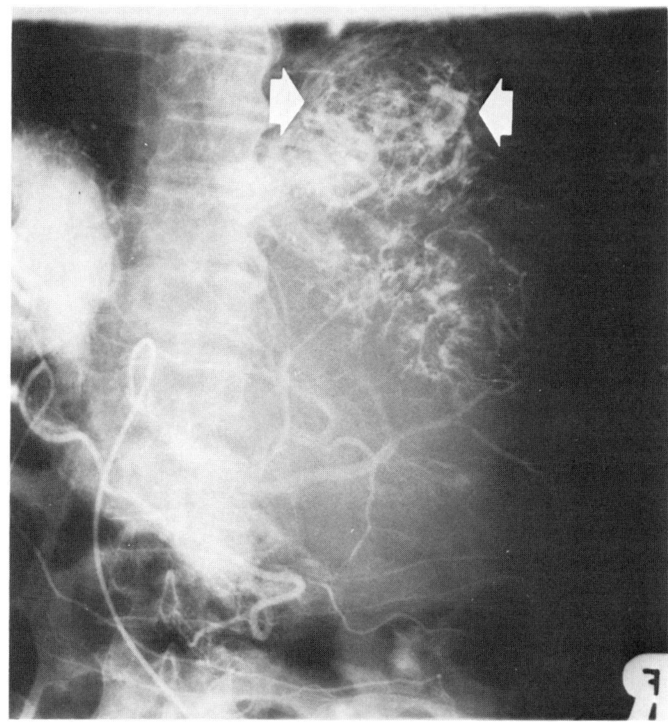

FIGURE 5. (**A**) Arteriographic study of a ferritin positive hepatoma. (**B**) Technitium^{99} scan of the same patient's hepatoma. (**C**) Gallium scan demonstrating gallium uptake in the tumor ferritin. (**D**) Computed tomogram (CT) of the patient's tumor (arrows) with central necrosis (the darkest region). (**E**) Before (a) and after (b) computer axial tomograms of the patient treated with ^{131}I antiferritin IgG, presently with the longest remission 3 years.

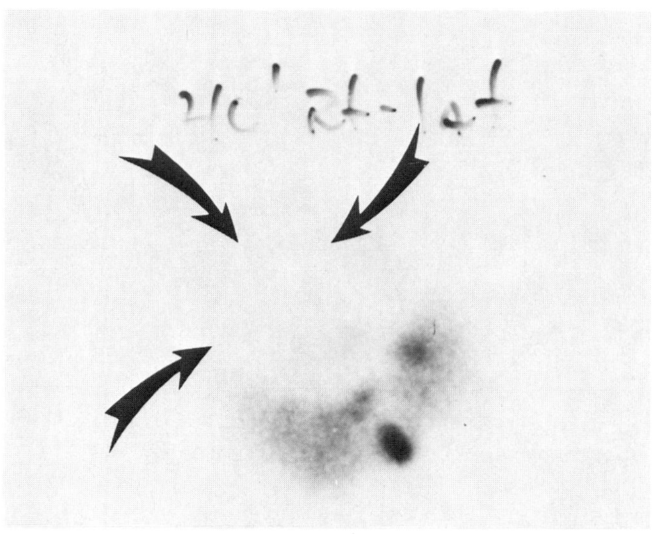

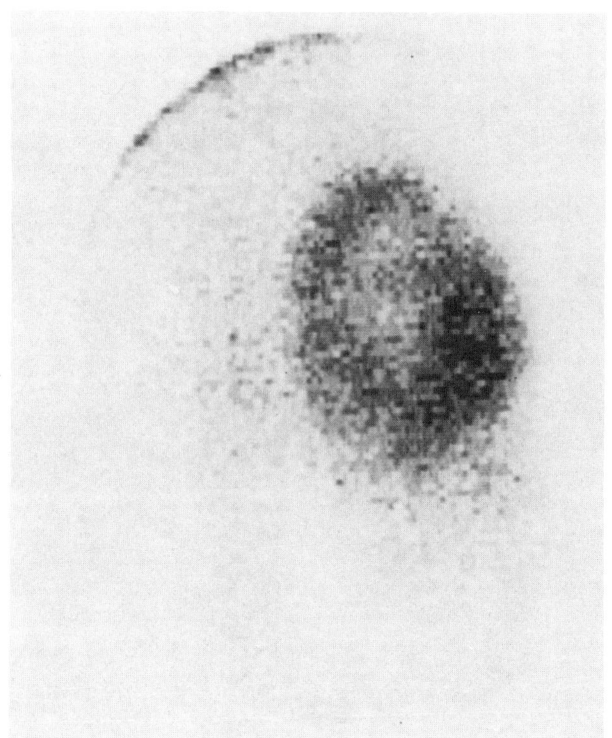

FIGURE 5.C

FIGURE 5.D

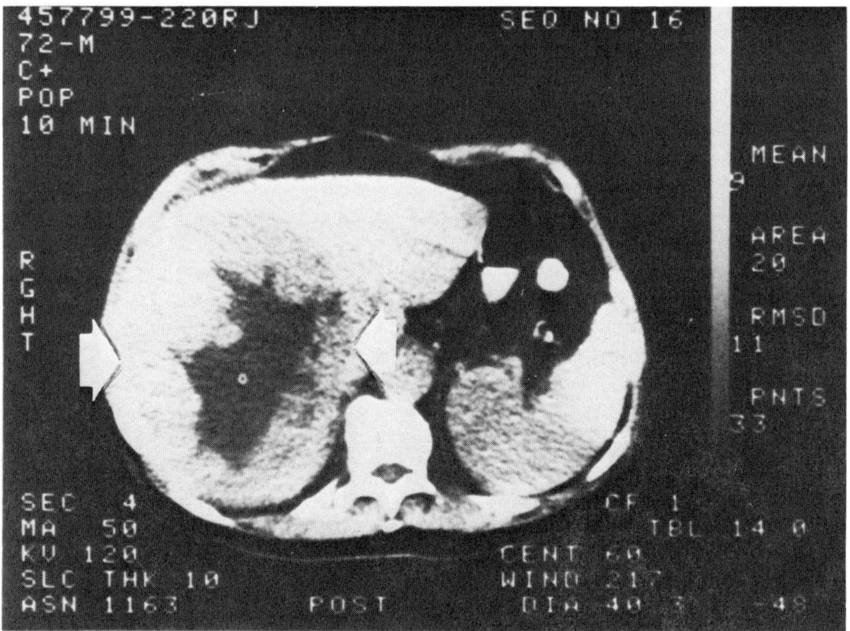

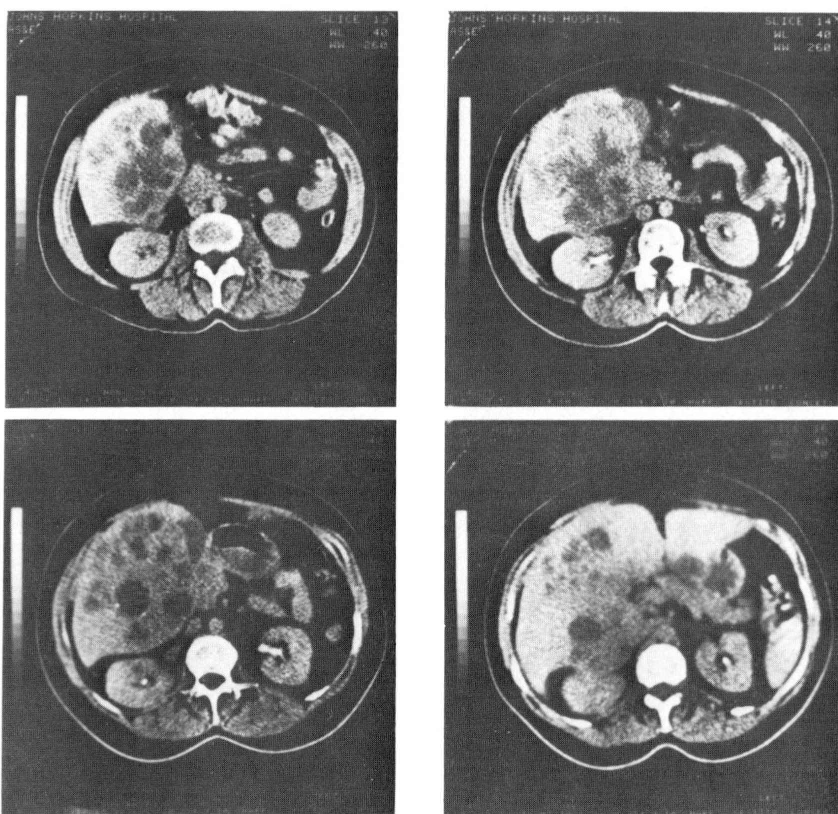

FIGURE 5.E (a)

Our studies have established the feasibility of cyclic radiolabeled antibody administration by altering species of origin. The "biologic window" that allows preferential radiolabeled antibody targeting to tumors probably consists of the neovasculature, which lacks smooth muscle; the slower circulation in tumors; and the high concentration of tumor-associated proteins (Order, 1982). The neovasculature was shown in a patient with hepatoma using arteriographic studies; the ^{99}Tc scan showed a defect caused by lack of tumor uptake, whereas the gallium scan demonstrates the spherical tumor mass (Figure 5). Gallium is deposited in tumor ferritin (Claussen et al., 1974). Therefore, the correlation of these special features of the malignancy, namely neovasculature, increased ferritin concentration, and slow blood flow, aid in understanding the dynamics of preferential tumor binding by radiolabeled antiferritin.

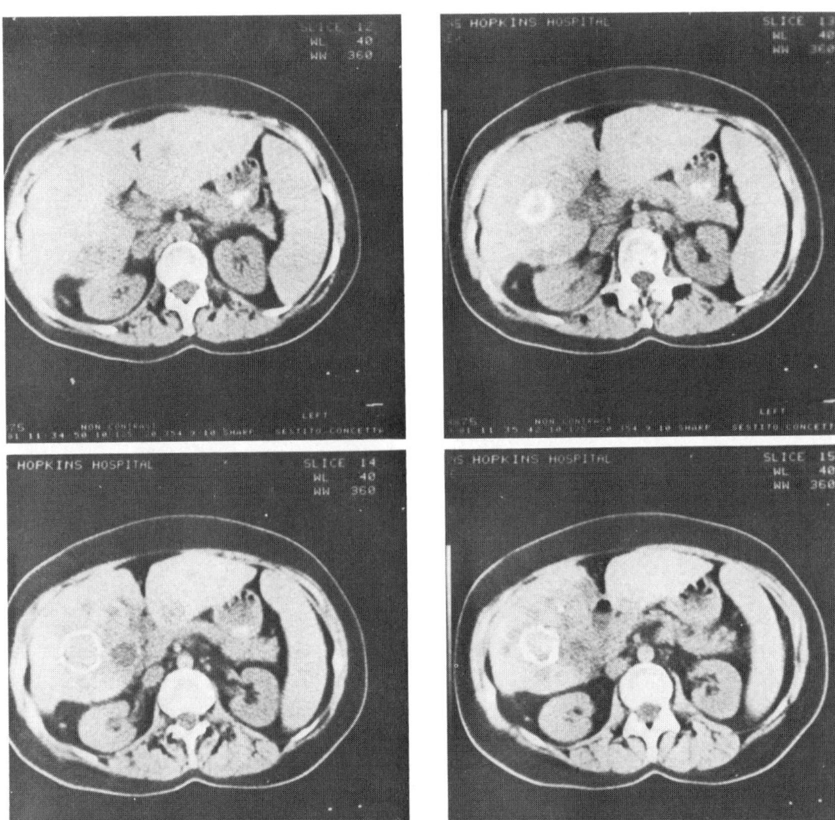

FIGURE 5.E (b)

NEW APPROACHES

Our next studies prior to the randomized phase III trial seek to take advantage of the potentiation of radiation by Adriamycin (Sherman et al., 1982), an active agent in the treatment of hepatoma, and 5-fluorouracil, a cytotoxic agent often additive in its effect with external irradiation. Dose escalation of Adriamycin and 5FU with fixed doses of radiolabeled antiferritin is now being studied. New isotopic labels are being explored and if successful could replace the present ^{131}I label.

Monoclonal antibody directed against ferritin when radiolabeled with ^{131}I unfortunately dehalogenates the label (Order, 1982). The same was true for monoclonal antiCEA when labeled with ^{131}I. New monoclonal antibody labels are presently being investigated. The chief advantage of monoclonal antibody could be the potential increase in antibody deposition. However, restriction as to the number of times monoclonal antibody may be administered has recently been shown by Sears and Coworkers (1982), where monoclonal sensitization against immune IgG occurred in three-fourths patients after 1 week of administration. Unfortunately, multispecies-derived monoclonal antibodies are not available, although they may be in the future.

Our conclusions to date are that radiolabeled antibody represents a new and important opportunity in cancer therapy that has shown preliminary effectiveness in hepatoma. The new developments outlined represent just a few of the approaches that will be brought to bear in treating hepatoma and primary intrahepatic biliary cancer. The principles learned in the treatment of hepatoma may result in newer approaches in other gastrointestinal malignancies, including liver metastases, as more is learned about the use of radiolabeled antibody in cancer therapy.

Supported by National Institute of Health, National Cancer Institute grant CA-06973-18, Radiation Therapy Oncology Group (Luther Brady, Chairman, CA-21661).

REFERENCES

Beck G, Bollack C (1974) Synthesis of ferritin in cultured hepatoma cells. Fed Exp Biol Soc 47:314–317.

Claussen J, Edeling CJ, Fogh J (1974) Ga binding to human serum proteins and tumor components. Cancer Res 34:1931–1937.

Davies DAL, O'Neill GJ (1973) In vivo and in vitro effects of tumor specific antibodies with chlorambucil. Br J Cancer 28:285–298.

Ettinger DS, Dragon LH, Klein J, et al. (1979) Isotopic immunoglobulin in an integrated multimodal treatment program for a primary liver cancer: A case report. Cancer Treatm Rep 63:131–134.

Ettinger DS, Order SE, Wharam MD, et al. (1982) Phase I–II study of isotopic immunoglobulin therapy for primary liver cancer. Cancer Treatm Rep 66:289–297.

Friedman M, Cassiday M, Levine M, et al. (1979) Combined modality treatment of hepatic metastases. Cancer 44:906–913.

Ghose T, Blair AA (1978) Antibody-linked cytotoxic agents in the treatment of cancer. Current status and future projects. J Natl Cancer Inst 61:651–676.

Hann HL, Levy HM, Evans AE, Drysdale JW (1979) Serum ferritin and neuroblastoma. Proc Am Soc Clin Oncol 20:126.

Humphrey RL, Frondoza CG, Trivedi SM, et al. (1982) Synthesis—secretion of ferritin by human and mouse myeloma tumor cells. FASEB. Abstract 1660.

Kim EE, Deland FH, Nelson MO, et al. (1980) Radioimmunodetection of cancer with radiolabeled antibodies to alpha-fetoprotein. Cancer Res 40:3008–3012.

Leichner PK, Klein JL, Garrison JR, et al. (1981) Dosimetry of I-131 labeled anti-ferritin in hepatoma: A model for radioimmunoglobulin dosimetry. Int J Radiat Oncol Biol Phys 7:323–333.

Mach JP, Carrel S, Forni M, et al. (1980) Tumor localization of radiolabeled antibodies against carcinoembryonic antigen in patients with carcinoma: A critical evaluation. N Eng J Med 303:5–10.

Matsumoto Y, Suziki T, Asad I et al. (1982) Clinical classification of hepatoma in Japan according to serial changes in serum alpha-fetoprotein levels. Cancer 49:354–360.

Order SE (1982) Monoclonal antibodies potential role in radiation therapy and oncology. Int J Radiat Oncol Biol Phys 8:1193–1201.

Order SE, (1984) Radioimmunoglobulin therapy of cancer. Compr Ther 9–18.

Order SE, Leibel SA (1982) Combined hepatic irradiation and misonidazole for palliation of liver metastases. In: Weiss L, Gilbert H, eds., Liver Metastasis. Boston: G. K. Hall, pp. 629–636.

Order SE, Donahue V, Knapp R (1973) Immunotherapy of ovarian carcinoma: An experimental model. Cancer 32:573–579.

Order SE, Kirkman R, Knapp R (1974) Serologic immunotherapy: Results and probable mechanism of action. Cancer 34:175–183.

Order SE, Klein JL, Ettinger D, et al. (1980) Phase I–II study of radiolabeled antibody integrated in the treatment of primary hepatic malignancies. Int J Radiat Oncol Biol Phys. 6:703–710.

Order SE, Klein JL, Leichner P (1981a) Antiferritin IgG antibody for isotopic cancer therapy. Oncology 38:154–160.

Order SE, Rosenshein J, Klein JL, et al. (1981b) The integration of new therapies and radiation in the management of ovarian cancer. Cancer 48:604–606.

Pino y Torres J, Hernandez E, Rosenshein N, et al. (1982) Multimodality treatment of advanced ovarian carcinoma. Int J Radiat Oncol Biol Phys. 8:1671–1677.

Rostock RA, Klein JL, Leichner PK, et al. (1983) Selective tumor localization in hepatoma by radiolabeled antiferritin. Int J Radiat Oncol Biol Phys 9:1345–1350.

Sarcione EJ, Smalley JR, Lenia MJ, Stutzman L (1977) Increased ferritin synthesis and release by Hodgkin's disease peripheral blood lymphocytes. Int J Cancer 20:339–346.

Sears HF, Mattis J, Herlyn, et al. (1982) Phase I clinical trial of monoclonal antibody in treatment of gastrointestinal tumors. Lancet 762–765.

Sherman D, Weichselbaum R, Order SE, et al. (1978) Palliation of hepatic metastasis. Cancer 41:2013–2017.

Sherman DM, Carabell SC, Belli JA, Hellman S (1982) The effects of dose rate and adriamycin on the tolerance of thoracic radiation in mice. Int J Radiat Oncol Biol Phys 8:45–51.

White GP, Worwood M, Parry DH, Jacobs A (1974) Ferritin synthesis in normal and leukemic leukocytes. Nature 250:584–586.

Wright T, Sinanan M, Harrington D, et al. (1979) Immunoglobulin: Applications to scanning and treatment. Appl Radiol 120–124.

THE ROLE OF HEPATITIS B VIRUS IN PRIMARY HEPATOCELLULAR CARCINOMA

ARIE J ZUCKERMAN, M.D., D.Sc., F.R.C.P., F.R.C.Path.

The role of viral hepatitis in the pathogenesis of chronic liver disease has been debated for many years. After the development of specific laboratory tests for markers of infection with hepatitis B virus, an association between hepatitis B macronodular cirrhosis and primary hepatocellular carcinoma became apparent. Zuckerman (1974) noted that the epidemiology of liver cancer does not display the properties of an infectious disease and outlined the criteria that were required to establish the progression of hepatitis B to primary hepatocellular carcinoma since hepatitis B is ubiquitous, particularly in Africa and southeast Asia.

The problem is whether the virus is the driver or the passenger. The evidence needed must show that infection precedes the development of cancer, that the tumor cells contain virus-specific molecules or antigens, that the malignant cells produce the agent, and that the virus can transform cells in culture or induce liver cancer in experimental animals. Most importantly, it must be shown that immunization against the infectious agent will lower the incidence of cancer.

Most of these criteria have now been largely met. The currently available evidence for the implication of hepatitis B virus in the pathogenesis of hepatocellular carcinoma is based on epidemiologic and geographic observations of a strong correlation between hepatitis B infection and primary liver cancer. These include a relatively constant risk of developing primary hepatocellular carcinoma in both endemic and nonendemic areas among male persistent carriers of hepatitis B surface antigen where infection precedes and may accompany the development of cancer, usually in a liver with chronic damage or macronodular cirrhosis. Hepatitis B antigens are present in the malignant tis-

From the Department of Medical Microbiology, and WHO Collaborating Centre for Reference and Research on Viral Hepatitis, London School of Hygiene and Tropical Medicine (University of London).

sue, and there is evidence of covalent integration of the genome of hepatitis B virus into the DNA of the tumor cells.

Several cell lines derived from primary hepatocellular carcinoma secrete hepatitis B surface antigen in culture, and DNA has been shown to be integrated into the genome of these cells as well as in RNA molecules containing specific sequences of hepatitis B virus. At least one of these cell lines has been shown to be heterotransplantable. The final piece of evidence is the finding of chronic liver damage and primary liver cancer in several animal species infected with viruses that are phylogenetically related to human hepatitis B virus.

PROPERTIES OF HEPATITIS B VIRUS AND SEROLOGIC MARKERS OF INFECTION

Examination by electron microscopy of serum containing hepatitis B surface antigen reveals the presence of small spherical particles measuring about 22 nm in diameter, tubular forms of varying length with a diameter close to 22 nm, and large double-shelled or solid particles approximately 42 nm in diameter (Figure 1). The large particles contain a core or nucleocapsid about 28 nm in diameter. The 42-nm particle is the hepatitis B virus (Dane particle), whereas the small 22-nm particles and the tubules are noninfectious surplus virus coat protein.

The core of the virus contains a DNA-dependent DNA polymerase, which is closely associated with a DNA template. Double-stranded circular DNA has been extracted from circulating virus and also from cores of the virus isolated from the nuclei of infected hepatocytes. The molecular weight of the DNA is about 2.3×10^6, and the DNA is approximately 3200 nucleotides in length, containing a single-stranded gap varying from 600 to 2100 nucleotides. The endogenous DNA polymerase appears to repair the gap.

Infection with hepatitis B virus results in the appearance in the plasma during the incubation period of hepatitis B surface antigen about 2 to 8 weeks before biochemical evidence of liver dysfunction or the onset of jaundice. The surface antigen persists during the acute illness; it is usually cleared from the circulation during convalescence. Next to appear in the circulation is a specific hepatitis B DNA polymerase associated with the core of the virus. At about the same time another antigen, the e antigen, becomes detectable, again preceding serum aminotransferase elevations. The e antigen is a distinct soluble antigen that is located within the core and correlates closely with the number of complete virus particles and relative infectivity.

Antibody to the hepatitis B core antigen is found in the serum 2 to 4 weeks after the appearance of the surface antigen. It is always detectable during the early acute phase of the illness. Core antibody of the IgM class becomes undetectable within some months of the onset of uncomplicated acute infection, but IgG core antibody persists after recovery for many years, and possibly for life. The next antibody to appear in the circulation is directed against the e antigen. There is evidence that anti-e indicates relatively low infectivity of serum (McCollum and Zuckerman, 1981). Antibody to the surface antigen component, hepatitis B surface antibody, is the last marker to appear late in convalescence

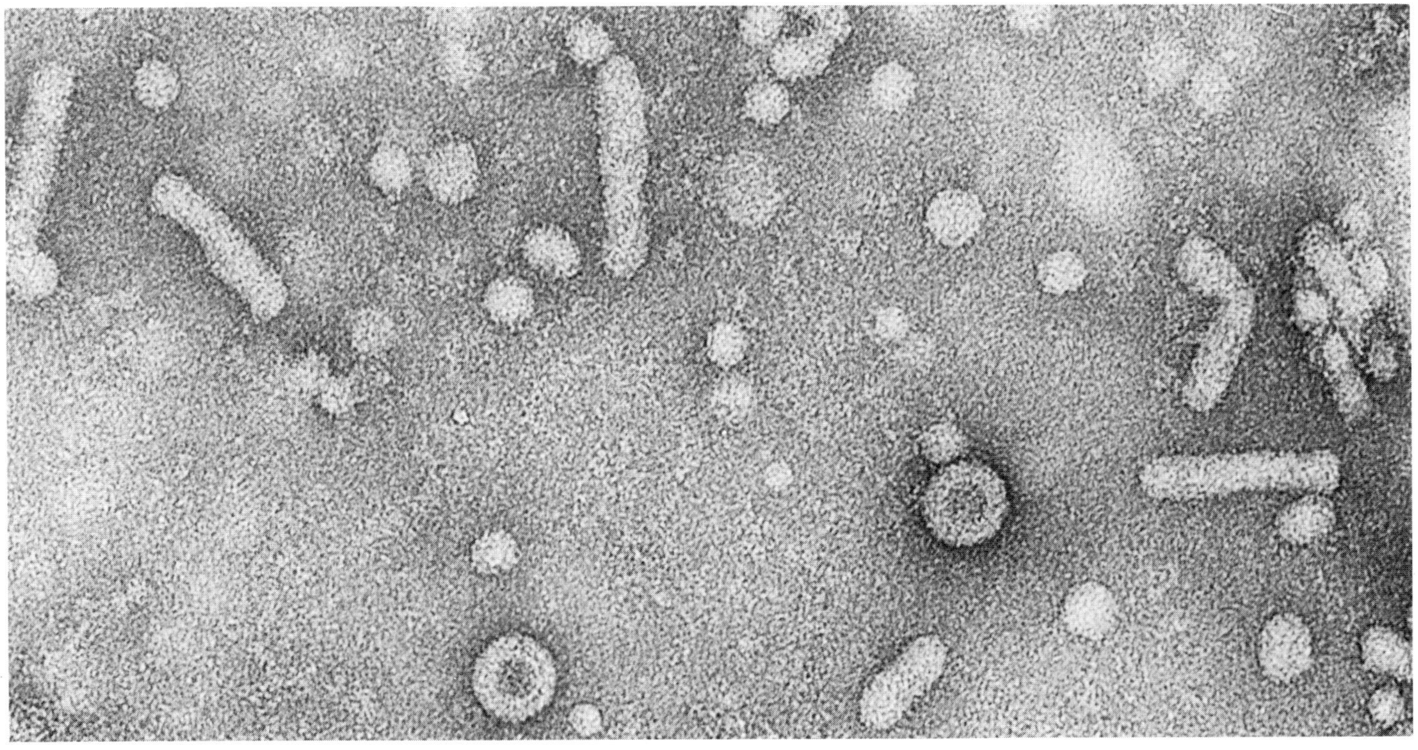

FIGURE 1. Electron microscopy of serum containing hepatitis B virus and surface antigen. Three distinct morphologic entities are present: small pleomorphic spherical particles (20–25-nm diameter), tubular forms of varying length, and large spherical particles (approximately 42-nm diameter), some of which are penetrated by negative stain to reveal an inner core of 28-nm diameter. (Negative stain, ammonium molybdate; final magnification × 252,000.) *Source:* Reproduced with permission from Zuckerman (1975).

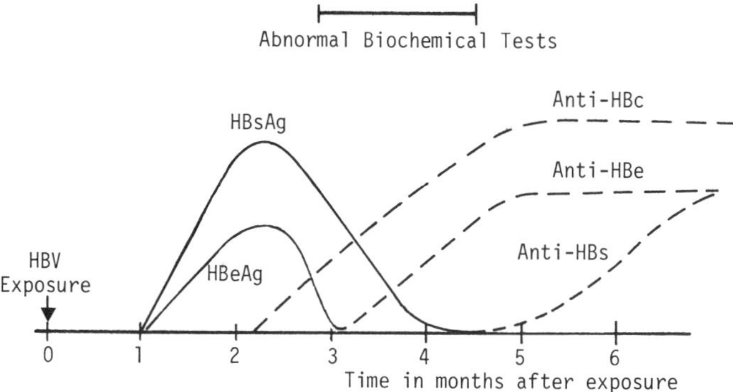

FIGURE 2. Serological course of uncomplicated acute hepatitis B with recovery. *Source:* McCollum and Zuckerman (1981).

(Figure 2). Precipitating antibodies reacting with antigenic determinants on the complete virus particle have also been described. These antibodies may be important for clearing circulating hepatitis B virions. Their absence in patients with chronic active hepatitis may explain why the infection persists. Cell-mediated immunity also appears to be important in terminating hepatitis B infection and possibly in promoting liver damage and in the genesis of autoimmunity.

THE CARRIER STATE OF HEPATITIS B VIRUS

Survival and persistence of hepatitis B virus in the population on a global scale is ensured by a huge reservoir of carriers, estimated conservatively to number between 175 and 200 million. Prolonged "shedding" of the virus occurs in a proportion of carriers by varied mechanisms and routes of transmission, including perinatal infection, and the virus is relatively stable in the environment (reviewed by Zuckerman, 1982).

As a result of longitudinal studies of patients with hepatitis B, the persistent carrier state is defined as the presence of hepatitis B surface antigen in blood for more than 6 months (WHO Report, 1977). Such a carrier state may be associated with liver damage ranging from minor changes in the nucleus of the hepatocytes to chronic persistent hepatitis, chronic active hepatitis, and cirrhosis, with persistence of the viral component in the hepatocytes.

Extensive seroepidemiologic surveys in many parts of the world have shown that the prevalence of hepatitis B surface antigen in apparently healthy persons varies from 0.1% to 20%. Europe may be roughly divided into three regions, with a low prevalence area of about 0.1% or less in northern countries, 0.1 to 3% in some central and eastern European countries, and about 5% and even higher in some countries bordering the Mediterranean. The prevalence in North America and Australia is 0.1% or less, 3–5% or higher in Asia, and 15–20% or more in several tropical countries. It should be noted, however, that the information on the global distribution of hepatitis B surface antigen is incomplete and standardized techniques and reagents have not been uniformly used.

Several risk factors have been identified that increase the risk of developing the carrier state. It is more common in males, more likely to follow infections acquired in childhood than those acquired in adult life, and the carrier state is more likely to occur in patients with natural or acquired immune deficiencies.

In countries in which infection with hepatitis B virus is relatively uncommon, the highest prevalence of the surface antigen is found in the 20 to 40 years age group. The prevalence of surface antibody increases steadily with age. In countries where infection with hepatitis B virus is common, the highest prevalence of the surface antigen is observed in children 4 to 8 years old, with declining rates among older age groups. The decline in antigen carriage rates with age suggests that the carrier state is not invariably lifelong.

The carrier state of hepatitis B is characterized serologically by persistence of hepatitis B surface antigen, with or without detectable complete virion and generally in the absence of measurable surface antibody. Core antibody is present, often in high titer, and in some persistent carriers IgM core antibody remains detectable. In some carriers, hepatitis B DNA polymerase is found, often with fluctuating levels, and hepatitis B e antigen persists. In other carriers, specific DNA polymerase is not detectable and anti-e is present. Hepatitis B e antigen has been found more commonly in young than in adult carriers, while the prevalence of anti-e seems to increase with age. These observations suggest that young carriers may be the most infective.

EPIDEMIOLOGIC AND GEOGRAPHIC CORRELATIONS BETWEEN HEPATITIS B INFECTION AND PRIMARY HEPATOCELLULAR CARCINOMA

Many studies in different parts of the world, particularly in Africa, Asia, and the Mediterranean region (especially in Greece), show a highly significant excess of surface antigen, core antibody, and surface antibody in patients with primary hepatocellular carcinoma (reviewed by Szmuness, 1978; Maupas and Melnick, 1981). It has been suggested that an important factor in the possible etiologic association between hepatitis B and liver cell carcinoma may lie in an early age of infection. In areas of the world where the prevalence of macronodular cirrhosis and primary hepatocellular carcinoma is high, infection with hepatitis B virus and development of the persistent carrier state occur most frequently in infants and children. Of the many published reports, the following two surveys have been selected as examples:

A case-control study of patients with primary hepatocellular carcinoma and their families was carried out in Dakar, Senegal, by Larouze and colleagues (1976). Nearly all the 28 patients with hepatocellular carcinoma (96%) and most of the 28 matched controls (93%) had some serologic evidence of infection with hepatitis B virus, but the patients with carcinoma were less likely to have surface antibody. Seventy-one percent of the mothers of the patients were positive for the surface antigen, whereas only 14.3% of the mothers of the control subjects were antigen-positive. Similar observations have also been made in Taiwan (see Szmuness, 1978). These observations suggest that the patients with carcinoma acquired the infection early in life and probably from their mothers during the perinatal period (see Zuckerman, 1974).

The results of a large survey were reported by Beasley and coworkers (1981). Between 1975–1978, 22,707 male Chinese civil servants in Taiwan were enrolled in a prospective study to determine the relative risk of primary hepatocellular carcinoma among carriers of hepatitis B surface antigen and to determine whether the carrier state precedes the development of this neoplasm. Among the subjects, 81.6% were aged between 40 and 59 years and 3,454 (15.2%) were carriers of the antigen. The carrier rate is the same as that in other groups of men of the same age in Taiwan, and the mortality rate from primary liver cancer and cirrhosis is approximately the same as that in the general population.

Active surveillance involved annual completion of a health questionnaire and retesting for markers of hepatitis B infection. Adherence to the follow-up program average 95% annually, and the cause of death was unknown in only 0.3% of the original recruits. By the end of 1980, approximately 75,000 man-years of follow-up were carried out, an average of 3.3 years per man. There was a marked excess of deaths from primary hepatocellular carcinoma and cirrhosis in carriers of hepatitis B surface antigen on recruitment. Forty out of the 41 men who died of primary hepatocellular carcinoma were in the group of 3454 antigen carriers and only one was in the group of 19,253 antigen-negative men, giving a relative risk of 223. Thus, the incidence of primary liver cancer among carriers of the surface antigen was 1158 per 100,000, whereas it was 5 per 100,000 among noncarriers during 75,000 man-years of follow-up. There was also a large excess mortality from cirrhosis among antigen-positive men—17 out of 19 men who died from cirrhosis were antigen-positive. Primary liver cancer and cirrhosis together accounted for 57 out of 105 deaths among the antigen-positive men (54.3%), compared with 3 out of 202 deaths among those without the antigen (1.5%). Together, primary hepatocellular carcinoma and cirrhosis accounted for 20% of all deaths in this study. The results of this prospective study also clearly establish that the carrier state of hepatitis B surface antigen commonly precedes primary hepatocellular carcinoma in Chinese men. The very high relative risk found in this study, and the many case-control studies in various parts of the world, suggest that hepatitis B virus is closely associated with the process leading to primary liver cancer and that it is not simply a risk factor.

PRODUCTION OF HEPATITIS B SURFACE ANTIGEN BY CELL LINES DERIVED FROM HUMAN HEPATOCELLULAR CARCINOMA

The failure to cultivate hepatitis B virus in tissue culture and the lack of susceptibility of available laboratory animals (other than chimpanzees) to infection with this virus have made it difficult to study many aspects of the biology of hepatitis B. However, the establishment of continuous cell lines from human hepatocellular carcinoma that produce hepatitis B surface antigen provide a laboratory model system. The first of these cell lines, the PLC/PRF/5 cell line described by Alexander and coworkers (1976) and Macnab and coworkers (1976), produces hepatitis B surface antigen similar in size, morphology, and polypeptide composition to the form that occurs in the serum of naturally infected individuals (Stannard and Alexander, 1977; Skelly et al., 1979). Hepatitis B core antigen, e antigen, and DNA polymerase have not been detected in the cells and the media of these cultures. Aden and coworkers (1979) described the second hepatitis B surface antigen-producing cell line, Hep 3B, which differs in some ways from the PLC/PRF/5 cells. A third hepatocellular carcinoma cell line, DELSH-5, was established by Das and coworkers (1980). This cell line released hepatitis B surface antigen into the medium from the thirteenth passage onward and, like the Hep 3B cells, the cells synthesized albumin and alpha-fetoprotein.

INTEGRATION OF HEPATITIS B VIRAL DNA IN THE PLC/PRF/5 CELL LINE

Marion and colleagues (1980a) reported that the PLC/PRF/5 cells contained approximately four copies of viral DNA per haploid, mammalian cell DNA equivalent. Evidence was obtained that DNA from all regions of the viral genome is present in these cells, suggesting that the cells contain most, and possibly all, of the viral genome. Furthermore, the results indicated that the viral DNA is integrated in high molecular weight DNA at three different sites in the cells and that there is no viral DNA in an episomal form (DNA molecules outside the chromosome capable of independent replication). Cellular RNA radiolabeled with ^{32}P was found to hybridize with all restriction fragments of hepatitis B virus DNA, which suggests that most, and possibly all, of the viral DNA in these cells is transcribed.

Chakraborty and coworkers (1980) also presented evidence for integration of the DNA of hepatitis B virus into the host genome of the PLC/PRF/5 cells and for expression of three RNA molecules containing specific sequences of hepatitis B virus. In order to study the expression of viral RNA in this cell line, total cytoplasmic and nuclear RNAs were isolated and separated into poly $(A)^+$ (that is, fractions possessing a long track of polyadenosine at the terminal end of the molecule) and poly $(A)^-$ fractions (fractions lacking a polyadenosine tail), and hepatitis B virus sequences were identified by hybridization with a ^{32}P-hepatitis B virus probe. The total cytoplasmic poly $(A)^+$ RNA revealed two bands containing virus sequences. The sedimentation coefficient of these two bands was 21.5 S and 19.5 S. There were three bands in the total nuclear RNA: 27 S, 21.5 S, and 19.5 S. The 21.5 S and 19.5 S bands probably represent the same components found in the cytoplasm. The biologic activity and function of these viral RNAs are not known. The presence of poly (A) tail in the 21.5 S and 19.5 S RNA species suggests that they represent specific viral mRNAs. Either the 21.5 S or the 19.5 S poly $(A)^+$ viral RNA probably codes for hepatitis B surface antigen. The finished polypeptide of a molecular weight 25,000 may be derived by posttranslational processing of a larger precursor. Since the PLC/PRF/5 cells produce only one recognized viral protein, the surface antigen of hepatitis of B virus, the role of the other two viral specific RNAs is not known. These RNAs may code for nonstructural proteins that do not become incorporated into the mature virus as occurs in other viral infections.

Using a modification of the Southern blot-transfer hybridization technique and cloned hepatitis B virus DNA as a probe, Brechot and coworkers (1980) demonstrated the integration of viral DNA in the cellular genome of human hepatocellular carcinoma tissue and in the PLC/PRF/5 cell line. The results suggest the existence of a limited number of integration sites in the cellular DNA, which is consistent either with the development of the liver tumor from one clone with several integration sites or with its development from a few clones each having particular integration sites. Other observations suggest the presence of two or more whole viral genomes inserted in tandem head-to-tail. It was pointed out, however, that the demonstration of integrated DNA sequences of hepatitis B virus is not sufficient proof of the role of this virus in the etiology of human primary hepatocellular carcinoma, although this is an additional argument in favor of this view.

Edman and coworkers (1980) also showed that sequences of hepatitis B virus are integrated into a minimum of six different sites in the DNA of the PLC/PRF/5 cells. The results of the experiments suggest that the nicked cohesive end region of the DNA of hepatitis B virus (namely, the incomplete DNA possessing complimentary terminals that permit integration of the DNA) coincides with the region of integration of at least several viral fragments. It has been suggested that retroviruses, which are known integrating viruses, have a circular structure with terminally redundant ends that serve as the precursor to integration (see also Summers and Mason, 1982). Such a structure could be formed in hepatitis B virus by repair of the nicked region with the endogenous polymerase activity, resulting in a structure that contains a terminally redundant sequence. These authors also pointed out that integration of the hepatitis B virus in a malignant cell does not imply that the virus is the oncogenic agent. However, viral transformation is usually associated with the integration of viral sequences into host chromosomal DNA. If hepatitis B virus is an oncogenic virus, the transforming event producing the PLC/PRF/5 cells might have involved the expression of the hepatitis B surface antigen gene or be some function of the integration of the virus.

HETEROTRANSPLANTABILITY OF THE PLC/PRF/5 CELLS

Desmyter and coworkers (1980) induced tumors in 80% or more of nude mice (Pfd:NMRI/nu-nu) injected subcutaneously with 5–10 $\times$ 10^6 cells. The tumors usually became detectable after 2 weeks and grew up to 15 to 30% of the body weight of the mice. Metastases were not found. When the cells were inoculated intraperitoneally, multiple tumors developed in various abdominal organs. The histology of the tumors was that of a well-differentiated human hepatocellular carcinoma. Hepatitis B surface antigen was demonstrated by immunofluorescence in 0.1 to 10% of the tumor cells. Hepatitis B surface antigen, but no other serologic marker of the virus, was found in the serum of the tumor-bearing mice. Newborn and weanling nude mice were equally susceptible.

The tumors were serially transplantable three to five times, but the take rates decreased with each passage, although there were no obvious differences between first-passage and later-passage tumors. The take rates were better when pieces of tumor were transplanted rather than trypsinized tumor cells. It was also possible to clone cells from the tumors, and their progeny induced tumors.

Similar tumors were obtained in nude, athymic rats (Rowett Pfd:WIST-rnu-

rnu), although the rats were less susceptible than nude mice. Similar results have been reported by Bassendine and colleagues (1980) and by other investigators.

INTEGRATION OF HEPATITIS B VIRUS DNA INTO THE GENOME OF LIVER CELLS

Lutwick and Robinson (1977) and Summers and colleagues (1978a) reported the finding of hepatitis B virus DNA in primary hepatocellular carcinoma tissue. The application of recombinant DNA and molecular hybridization techniques has allowed more precise analysis of DNA sequences in living cells. DNA restriction enzyme mapping, radiolabeling of purified recombinant DNA probes of high specific activity, and improved techniques of gel electrophoresis allow the detection of specific DNA sequences in amounts smaller than 1 pg, that is, less than 0.1 copy per haploid genome equivalent. Furthermore, on a weight comparison basis, molecular hybridization is approximately 1000 times more sensitive than radioimmunoassay. Hybridization may therefore also provide a more sensitive and direct test for detecting hepatitis B virus in serum, blood product, body fluids, and vaccines.

Shafritz and Kew (1981) examined extracts of DNA from hepatocellular carcinomas from 13 patients for hepatitis B Virus (HBV) DNA sequences by molecular hybridization using ^{32}P-labeled recombinant, cloned, and purified HBV-DNA. Hepatitis B surface antigen was present in the serum of eight of these patients, and HBV-DNA sequences were found to be integrated into the host genome in carcinomatous tissues in each patient. The integration pattern was unique for each tumor. Hepatitis B virus DNA was not found in DNA extracts from the tumors of five patients who were not carriers of the surface antigen. Brechot and coworkers (1981a) used the Southern blot-transfer hybridization technique to examine tissue extracted DNA immobilized on nitrocellulose paper by hybridization with cloned hepatitis B virus DNA (HBV-DNA) as a probe labeled with ^{32}P by the nick translation procedure.

Viral DNA was found to be integrated into cellular DNA in both liver tumor and nontumor tissue in patients with primary hepatocellular carcinoma as demonstrated by hybridization of high molecular weight DNA after digestion with *Hind* III and *Eco* R1 endonucleases. Integrated HBV-DNA was also found in patients with cirrhosis, with or without chronic active hepatitis. Free HBV-DNA was found in the liver in two patients with chronic persistent hepatitis and one patient with chronic active hepatitis. The intense smear in the gel with an upper limit at the 3.2 kb position after digestion with *Hind* III indicates large quanity of free HBV-DNA in the liver. This may be due to viral multiplication and molecular heterogeneity due to the single-stranded region of the viral DNA, which is of variable length. However, free viral DNA in large amounts may be trapped in the host DNA during electrophoresis, causing smearing throughout the track that may mask the presence of any small amount of integrated DNA. Restriction endonuclease patterns in two patients with acute hepatitis B strongly suggested HBV-DNA integration. If these findings are confirmed by the examination of a large number of patients with acute hepatitis B, then viral integration seems to occur early in the course of infection.

In a further study using the same technique, Brechot and coworkers (1981b) found two different types of persistent carriers of hepatitis B virus: The first type is characterized by viral multiplication, with free viral DNA in the liver and viral DNA and hepatitis B e antigen in the serum. Integrated HBV-DNA was also present, at least in some of these carriers. The second type of the persistent carrier state is characterized by the presence of only integrated HBV-DNA sequences in the liver; viral DNA and e antigen were not found in the serum. However, free viral DNA was found in the livers of two e antigen-negative patients, and HBV-DNA was also detected in the serum of one of these patients. The detection of HBV-DNA in the serum of this patient probably reflects the presence of the complete virion.

Shafritz and colleagues (1981) also used recombinant DNA techniques and gel electrophoresis for the detection of hepatitis B virus DNA in liver cells of patients with primary hepatocellular carcinoma and chronic liver disease. Integrated hepatitis B virus DNA (HBV-DNA) was found in patients with primary hepatocellular carcinoma in whom viral DNA sequences were present. (In several tumors, however, the hybridization signal was weak and integration was difficult to assess. When tumors and livers had extensive fibrosis, difficulty was experienced in detecting HBV-DNA sequences in known carriers of the surface antigen, probably because of dilution of HBV sequences by DNA from fibroblasts and stromal cells. DNA degradation also occurred sometimes, particularly in necrotic tissue, which occasionally resulted in loss of specific HBV-DNA integration bands).

When the extracted DNA was intact, virtually all HBV-DNA sequences were integrated into the host cell genome in hepatocellular carcinomas, and in each tumor the integration pattern was unique. In one patient with partial DNA degradation, low molecular weight extrachromosomal HBV-DNA was also present. In some specimens of liver tissue adjacent to tumors, extrachromosomal and integrated HBV-DNA were present. The presence of integrated HBV-DNA in nontumor tissue from patients with hepatocellular carcinoma suggests that integration precedes development of gross neoplasia. Integrated HBV-DNA was present in tumors from all patients whose serum was positive for the surface antigen and also in three patients in whose serum surface antibody was present but who were serologically negative for the antigen. This finding indicates that there is no simple correlation between serum markers of hepatitis B virus and HBV-DNA in the tumor.

In carriers of hepatitis B virus with or without histologic evidence of chronic liver disease, HBV-DNA was present in liver specimens in two forms, either as the full length double-stranded HBV-DNA or as double-stranded DNA with a gap in one strand (as in the circulating virus). Integrated DNA was not found in most of the carriers with relatively recent history of liver disease. However, in two patients who were long-term carriers, there was diffuse hybridization in the high molecular weight regions of the gel. Free viral DNA was not identified. In these cases, it is possible that HBV-DNA is integrated diffusely throughout the host genome. Such integration might precede a stage in persistent infection with hepatitis B virus during which a specific subpopulation of hepatocytes undergoes cellular division into a clonal focus containing integrated HBV-DNA in one of a few specific sites. Additional factors may then be involved, perhaps years later, in the development of neoplasia from such a clonal focus.

Although many questions remain to be answered (reviewed by Prince, 1981), molecular biology is providing definitive evidence for covalent integration of the genome of hepatitis B virus into the cellular DNA in hepatocellular carcinomatous tissue, suggesting a possible sequence of events of infections of hepatocytes culminating in malignant transformation.

ANIMAL VIRUSES THAT ARE PHYLOGENETICALLY RELATED TO HUMAN HEPATITIS B VIRUS

Snyder (1968) reported the presence of liver cancer in 22 out of 76 eastern woodchucks *(Marmota monax)* that lived longer than 4 years in an established colony. In addition, the lesions of chronic active hepatitis and sometimes cirrhosis were usually found in the nontumor tissue. Examination by electron microscopy of sera collected from the captive woodchucks revealed virus particles that closely resemble human hepatitis B virus (Summers et al., 1978b). Human hepatitis B virus and the woodchuck hepatitis virus share the following characteristics. Infection with either virus results in the accumulation in blood of large amounts of excess virus coat protein in the form of spherical and tubular particles measuring 20 to 25 nm in diameter. Both are 40- to 50-nm double-shelled or solid particles with a nucleocapsid or core containing double-stranded circular DNA with a gap, and both contain a viral DNA polymerase. Each virus is associated with chronic hepatitis and primary hepatocellular carcinoma. Werner and coworkers (1979) identified a high degree of antigenic cross-reactivity between the cores of the two viruses but only minor common antigenic determinants on the virus surface protein. A small region of 100 to 150 base pairs of nucleic acid homology, measured by liquid hybridization, was found in the genomes of the two viruses. It seems likely that this 3 to 5% of nucleic acid homology represents one or two regions of nearly identical nucleotide sequence.

This degree of nucleic acid homology has been detected among papovaviruses, for example between SV40 and BK virus. Cummings and coworkers (1980) cloned the DNA of human hepatitis B virus and the DNA of woodchuck hepatitis virus in the vector lambda-gtWES. This was then subcloned into the kanamycin-resistant plasmid pA01. Comparison of the recombinant DNAs with authentic virus DNAs by specific hybridization, size, and restriction enzyme analysis indicated that the recombinants contained the complete genome of each virus. The nucleic acid homology between the two viral DNAs was confirmed with the cloned DNAs. Thus the woodchuck hepatitis virus and the human hepatitis B virus are phylogenetically related. The analogy between the two viruses is even closer when judged by their adaptation in their respective hosts causing persistent infection and close association with chronic liver disease and primary liver cancer.

Another virus related to human hepatitis B has been described in Beechey ground squirrels *(Spermophilus beecheyi)* in northern California (Marion et al., 1980b). Common features with the human hepatitis B virus include virus morphology, size and structure of the viral DNA, a virion DNA polymerase that repairs a single-stranded region in the double-stranded circular genome, cross-reacting surface viral antigens, antigen-antibody systems similar to hepatitis B e antigen and the core antigen, and persistent infection with viral antigen present continuously in the blood. Because the ground squirrels were only bled and then released, it was not possible to observe a disease accompanying this virus in the ground squirrel. Antigenic and structural relationships between the surface antigens of the human hepatitis B virus, the ground squirrel hepatitis virus, and the woodchuck hepatitis virus have been described more recently (Feitelson, 1981).

A fourth possible member of this class of viruses was described by Snyder (1979) in black-tailed prairie dogs *(Cynonys ludoviccianus)* of the family Sciuridae, a close relative of the woodchuck. Hepatitis and hepatocellular carcinoma were found in prairie dogs, and positive orcein staining of liver cells implies a surface antigen similar to human hepatitis B virus. Virologic studies, however, have not yet been reported. A fifth member of this virus group is being investigated in Pekin ducks *(Anas domesticus)* in the People's Republic of China and in commercial flocks of ducks in the United States originally imported from China many years ago. This species of duck develops primary liver cancer, and a DNA virus similar morphologically to human hepatitis B virus has been identified. The viral genome is circular and partially single-stranded. An endogenous DNA polymerase can convert the DNA genome to a complete double-stranded circular form with a size of approximately 3000 base pairs. Examination for viral DNA in the organs of infected birds revealed preferential localization in the liver. The virus is transmitted vertically, and infected ducklings may develop persistent viraemia (Mason, et al., 1980).

More recently, it was found that the DNA genome of hepatitis B-like viruses is reverse transcribed through an RNA intermediate. There are differences and similarities to the strategy of replication of the retroviruses, and it has been proposed that hepatitis B viruses are a group of reverse transcribing viruses differing from all known retroviruses (Summers and Mason, 1982).

In summary, therefore, various studies have established that there is a strong and specific association between persistent hepatitis B virus infection and primary hepatocellular carcinoma, and it is likely that this association is causal (McCollum and Zuckerman, 1981). However, factors other than hepatitis B virus are implicated. It is possible that primary liver cancer is the cumulative result of several cofactors or hepatocarcinogens including genetic, immunologic, nutritional, and hormonal factors, mycotoxins, chemical carcinogens and other environmental influences, and that hepatitis B virus acts either as a carcinogen or as a cocarcinogen in persistently infected hepatocytes (Zuckerman, 1978).

REFERENCES

Aden, DP, Fogel A, Plotkin S, et al. (1979) Controlled synthesis of HBsAg in a differentiated human liver carcinoma-derived cell line. Nature 282:615–616.

Alexander JJ, Bey EM, Geddes EW, Lecatsas G (1976) Establishment of a continuously growing cell line from primary carcinoma of the liver. S Afr Med J 50:2124–2128.

Bassendine MF, Arborgh BAM, Shipton N, et al. (1980) Hepatitis B surface antigen and alpha-fetoprotein secreting human primary liver cancer in athymic mice. Gastroenterology 79:528–532.

Beasley, RP, Hwang L-Y, Lin C-C, Chien C-S (1981) Hepatocellular carcinoma and hepatitis B virus: A prospective study of 22,707 men in Taiwan. Lancet 2:1129–1133.

Brechot C, Pourcel C, Louisa A, et al. (1980) Presence of integrated hepatitis B virus DNA sequences in cellular DNA of human hepatocellular carcinoma. Nature 286:533–535.

Brechot C, Hadchouel M, Scotto J, et al. (1981a) State of hepatitis B virus DNA in hepatocytes of patients with hepatitis B surface antigen-positive and -negative liver diseases. Proc Nat Acad Sci USA 78:3906–3910.

Brechot C, Hadchouel M, Scotto J, et. al. (1981b) Detection of hepatitis B virus DNA in liver and serum: A direct appraisal of the chronic carrier state. Lancet 2:765–768.

Chackraborty PR, Ruiz-Opazo N, Shouval D, Shafritz D (1980) Identification of integrated hepatitis B virus DNA and expression of viral RNA in an HBsAg-producing hepatocellular carcinoma cell line. Nature 286:531–533.

Cummings IW, Browne JK Salser WA, et al. (1980) Isolation, characterisation and comparison of recombinant DNAs derived from genomes of human hepatitis B virus and woodchuck hepatitis virus. Proc Nat Acad Sci USA 77:1842–1846.

Das PK, Nayak NC, Tsiquaye KN, Zuckerman AJ (1980) Establishment of a human hepatoma carcinoma cell line releasing hepatitis B surface antigen. Br J Exp Pathol 61:648–654.

Desmyter J, de Groote J, Ray MB, et al. (1980) HBsAg-producing human hepatoma cell line: Tumours in nude mice and interferon properties. In: Bianchi L, Gerok W, Sinkinger K, Stalder GA, eds., Virus and the Liver. Lancaster, Eng.: MTP Press, pp. 217–221.

Edman, JC, Gray P, Valenzuela P, et al. (1980) Integration of hepatitis B virus sequences and their expression in a human hepatoma cell. Nature 286:535–538.

Feitelson MA, Marion PL, and Robinson WS (1981) Antigenic and structural relationships of the surface antigens of hepatitis B virus, ground squirrel hepatitis virus, and woodchuck hepatitis virus. J Virol 39:447–454.

Larouze B, London WT, Saimot G, et al. (1976) Host responses to hepatitis B infection in patients with primary hepatic carcinoma and their families: A case-control study in Senegal, West Africa. Lancet 2:534–538.

Lutwick LI, Robinson WS (1977) DNA synthesized in the hepatitis B Dane particle DNA polymerase reaction. J Virol 21:96–104.

McCollum RW, Zuckerman AJ (1981) Viral hepatitis: Report on a WHO informal consultation. J Med Virol 8:1–29.

Macnab GM, Alexander JJ, Lecatsas G, et al. (1976) Hepatitis B surface antigen produced by a human hepatoma cell line. Br Cancer 34:509–515.

Marion PL, Salazar FH, Alexander JJ, Robinson WS (1980a) State of hepatitis B viral DNA in a human hepatoma cell line. J Virol 33:795–806.

Marion PL, Oshiro L, Regnery DC, et al. (1980b) A virus in Beechey ground squirrels which is related to hepatitis B virus of man. Proc Nat Acad Sci USA 77:2941–2945.

Mason WS, Seal G, Summers J (1980) Virus of Pekin ducks with structural and biological relatedness to human hepatitis B virus. J Virol 36:829–836.

Maupas PH, Melnick JL, Eds. (1981) Hepatitis B virus and primary hepatocellular carcinoma. Prog. Med Virol 27:1–210.

Prince AM (1981) Hepatitis B virus and hepatocellular carcinoma molecular biology provides further evidence for an etiologic association. Hepatology 1:73–75.

Shafritz DA, Kew MC (1981) Identification of integrated hepatitis B virus DNA sequences in human hepatocellular carcinomas. Hepatology 1:1–8.

Shafritz DA, Shouval D, Sherman HI, et al. (1981) Integration of hepatitis B virus DNA into the genome of liver cells in chronic liver disease and hepatocellular carcinoma studies in percutaneous liver biopsies and post-mortem tissue specimens. N Eng J Med 305:1067–1073.

Skelly J, Copeland JA, Howard CR, Zuckerman AJ (1979) Hepatitis B surface antigen produced by a human hepatoma cell line. Nature 282:617–618.

Snyder RL (1968) Hepatomas of captive woodchucks. Am J Pathol 52:32.

Snyder RL (1979) Hepatitis and hepatocellular carcinoma in captive prairie dogs (*Cynomys ludovicianus*). In: Sonderdruck aus Verhandlungsbericht des XXI, International Symposiums über die Erkrankungen der Zootiere. Berlin: Akademie Verlag, pp. 325–328.

Stannard LM, Alexander J (1977) Electron microscopy of HBsAg from human hepatoma cell line. Lancet 2:713.

Summers J, Mason WS (1982) Properties of hepatitis B-like viruses related to their taxonomic classification. Hepatology 2 (Suppl):61S–66S.

Summers J, O'Connell A, Maupas P, et al. (1978a) Hepatitis B virus DNA in primary hepatocellular carcinoma. J Med Virol 2:207–214.

Summers J, Smolec MJ, Snyder RL (1978b) A virus similar to human hepatitis B virus associated with hepatitis and hepatoma in woodchucks. Proc Nat Acad Sci USA 75:4533–4537.

Szmuness W (1978) Hepatocellular carcinoma and the hepatitis B virus: Evidence for a causal association. Prog Med Virol 24:40–69.

Werner BG., Smolec JM, Snyder RL, Summers J (1979) Serological relationship of woodchuck hepatitis virus to human hepatitis B virus. J Virol 32:314–322.

WHO Report (1977) Advances in viral hepatitis. Report of the WHO Expert Committee on Viral Hepatitis. Technical Report Series, No. 602, Geneva.

Zuckerman AJ (1974) Viral hepatitis, the B antigen and liver cancer. Cell 1:65–67.

Zuckerman AJ (1975) Human Viral Hepatitis. Amsterdam, Elsevier.

Zuckerman, AJ (1978) Hepatocellular carcinoma and hepatitis B. Trans Soc Trop Med Hyg 71:459–461.

Zuckerman AJ (1982) Persistence of hepatitis B virus in the population. In: Mahy BWJ, Minson AC, Darby, GK, eds., Virus persistence. Cambridge, Eng.: Cambridge University Press, pp. 39–56.

MECHANISMS OF ADENOMA FORMATION IN THE COLON

ALAIN P MASKENS, M.D.

The sequence of events from normal epithelial cells to a fully developed adenoma is incompletely understood. Yet, from the many classic or more recent works devoted to this question, it is now possible to give a rather detailed account of the successive phases that characterize this process. Such a description will in turn clarify some of the mechanisms involved, while pointing to new and challenging questions.

Until 1962, our information in this field was essentially based on histologic analyses of minute polyps. In 1962, Deschner and coworkers introduced a means of incorporating tritiated thymidine (3H-TdR) into colorectal biopsies in vitro, enabling subtle proliferative defects preceding the emergence of adenomas to be traced.

THE TUBULAR ADENOMA

Benign neoplasms originating in the colorectal epithelium constitute frequent findings in patients from Western countries. In autopsy studies, their prevalence can be as high as 37 to 51% of the population aged 50 or more (Day, 1982).

Two main histologic types can be recognized. The tubular adenoma is characterized by an accumulation of irregular neoplastic glands primarily in the upper aspect of the mucosa, which becomes thicker. Epithelial cells are crowded and more deeply stained, with hyperchromatic nuclei. The typical tubular adenoma appears as a small sessile or pedunculated nodule. In a large surgical series, 76.6% of the tubular adenomas were less than 1 cm, and only 3.7% were larger than 2 cm (Muto et al., 1975). In familial polyposis coli (FPC) specimens, 89% of the polyps were less than 0.5 cm, and only 1% were more than 1 cm (Bussey, 1975). Foci of carcinoma are rare in the small tubular ade-

From the Groupe de Recherche Alimentation et Cancer, Brussels.

nomas, with an occurrence of about 1% in surgical or endoscopic series (Haot et al., 1979; Muto et al., 1975). In untreated FPC patients, the yearly rate of cancer incidence, as computed from Bussey's observations (Bussey, 1975), is about 3%, or a transformation rate of 1 per 33,000 polyps per annum (Maskens, 1982).

The main features of villous tumors are in sharp contrast to those of tubular adenomas. They are essentially constituted by villi, crests, and other projecting structures that develop from the mucosal surface into the lumen. These tumors are usually sessile and reach very large sizes. In the surgical series of Muto and coworkers (1975), 60.3% of the villous tumors had a size greater than 2 cm. Also, the frequency with which foci of cancer are found in such lesions is very high, ranging from 13% (Haot et al., 1979) to 55% (Enterline et al., 1962). In some polyps, the coexistence of glandular and villous elements on histologic examination can make the distinction between tubular and villous adenomas quite difficult. While some investigators refer to "villoglandular" (Morson and Dawson, 1972), "intermediate" (Muto et al., 1975), or "tubulovillous" (WHO, 1976) polyps, others prefer to classify them together with the villous tumors (Haot et al., 1979) because they behave rather similarly with respect to size and cancer risk (Fung and Goldman, 1970; Kurzon et al., 1974; Muto et al., 1975).

Among the two main types of neoplastic colorectal polyps, the tubular adenomas are much more frequent. In surgical series, they can represent 75% of the observed lesions compared with 9% for the villous tumors and 16% for "intermediate" histologic types (Muto et al., 1975). In patients suffering from FPC, an average of about 1000 tubular adenomas can be found per patient, while villous tumors remain rare (Bussey, 1975).

In the present study, the analysis will be restricted to the small tubular adenoma, which, as just seen, forms a well-defined pathologic entity and represents the most frequent colonic neoplasm.

SUCCESSIVE PHASES IN THE EMERGENCE OF A TUBULAR ADENOMA

The Normal Crypt

The colorectal mucosa is essentially composed of a regular succession of cylindrical glands perpendicular to the intestinal lumen, the "crypts of Lieberkuhn." These glands are lined by epithelial cells exhibiting an increasing degree of maturation from base to neck of the crypts. Two main cell lines can be distinguished: absorptive (columnar) and goblet cells. Occasionally, argentaffin and, more rarely, Paneth cells can be recognized at the bottom of crypts (Deschner and Lipkin, 1966, 1978). The layer of epithelial cells is tightly surrounded by a "pericryptal sheath" (Kaye et al., 1968; Maskens et al., 1979), consisting of the epithelial basement lamina, on which all epithelial cells are attached, as well as collagen fibers and fibroblasts. The latter appear as fusiform cells closely lining the outside of the crypt. The pericryptal sheath is in continuity with the lamina propria, a loose network of connective fibers filling the spaces between crypts and containing reticular cells, macrophages, lymphocytes, other inflammatory cells, and blood capillaries.

In normal adults, the epithelium is actively renewing, with a turnover time

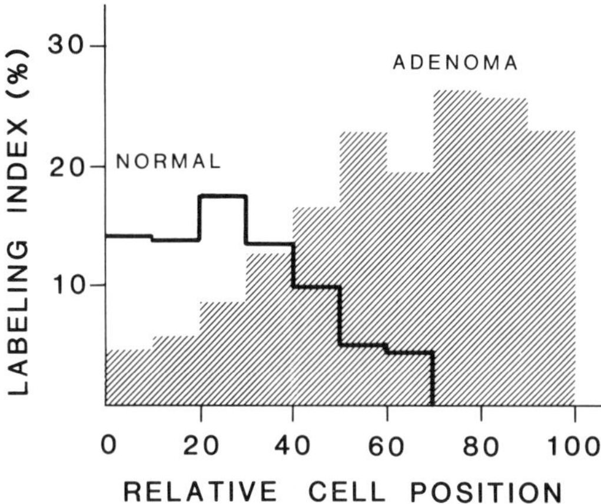

FIGURE 1. Tritium labeling index (LI) at various levels of normal and adenomatous human colon crypts, as observed on autoradiographic preparations after in vitro incorporation of tritiated thymidine (3H-TdR). Cell positions are counted from gland base to luminal surface; glands are normalized to 100 cell positions, so that position 0 represents the base of the gland and position 100 the junction between crypt and surface epithelium. In normal crypts, cell proliferation is restricted to the lower two thirds of crypt height. Adenomatous crypts are characterized by an increased LI and an upward shift of the proliferative compartment, which predominates in their upper aspect.

of about 3 to 8 days (Cole and McKalen, 1961; Lipkin et al., 1963; McDonald et al., 1964). Of importance is the constant observation that DNA synthesis activity is always confined to the lower two thirds of the crypts, with a clear preponderance in the lower third (Figure 1). As newly produced cells migrate upward, the probability of entering a new mitotic cycle rapidly declines. In the upper third of crypts, this probability is very low (Deschner et al., 1963; Maskens and Deschner, 1977; Maskens, 1978b; Deschner, 1980; Deschner and Maskens, 1982). Rather, the cells become fully mature and eventually die and/or desquamate.

The crypts can therefore be regarded as isolated units under a primary control mechanism. Cell production will always be followed by an equivalent amount of cell loss, provided the pericryptal sheath does not expand and the epithelial cells mature normally. Primary control can be modulated by additional factors (for example, neural or hormonal), resulting in variations in the size of crypt cell populations, turnover time, and possibly other proliferative parameters (Tutton and Barkla, 1982). Under given conditions, variation from crypt to crypt is also present, in both 3H-TdR labeling index (Deschner and Maskens, 1982) and extension of the proliferative compartment (Figure 2). Temporal fluctuation within single crypts, although impossible to demonstrate, is probably also present.

During the normal growth phase of the large intestine, a large number of new crypts are being produced. In the rat, where this process has been analyzed in detail, the total number of crypts in the colon and rectum is multiplied

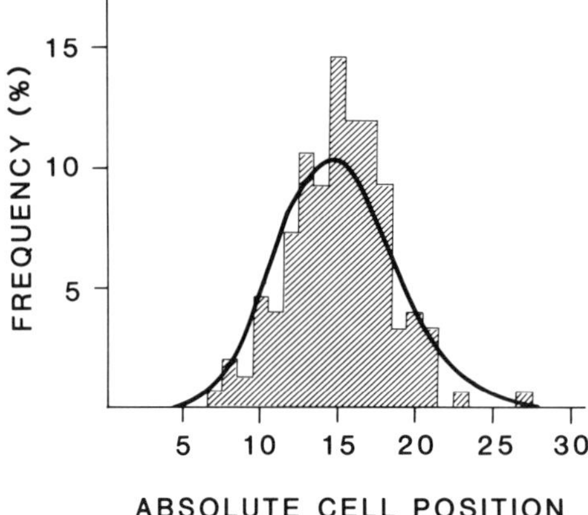

FIGURE 2. Illustration of the fluctuation of the upper limit of the proliferative compartment in normal colon crypts. In this experiment, the labeling of DNA synthesizing cells has been observed in normal adult BD IX rats, after in vivo incorporation of 3H-TdR. A large number of crypts (150) have been analyzed. The figure shows the frequency distribution of the position of the highest labeled cell per crypt section. The line gives the corresponding Poisson distribution.

by a factor of about 100 between birth and adulthood (Maskens and Dujardin-Loits, 1981). Of interest, even during this intense growth activity, cell proliferation remains confined to the lower regions of the crypts, and new crypts are being produced by a mechanism of fission, or bifurcation starting at their base (Maskens, 1978a).

Adenoma Genotype in the Histologically Normal Crypt

The very first abnormality in adenoma formation is a histologically normal crypt with a normal proliferative pattern, but which harbors the adenoma genotype.

It is possible that all adenomas are the expression of a genetic defect. Hereditary conditions exist that are characterized by the development of thousands of adenomas in the colon and rectum of the affected patients. These conditions—FPC and Gardner syndrome (GS)—are inherited in an autosomal dominant manner controlled by a single gene (Bussey, 1975; Lynch and Lynch, 1978; McConnell, 1980; Gardner et al., 1982). By analogy, it is usually believed that isolated, nonhereditary adenomas probably result from somatic mutation (Hill et al., 1978). In favor of this view are experimental observations that multiple adenomas can be induced in the large intestine of mice following treatment with symmetrical 1,2-dimethylhydrazine (DMH), a mutagenic (Moriya et al., 1978; Wilpart et al., 1982) and carcinogenic (Druckrey et al., 1967; Druckrey, 1970) chemical.

In FPC and its variant GS, all enterocytes must share the common genetic abnormality responsible for the development of adenomas. Yet, while only a few thousand polyps may be present, there will be millions of crypts not expressing their capacity to become adenomatous. On histologic examination, such crypts are undistinguishable from crypts of unaffected subjects. In addition, 3H-TdR incorporation studies have shown that a proportion of these crypts have a normal proliferative pattern (Deschner and Lipkin, 1975). We must therefore conclude that, even in situations where all cells in a crypt are affected by the dominant gene responsible for the development of an adenoma, the probability that abnormal proliferative behavior will be observable at the crypt level is much less than 100%; the probability that an adenoma will actually develop is in fact very low.

Histologically Normal Crypt with an Abnormal Proliferative Pattern

Investigation of the incorporation of 3H-TdR in normal-looking crypts from adenoma-prone patients shows a progressive series of abnormalities. Three stages have been described.

Stage I Abnormality. The first proliferative abnormality in histologically normal crypts from FPC patients was described by Deschner and coworkers in 1966. It is characterized by the appearance of DNA-synthesizing cells in the upper third of the affected crypts, although the major proliferative zone remains confined to their lower third. These changes were also found in patients with isolated adenomas or colon cancer and in asymptomatic relatives of patients with familial polyposis (Deschner, 1980). Lipkin (1974) called this "phase I" abnormality. In the same paper, Lipkin called "phase II" a stage in which the cells accumulate in the mucosa in increasing numbers. Two additional stages preceding this "phase II" have since been described and will be referred to here as stages II and III.

State II Abnormality. Although only recently fully characterized, this second abnormality was described in the original study by Deschner and coworkers in 1966. In this stage, the major zone of DNA synthesis is no longer restricted to the lower third of crypts: it is shifted upward to the middle and upper third (Maskens and Deschner, 1977). This abnormality has been observed in a variety of conditions characterized by a high risk of developing colorectal adenomas but was much less frequent than the stage I defect (Deschner, 1980).

Stage III Abnormality. It was recently shown in a group of patients with colon cancer or isolated adenomas that some individual crypts may exhibit a higher than normal thymidine labeling index (LI) (Deschner and Maskens, 1982). Such crypts are affected by the stage II abnormality to a greater extent than crypts with a normal LI. This combination of an upward shift in the major proliferative zone and an increased LI in crypts with a normal histologic appearance probably represents the state immediately preceding the frank adenomatous stage; Deschner (1982) called it "stage III" (Figure 3).

These abnormalities were confirmed by the analysis of 3H-TdR incorporation patterns in histologically normal crypts from DMH-treated mice, before appearance of the adenomas. As in the human material, all three stages could be observed (Deschner and Maskens, 1982).

Whether these stages are specific to the adenoma-formation process is, however, not entirely elucidated. Stage I abnormality is certainly not specific, as it has been reported to occur in control subjects and patients with inflammatory bowel diseases (Bleiberg et al., 1970; Deschner, 1980; Biasco et al., 1982). It is therefore suggested that this abnormality might in such situations reflect regen-

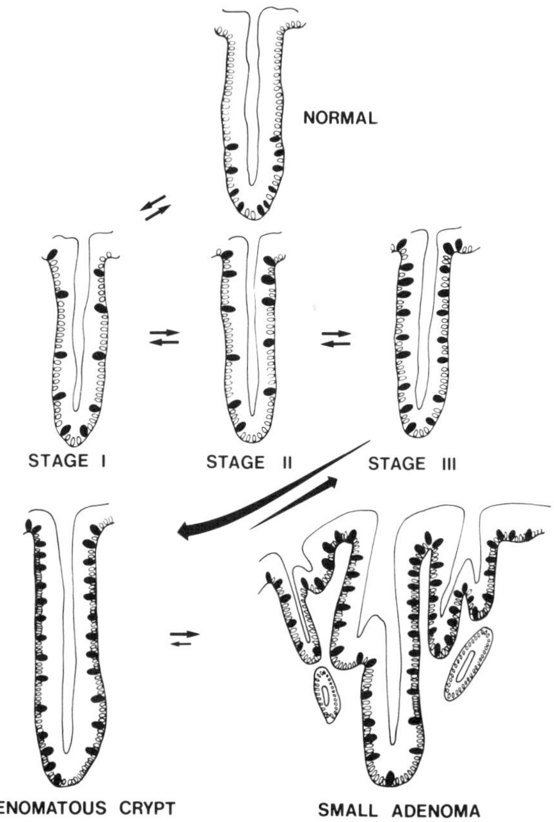

FIGURE 3. Schematic representation of the successive stages leading from a normal colon crypt to an adenoma. The large, black nuclei represent DNA-synthesizing cells.

erative activity of the mucosa. Stage II abnormality appears to be much more specific; it was reported only in patients at risk for developing colon neoplasms, either adenomas or carcinomas (Maskens and Deschner, 1977, 1980; Biasco et al., 1981). The stage III abnormality needs to be further documented before its degree of specificity can be established.

The Isolated Adenomatous Crypt

At this stage, histologic observation clearly reveals the adenomatous pattern of the crypt: the diameter of the crypt is enlarged and the cells are crowded, indicating a significant increase in the crypt cell population. Most cells are poorly differentiated, and mitotic figures, in increased number, can be observed over the entire crypt height (Figure 1). Such isolated adenomatous crypts are frequent findings in sections of flat colorectal mucosa from FPC patients (Bussey, 1975; Maskens, 1979). They have also been recently described in the mucosa of patients with isolated adenomas (Woda et al., 1977; Dohara et al., 1981).

The Adenoma

On observation of small adenomas, several features indicate the mechanism by which new glands are being produced around the initial adenomatous crypt (Maskens, 1979). Adenomatous crypts accumulate mainly in the upper aspect of the mucosa, in and around normal crypts. The number of gland openings along the surface of the adenomas is larger than the number of gland bases along the corresponding portion of the muscularis mucosae, a difference that increases with increasing polyp size. In contrast to normal mucosa, bifurcation of the bases of crypts is not found. However, branching is frequently observed, mainly in the upper portion. It is in this area, as well as along the mucosal surface, that DNA synthesis also clearly predominates.

From these observations, it appears that two mechanisms are responsible for the accumulation of new, neoplastic crypts: downward infolding of the surface epithelium, as well as branching along the upper aspect of adenomatous crypts (Wiebecke et al., 1974; Maskens, 1979). Of interest, such a phenomenon could represent the simple mechanical consequence of cell crowding along the epithelial basement membrane. Lipkin (1974) suggested that DNA-synthesizing cells tend to adhere more on the epithelial basement membrane than do the differentiated cells.

MECHANISMS OF ADENOMA FORMATION

The Fundamental Abnormality at the Cell Level

From the observations just summarized, the following can be concluded: a permanent decrease in the repression of DNA synthesis while cells migrate upward in the crypts can explain the sequence of events leading to the development of an adenoma. Production of immature elements higher in the crypt (stage I) will progressively result in an upward shift of the major proliferative zone (stage II) and an increase in the size of the proliferative pool (stage III). As more and more immature elements reach the surface where cells are shed, the balance between cell production and cell loss is altered. Crowding of undifferentiated cells in the affected crypt will ensue, followed by surface extension of the adenomatous cell population and formation of additional neoplastic crypts via the infolding and branching mechanisms.

Reversibility of the Stages

The question then immediately arises whether the intermediate stages are stable and/or irreversible. In other terms, once a stage I abnormality is present, is the crypt necessarily committed to become an adenoma? Can crypts remain at any given intermediate stage for prolonged periods? Can abnormal crypts regress to a normal stage?

Precise answers to these questions would necessitate extensive quantitative analyses of crypts from FPC patients, in order to obtain estimates of the proportion of crypts affected by each of the successive stages, including the number of isolated adenomatous crypts and small adenomas. Although such an approach is probably beyond our present technical possibilities, rough conclusions can be reached on the basis of a few simple observations.

First, the probability of proceeding from the first stages to the adenomatous crypt seems to be rather low. In some FPC patients, random sampling of crypts reveals that a majority can be affected by the stage I or II defects (Deschner et al., 1966; Deschner and Maskens, 1982). Yet, the proportion of isolated adenomatous crypts does not seem to exceed 1 per 100 histologically normal crypts (Bussey, 1975). This last figure also indicated that a proportion only of the adenomatous crypts will evolve into an adenoma, because the total number of adenomas in FPC patients does not exceed a few thousands.

Second, some degree of reversibility of the various stages must be accepted. It seems unlikely that the small disturbances observed in the earliest stages of the process could remain perfectly stable for prolonged periods, because of the natural variability of the proliferative activity of normal crypts under physiologic conditions (see Figure 2), and because all crypts undergo renewal every few days. Fluctuation between stages should thus be considered. Because evolution to an adenoma is probably relatively uncommon, reversal of any of these stages may also occur. Even in the later stages (isolated adenomatous crypt, small adenoma), some minor degree of reversibility cannot be excluded. That fully developed rectal adenomas can regress is a classic observation in FPC patients submitted to colectomy with ileorectal anastomosis (Pickens and Farringer, 1969; Shepherd, 1971). In addition, the reversibility of benign neoplasms is well established in experimental tumor systems such as skin papillomas (Burns et al., 1978) and preneoplastic liver nodules (Newberne, 1976; Pitot, 1977).

The Fluctuation Model

The working hypothesis proposed is as follows:

The adenoma-prone cells have a genetic defect that makes them slightly less susceptible to engage in irreversible differentiation.

In crypts composed of such cells, as is the case of FPC, the chance that some elements continue synthesizing DNA while migrating in their upper portion is rather high, but is almost nonexistent in normal crypts under physiologic conditions.

This creates a small probability that, due merely to random sample distribution laws, some crypts will occasionally have a high number of abnormally located proliferating cells.

These changes may result in a further disruption in the equilibrium between cell production, orderly migration, cell differentiation, and cell loss. The stage of the adenomatous crypt is now reached.

It is interesting to remember here that the normal crypts also show random fluctuation of the individual values of the limits of the proliferative compartment (Figure 2). It is similarly proposed that adenoma-prone crypts fluctuate at a slightly higher level. Here, in extreme cases, crypt conditions can be reached that will lead to a new status, the adenomatous crypt, rather than reverting to normal values. As in normal epithelium, some factors extrinsic to the crypt may modify this fluctuation level, some of them greatly enhancing the probability of adenoma formation. This view is in agreement with the model proposed by Hill and coworkers (1978).

When the genetic defect is acquired by a somatic mutuation ("isolated adenoma"), it is likely that the abnormal cell and its progeny will have to replace a large proportion of the normal cells in the crypt progressively before a real risk of adenomatous transformation becomes present.

SUMMARY AND CONCLUSIONS

Our present hypothesis on the mechanisms of adenoma formation is summarized in Figure 3. The adenomatous epithelium is characterized by cell overpopulation, increased labeling index, and upward shift of the proliferative compartment, which predominates in the upper aspect of the crypts. The most conspicuous intermediate between a normal crypt and an adenoma is the isolated adenomatous crypt, a finding reported by several authors.

In conditions associated with a high risk of adenoma formation, crypts have been observed that exhibit proliferative patterns intermediate between the normal and adenomatous elements, in spite of a histologically normal appearance. Three stages have been described. In stage I, some cells continue to synthesize DNA while migrating into the upper third of the crypts. In stage II abnormality, the major part of the proliferative compartment is now to be found in the upper two thirds of the crypts. In stage III abnormality, the upward shift of the proliferative compartment is accompanied by an increased labeling index.

It is quite reasonable to imagine that these three stages represent a sequence through which crypts will progress before attaining a frank adenomatous appearance. The question of the specificity, stability, and reversibility of these stages remains, however, to be answered. A "fluctuation" model is proposed here as a working hypothesis. This model implies that single crypts harboring the adenoma genotype can fluctuate between normal and abnormal levels. The probability of reaching a given stage, as well as its reversibility, decreases with increasing degree of abnormality.

REFERENCES

Biasco G, Miglioli M, Minarini A, Vallorani V, Morselli AM, Dalaiti A, Barbara L (1982) Renewal of the rectal epithelial cells in ulcerative colitis. Ital J Gastroenterol 14:76–79.

Bleiberg H, Mainguet P, Galand P, et al. (1970) Cell renewal in the human rectum—In vitro autoradiographic study on active ulcerative colitis. Gastroenterology 58:851–855.

Bleiberg H, Mainguet P, Galand P (1972) Cell renewal in familial polyposis: Comparison between polyps and adjacent healthy mucosa. Gastroenterology 63:240–245.

Burns FJ, Vanderlaan M, Snyder E, Albert RE (1978) Induction and progression kinetics of mouse skin papillomas. In: Slaga TJ, Sivak A, Boutwell RK, eds., Carcinogenesis, Vol. 2 mechanisms of tumor promotion and cocarcinogenesis. New York: Raven Press, pp. 91–96.

Bussey HJR (1975) Familial polyposis coli. Baltimore: The Johns Hopkins University Press.

Cole JW, McKalen A (1961) Observations of cell renewal in human rectal mucosa in vivo with thymidine-H3. Gastroenterology 41:122–125.

Day DW (1982) Epidemiology of colorectal cancers. In: Malt RA, Williamson RCN, eds., Colonic Carcinogenesis. Lancaster, Eng.: MTP Press Limited, pp. 135–144.

Deschner EE (1980) Cell proliferation as a biological marker in human colorectal neoplasia. In: Winawer S, Schottenfeld D, Sherlock P, eds., Colorectal cancer: Prevention, epidemiology, and screening. New York: Raven Press, pp. 133–142.

Deschner EE (1982) Relationship of altered proliferation to colonic neoplasia. In: Malt RA, Williamson RCN, eds., Colonic carcinogenesis. Lancaster, Eng.: MTP Press Limited, pp. 25–30.

Deschner EE, Lipkin M (1966) An autoradiographic study of the renewal of argentaffin cells in human rectal mucosa. Exp Cell Res 43:661–665.

Deschner EE, Lipkin M. (1978) Proliferation and differentiation of gastrointestinal cells in health and disease. In: Lipkin M, Good R, eds. Gastrointestinal tract cancer. New York: Plenum Press, pp. 3–27.

Deschner EE, Maskens AP (1982) Significance of the labelling index and labelling distribution as kinetic parameters in colorectal mucosa of cancer patients and DMH treated animals. Cancer 50:1136–1141.

Deschner EE, Lewis CM, Lipkin M (1962) In vitro H3-thymidine incoporation into human rectal mucosa. Clin Res 10:189.

Deschner EE, Lewis CM, Lipkin M (1963) In vitro study of human rectal epithelial cells. I. Atypical zone of H3 thymidine incorporation in mucosa of multiple polyposis. J Clin Invest 42:1922–1928.

Deschner EE, Lipkin M, Solomon C (1966) Study of human rectal epithelial cells in vitro. II. H3-Thymidine incorporation into polyps and adjacent mucosa. J Natl Cancer Inst 36:849–857.

Deschner EE, Lipkin M (1975) Proliferative patterns in colonic mucosa in familial polyposis. Cancer 35:413–418.

Druckrey H (1970) Production of colonic carcinomas by 1,2-dialkylhydrazines and azoxyalkanes. In: Burdette WJ, ed., Carcinoma of the colon and antecedent epithelium. Springfield, Ill: Charles C Thomas, pp. 267–279.

Druckrey H, Preussmann R, Matzkies F, Ivankovic S (1967) Selektieve Erzeugung von Darmkrebs bei Ratten durch 1,2-Dimethylhydrazin. Naturwissenschaften 54:285–286.

Enterline HT, Evans GW, Mercado-Lugo R, Miller L, Fitts WT Jr. (1962) Malignant potential of adenomas of colon and rectum. JAMA 179:322–330.

Fung CHK, Goldman H (1970) The incidence and significance of villous change in adenomatous polyps. Am J. Clin Pathol 53:21–25.

Gardner EJ, Woodward SR, Burt RW, Neff LK (1982) In vitro characterization of Gardner syndrome, familial polyposis coli, hereditary discrete colorectal polyps and carcinoma. In: Malt RA, Williamson RCN, eds., Colonic carcinogenesis. Lancaster, Eng.: MTP Press Limited, pp. 13–23.

Haot J, Rahier J, Maskens AP (1979) Colorectal polyps—Contribution of the anatomopathological analysis to the detection of intestinal tumours. Acta Endoscop 9:161–173.

Hill MJ, Morson BC, Bussey HJR (1978) Aetiology of adenoma—carcinoma sequence in large bowel. Lancet 1:245–247.

Kaye GI, Lane N, Pascal RR (1968) Colonic pericryptal fibroblast sheath: Replication, migration, and cytodifferentiation of a mesenchymal cell system in adult tissue. II. Fine structural aspects of normal rabbit and human colon. Gastroenterology 54:852–865.

Kurzon RM, Ortega R, Rywlin AM (1974) The significance of papillary features in polyps of the large intestine. Am J Clin Pathol 62:447–454.

Lipkin M (1974) Phase I and phase II proliferative lesions of colonic epithelial cells in diseases leading to colonic cancer. Cancer 34:878–888.

Lipkin M, Bell BM, Sherlock P (1963) Cell proliferation kinetics in the gastrointestinal tract of man. I. Cell renewal in colon and rectum. J Clin Invest 42:767–776.

Lynch HT, Lynch PM (1978) Heredity and gastrointestinal tract cancer. In: Lipkin M, Good R, eds., Gastrointestinal tract cancer. New York: Plenum Press, pp. 241–274.

McConnell RB (1980) Genetics of familial polyposis. In: Winawer S, Schottenfeld D, Sherlock P, eds., Colorectal cancer: Prevention, epidemiology, and screening. New York: Raven Press, pp. 69–71.

McDonald WC, Trier JS, Everett NB (1964) Cell proliferation and migration in the stomach, duodenum, and rectum of man: Radioautographic studies. Gastroenterology 46:405–417.

Maskens AP (1978a) Histogenesis of colon glands during postnatal growth. Acta Anat 100:17–26.

Maskens AP (1978b) Distribution du compartiment proliferatif dans la muqueuse recto-colique normale, preneoplasique et neoplasique. Acta Gastro-Ent Belg 41:226–240.

Maskens AP (1979) Histogenesis of adenomatous polyps in the human large intestine. Gastroenterology 77:1245–1251.

Maskens AP (1982) Adenomas and carcinomas of the large bowel: Distinct diseases possibly sharing common aetiologic factors? Acta Gastro-Ent Belg 45:158–164.

Maskens AP, Deschner EE (1977) Tritiated thymidine incorporation into epithelial cells of normal-appearing colorectal mucosa of cancer patients. J Natl Cancer Inst 58:1221–1224.

Maskens AP, Dujardin-Loits RM (1981) Kinetics of tissue proliferation in colorectal mucosa during postnatal growth. Cell Tissue Kinet 14:467–477.

Maskens AP, Rahier JR, Meersseman FP, et al. (1979) Cell proliferation of pericryptal fibroblasts in the rat colon mucosa. Gut 20:775–779.

Moriya M, Kato K, Watanabe K, et al. (1978) Detection of mutagenicity of the colon carcinogen 1,2-dimethylhydrazine by the host-mediated assay and its correlation to carcinogenicity. J Natl Cancer Inst 61:457–460.

Morson BC, Dawson IMP (1972) Gastrointestinal pathology. Oxford: Blackwell Scientific Publications.

Muto T, Bussey HJR, Morson BC (1975) The evolution of cancer of the colon and rectum. Cancer 36:2251–2270.

Newberne PM (1976) Experimental hepatocellular carcinogenesis. Cancer Res 36:2573–2578.

Oohara T, Ogino A, Tohma H (1981) Histogenesis of microscopic adenoma and hyperplastic (metaplastic) gland in nonpolyposis coli. Dis Colon Rectum 24:375–384.

Pickens DR Jr., Farringer JL Jr. (1969) Familial polyposis and the spontaneous regression of polyps. Am Surg 35:361–365.

Pitot HC (1977) The natural history of neoplasia. Am J Pathol 89:401–412.

Shepherd JA (1971) Familial polyposis of the colon with special reference to regression of rectal polyps after subtotal colectomy. Br J Surg 58:85–91.

Tutton PJM, Barkla DH (1982) Neural control of cell proliferation in colonic carcinogenesis. In: Malt RA, Williamson RCN, eds., Colonic carcinogenesis. Lancaster, Eng.: MTP Press Limited, pp. 283–295.

Wiebecke B, Brandts A, Eder M (1974) Epithelial proliferation and morphogenesis of hyperplastic adenomatous and villous polyps of the human colon. Virchows Arch A Pathol Anat Histol 364:35–49.

Wilpart M, Mainguet P, Maskens AP, Roberfroid M (1983) Mutagenicity of 1,2-dimethylhydrazine towards Salmonella Typhimurium: Co-mutagenic effects of secondary biliary acids. Carcinogenesis 4:45–48.

Woda BA, Forde K, Lane N (1977) A unicryptal colonic adenoma, the smallest colonic neoplasm yet observed in a non-polyposis individual. Am J Clin Pathol 68:631–632.

World Health Organization (1976) Histological typing of intestinal tumors. Morson BC, Sabin LH, eds. Geneva: World Health Orgnaization.

ADJUVANT CHEMOTHERAPY AND IMMUNOTHERAPY OF GASTROINTESTINAL CANCER

JOHN Y KILLEN, JR., M.D.,
AND SUSAN S ELLENBERG, PH.D.

PRINCIPLES OF ADJUVANT THERAPY OF CANCER

Adjuvant therapy can be succinctly defined as the addition of one or more modalities of treatment to other commonly accepted curative therapy. The latter is most often surgery in the case of adult nonhematologic malignancies. A familiar example of this would be the administration of chemotherapy to women with resectable breast cancer following mastectomy. The concept of adjuvant therapy is based on several fundamental aspects of cancer biology and treatment. First is the observation that surgery alone does not cure all patients whose cancer has been determined to be localized using available methods of detection. Second, a sizable proportion of these patients relapse at sites distant from the primary tumor in the absence of local recurrence, implying that the cancer disseminated either before or during operation. This has given rise to the concept of "micrometastases"—clinically undetectable microscopic deposits of metastatic tumor. Finally, most modalities of therapy used in the treatment of cancer are more effective in treating minimal disease. This is clearly the case for cytotoxic drugs and radiation therapy both in animal models and in human cancer; it may also be true of immunotherapy (Shabel, 1976).

Hence, it is sensible to suppose that the application of effective systemic therapy in the postoperative setting of micrometastases (that is, minimal disease) should increase the likelihood of cure. Obviously, the most attractive modalities or agents to be tested would be those known to be active against the specific cancer. The development of effective adjuvant programs thus follows a logical course. Because of their inherent toxicity, agents or combinations of drugs are first tested in patients with advanced disease where the potential for cure using "local" therapy (for example, surgery or radiotherapy) is low. Fol-

From the Cancer Therapy Evaluation Program, Division of Cancer Treatment, National Cancer Institute, Bethesda, Maryland.

lowing a rational series of clinical trials that establish efficacy in this setting, a given treatment is then applied to patients treated surgically for cure but at high risk for relapse. Of course it is imperative that the design of a clinical trial to evaluate the efficacy of a new adjuvant therapy must be meticulous, especially with respect to the choice of control group. Before such trials are initiated, one must also take into account the risk of relapse for a given patient, the possible complications of the proposed treatment, and some assessment of the potential for benefit.

A number of parameters are employed in assessing the results of an adjuvant study. The crude recurrence rate can be used, but it fails to take into account a number of factors, including the length of patient follow-up (which may be very important for diseases with long recurrence-free periods) or loss of patients to follow-up prior to recurrence (due to treatment-related or even unrelated causes). More useful are actuarial measures of disease-free and overall survival. The former is usually measured as the time from initiation of treatment to the first detection of recurrence and the latter from the same starting point until death. The ultimate measure, "cure rate," is not easily estimated because of such factors as the length of follow-up required and the morbidity and mortality of coexistent disease.

The remainder of this chapter will present an overview of the status of adjuvant chemotherapy and immunotherapy of various gastrointestinal cancers, with emphasis on data derived from properly designed and controlled clinical trials. The reader should begin this chapter cognizant of the generalization that surgery is the single modality with established curative potential in any gastrointestinal cancer.

GASTRIC CANCER

As described by Dr. Smith and his colleagues in their chapter "Chemotherapy of Advanced Gastrointestinal Malignancies," advanced adenocarcinoma of the stomach is the most responsive to chemotherapy of all the common gastrointestinal malignancies. Many drugs have been tested to date, and response rates ranging from 0 to 30% have been established for various single agents. The most active appear to be 5-fluorouracil (5-FU), doxorubicin (Adriamycin), mitomycin C, and the nitrosoureas. The resulting responses are of relatively brief duration, however, and there is minimal impact on overall survival. More recently, combinations of the active single agents have been studied including regimens of 5-FU plus a nitrosourea or mitomycin C with and without doxorubicin. Objective response rates between 35 and 50% have been frequently described (Macdonald et al., 1982).

During the mid-1970s, trials evaluating the role of adjuvant combination chemotherapy were initiated, following a series of largely negative results from earlier studies of single agents by the Veterans Administration Surgical Oncology Group (VASOG) and by the Stomach Cancer Study Group in Japan (Serlin et al., 1977; Koyama, 1978). The earliest and most extensively tested regimen, the combination of 5-FU plus methyl-CCNU, has prospectively been compared with surgery alone in randomized trials by the Gastrointestinal Tumor Study Group (GITSG), the VASOG, and the Eastern Cooperative Oncology Group (ECOG).

The GITSG trial was initiated in 1974 (GITSG, 1982). Patients who had undergone resection of gastric adenocarcinoma for cure were randomized to either surgery alone or surgery followed by 18 months of 5-FU plus methyl-CCNU. The study was stratified for type of surgery (proximal or total gastrectomy versus distal subtotal gastrectomy), tumor location (cardia versus other), extent of invasion (confined to the gastric wall versus invading adjacent tissues), lymph node status, and tumor histology (linitis plastica versus other). Rigid criteria for curative resection were established in the original protocol and eligibility was subsequently reviewed by a multidisciplinary committee blinded to treatment and outcome. The two treatment arms were well balanced with respect to all established and a number of possible prognostic variables.

Overall, the treatment was reasonably well tolerated. Seventy-one patients were randomized to the chemotherapy arm, and of these, eight (11%) had nine episodes of transient depression of the white blood cell count below $1000/mm^3$ or the platelet count below $50{,}000/mm^3$. Much less troublesome were vomiting, diarrhea, and dyspepsia. In a recently published report, recurrence rates were significantly lower and statistically significant survival superiority was found to exist for the patients randomized to adjuvant chemotherapy. Median survival could not be estimated reliably in the adjuvant group, but will exceed the current estimate of 33 months for the controls. This trend was present for patients with positive as well as negative lymph nodes and in both the total/proximal and the distal subtotal resection groups.

The trial by the ECOG was of almost identical design with respect to eligibility criteria, therapy, patient follow-up, and recurrence criteria. Nonetheless, a recent interim analysis failed to suggest any differences between treatment and control with respect to survival or disease-free survival (Engstrom and Lavin, 1983). At this time there is no obvious explanation for these differences in outcome between the ECOG and the GITSG studies. A joint evaluation of the data by the two groups is planned in the future when the data have become more mature.

The VASOG have also recently reported their findings from an adjuvant trial assessing the 5-FU + methyl-CCNU combination (Higgins et al., 1983). This group, too, failed to identify any benefit for the combination chemotherapy treatment in the subset of patients with no proven residual disease. However, important differences in trial design, especially with regard to eligibility criteria and drug treatment, make comparisons with either the GITSG or ECOG results extremely difficult. There are obvious differences in demographic characteristics—for example, the VASOG trial was restricted to male veterans. Moreover, from the VASOG report one cannot verify that the two treatment groups were well balanced with respect to important prognostic factors such as nodal status and serosal penetration within the subset of no residual disease. Finally, the survival of patients on both arms appears inferior to that reported by the GITSG.

Thus, the role of adjuvant chemotherapy in curatively resected gastric cancer patients is unsettled. On the basis of data from studies in advanced disease it now seems likely that 5-FU plus methyl-CCNU represents suboptimal treatment and that the chances of achieving meaningful improvement over surgery alone will be improved with the use of doxorubicin-containing combinations. Several such studies are currently active. The GITSG is evaluating the contribution of doxorubicin to the 5-FU methyl CCNU combination. A study by the North Central Cancer Treatment Group is comparing 5-FU plus doxorubicin with a surgery-alone control group. In studies by the Southwest Oncology Group and an international cooperative group, the FAM regimen (5-FU, doxorubicin, and mitomycin C) is being compared to surgery alone.

COLON CANCER

As discussed by Dr. Smith and colleagues in their chapter, the therapy of advanced colorectal cancer has, to date, been disappointing. Although the single agent 5-FU produces remissions in approximately 20% of patients and it is often stated that responders to 5-FU live longer than nonresponders, there is no apparent impact on the survival of the patient population as a whole (Sugarbaker et al., 1982). No other single agent has proven to be superior, and most produce more toxicity. Similarly, no tested combination has shown consistent and reproducible superiority to 5-FU alone. Nonetheless, adjuvant chemotherapy has been extensively tested, since up to 50% of the patients with this disease undergoing surgery die within 5 years of diagnosis (Sugarbaker et al., 1982).

The most extensively evaluated adjuvant chemotherapy consists of one of two fluorinated pyrimidines. In a series of three consecutive studies, the VASOG has evaluated: (1) 5-fluorodeoxy-uridine (FUDR) given at the time of surgery and in the immediate postoperative period; (2) 5-fluorouracil (5-FU) given in a similar manner; and (3) 5-FU given over an 18-month period following surgery ("prolonged intermittent therapy") (Higgins et al., 1978). In the latter two studies, patients were subdivided according to whether the resection was "curative" or palliative (histologically proven residual disease or tumor at the resected margin) and randomized separately. At the time, these patient subdivisions were considered separate studies. In all of the 5-FU studies, there was a slight trend toward better survival in the treated groups, but none of the differences were statistically significant.

In an attempt to clarify the possible benefit of postsurgical therapy with 5-FU further, the VASOG published an analysis in which the results of the separate 5-FU studies were aggregated, that is, treated as strata of a single study and in which the overall *P*-value thus obtained reached the conventional level of significance ($P = .05$) (Higgins et al., 1978). However, the rationale for combining these studies into a single analysis is somewhat questionable, having been formulated on the basis of the observed results. Further, there were major differences among the studies with regard to presence of residual disease and to treatment schedule and total dosage of 5-FU. While the VASOG studies are certainly consistent with the hypothesis that there is a very modest survival benefit to postresection therapy with 5-FU, it cannot be claimed that the pooled analysis conclusively demonstrates such benefit.

A major criticism of the VASOG trials is that suboptimal doses of 5-FU may have been administered. When drug-related toxicity is analyzed, it is apparent that the majority of patients could have received higher doses. Consequently, the Central Oncology Group initiated a study in which patients were randomized either to surgery alone or to surgery plus postoperative 5-FU administered to moderate toxicity and then on a weekly maintainance schedule (Grage et al., 1981). Fifty-four percent of 125 control patients compared with 62% of 108 treated patients were alive and free of disease at the last analysis. These proportions are not significantly different, nor are distributions of survival and disease-free survival times when adjusted for important prognostic factors such as location of lesion (colon or rectum) and Dukes' stage. For two subsets of patients—those with Dukes' C lesions or those with rectal cancer—a statistically significant benefit is reported. However, there are major problems with the analyses presented for this study, which lessen the reliability of the published conclusions. The follow-up period is very short (median follow-up time of 29 months), and the inevaluability rate is quite high (23%) with more patients apparently excluded from the treated than from the control arm. The analyses demonstrating benefit in subsets are unadjusted for the possible effect of other prognostic factors. Finally, the problems of interpreting positive results in subsets when multiple subsets are investigated and there is no significant effect overall are not discussed. For all these reasons, the results of the study must be considered with great caution; in particular, the positive findings in the Dukes' C and rectal patient subsets cannot be viewed as definitive, but rather as suggestions of benefit to be investigated further in other studies.

Because of the disappointing results achieved with single-agent therapy, more recent studies have explored the role of combination chemotherapy and/or immunotherapy in the adjuvant setting. In 1975, the GITSG began a study in which patients were randomized to one of four treatment arms: (1) surgery alone; (2) surgery plus chemotherapy consisting of 5-FU + methyl-CCNU administered in 6-week cycles over 18 months; (3) surgery plus nonspecific immunotherapy using the methanol extracted residue of BCG; and (4) combined chemotherapy and immunotherapy (GITSG, 1984). The choices of combination chemotherapy and immunotherapy were based on data available at the time, although subsequent evaluation has failed to confirm what were then preliminary observations. In a further departure from previous trials of adjuvant chemotherapy of colorectal cancer, patients with rectal cancer were treated on a separate protocol evaluating the roles of postoperative chemotherapy and pelvic irradiation. Eligibility criteria for the colon study included the presence of histologically confirmed, completely resected tumors (adenocarcinoma) of stage B2 (serosal penetration, nodes negative), C1 (1–4 positive nodes), or C2 (5 or more positive nodes), with no evidence of distant spread. This staging system was a slight modification of that described by Dukes and its subsequent Astler-Coller modification (Astler and Coller, 1954). Colon lesions were arbitrarily defined as those more than 12 cm proximal to the anal verge. The four arms were very well balanced with respect to known or a number of possible prognostic factors. In the recently published analysis of this trial, there were no statistically significant differences with regard to disease-free or overall survival among the four treatment arms. For the most part, treatment-related morbidity was tolerable, but one death related to myelosuppression and the recent development of seven cases of acute myelogenous leukemia or of severe myelodysplastic syndrome among the patients receiving methyl-CCNU are extremely disturbing, especially in light of the lack of treatment benefit.

Perhaps the most interesting information to emerge from this trial relates to outcome by tumor classification. Stage for stage, patients are doing substantially better than would have been anticipated on the basis of historical information available at the time of the study's design. For instance, approximately 40% of the stage C2 patients are alive at 3 years, and there is an apparent "plateau" on the survival curve. The reasons for this difference between expected and observed outcome are not clear at the present time, but most likely relate to more accurate "staging" performed during the course of initial evaluation and therapy, resulting in the inclusion of fewer patients with undetected metastastic disease. These data are corroborated by the findings from at least several other recent nonrandomized surgical series (Olson et al., 1980) and strongly underline the importance of the inclusion of appropriate controls in the design of clinical trials of adjuvant therapy. In the GITSG study, had reliance been placed on historical controls, one would have concluded that all three treatments prolonged life. The VASOG has also recently published the results of a trial comparing surgery alone with postoperative 5-FU plus methyl-CCNU (Higgins et al., 1984). Entry criteria for this study were somewhat different from those of the GITSG trial in that patients with no microscopic evidence of residual tumor but with evidence of disease spread (serosal penetration, invasion of perirectal fat, blood vessel or lymphatic invasion, regional lymph node metastasis, or cancer involving other organs included in the resection) were eligible. In addition, a group of patients with rectal cancer "who were not admitted to a concurrent trial of preoperative radiation therapy" were included. Finally, all patients in the VASOG study were male. The overall results of this trial were similar to those observed in previous VASOG studies; there was a trend favoring chemotherapy early in the follow-up period that did not reach statistical significance. As in the GITSG study, no important impact on patient survival was identified. In addition, it is interesting to note that the survival of patients in the VASOG study is inferior to that observed by the GITSG, especially when variations in the composition of the patient population, particularly tumor stage, are taken into account.

On the basis of an earlier unpublished observation from the GITSG, the VASOG also analyzed survival according to number of involved lymph nodes in the resection specimen, approximating the GITSG stage C1 and C2 categories. A highly statistically significant benefit favoring chemotherapy in the subset with 1 to 4 positive nodes was identified; in the groups with uninvolved or greater than 4 positive nodes, the treated patients actually did slightly worse than the control. The VASOG finding of a substantial improvement in median as well as long-term survival attributable to chemotherapy in the 1–4-positive node subset is not corroborated by current data from the GITSG trial (GITSG, unpublished results). It appears consistent with the observations of Grage et al., discussed earlier, although the long-term treatment comparison has yet to be made in that trial. Other investigators will want to consider this patient subset carefully in both the design and analysis of ongoing and future trials of adjuvant therapy of colon cancer.

Another trial currently in active follow-up was conducted by the Southwest Oncology Group. This study compared chemotherapy with 5-FU and methyl-CCNU to the same chemotherapy plus immunotherapy with BCG and to a surgery-only control group. Preliminary reports do not suggest that treatment benefits will be demonstrated (Panettiere and Chen, 1981).

Taylor and coworkers recently described a novel approach to adjuvant therapy of colorectal cancer (Taylor et al., 1979). Noting the frequency with which colorectal cancer recurs in the liver, and the established fact that very early metastases to the liver obtain their blood supply primarily from the portal vein, they randomized patients with Dukes' stage A, B, or C disease to receive either surgery alone or surgery plus postoperative chemotherapy consisting of a 7-day continuous infusion of 5-FU at a dose of 1 g/day administered into the portal vein via the umbilical vein. Five thousand units of heparin were also administered daily in the infusion. In a preliminary analysis of 90 patients, there had been 23 deaths in the 47 control patients compared to 7 of the 43 receiving adjuvant treatment. Hepatic metastases had developed in 13 and 2, respectively. The minimum follow-up time was 1 year, with an average of 25 months. Therapy was extremely well tolerated, with only minor complications observed. This study has generated some controversy due to reports of an unusually high rate of postoperative morbidity and mortality in both the treatment and the control groups. An additional difficulty is introduced by the inclusion of heparin in the infusate. Theoretical considerations and data from animal systems indicate that heparin may have a role in the prevention of the establishment of metastases by inhibiting the formation of "protective fibrin clots" around disseminated tumor cells lodged in capillary beds.

The logistics of carrying out such a trial (which would ideally include intraoperative pathologic staging and randomization) are very complicated and to date have prevented early confirmation of these results in a multiinstitution setting. Two studies are now under way, however, one by the North Central Cancer Treatment Group and a second by the NSABP. Other ongoing colon cancer adjuvant studies are shown in Table 1. Their outcome is awaited with interest.

TABLE 1. Ongoing or Unpublished Randomized Colon Cancer Adjuvant Trials

Group	Adjuvant treatment arms	Comment
ECOG	1. 5-FU + methyl-CCNU 2. 5-FU	No surgery-alone control
VASOG	1. Surgery alone 2. 5-FU 3. 5-FU + hydroxyurea	
NCCTG	1. Surgery alone 2. Levamisole 3. Levamisole + 5-FU	Based on Davis et al. (1982)
NCCTG	1. 5-FU by portal vein 2. Surgery alone	Attempt to replicate data of Taylor et al. (see text)
NSABP	1. Surgery alone 2. 5-FU + methyl-CCNU + vincristine 3. Cutaneous BCG	
GITSG	1. Hepatic irradiation plus 5-FU 2. Surgery alone	

In summary, no form of adjuvant chemotherapy or immunotherapy of colon cancer has been shown to be beneficial in properly controlled trials.

The existence of a small treatment benefit would not be inconsistent with the reported negative results of the previously discussed trials. However, such a benefit would have to be small indeed to have avoided statistical detection by any of these trials, several of which were quite large. The toxicity of chemotherapy, and in particular the association of the 5-FU + methyl-CCNU combination therapy with development of leukemia and other myelodysplastic disorders, requires that much stronger evidence of chemotherapeutic benefit be presented before adjuvant chemotherapy for colon cancer becomes standard practice. The use of a concomitantly randomized surgery-alone control group in trials evaluating adjuvant treatment remains essential. The routine use of adjuvant therapy outside of the research setting cannot be defended, and the entry of patients into properly designed clinical trials evaluating new treatment should be strongly encouraged.

RECTAL CANCER

Prior to the mid-1970s, most studies of adjuvant therapy for rectal cancer either involved radiotherapy alone or included these patients in chemotherapy trials for colon and rectal cancer. Data on the latter have been discussed earlier in this chapter. Dr. Gunderson and colleagues also discuss the role of radiation therapy in the following chapter.

In 1975, the Gastrointestinal Tumor Study Group initiated a trial of combination chemotherapy plus radiation therapy in rectal cancer (Mittelman et al., 1981). Patients were randomized to one of four treatment arms: (1) surgery alone; (2) postoperative irradiation to a total dose of 4400 to 4800 rad; (3) chemotherapy with a combination of 5-FU plus methyl-CCNU over 18 months; or (4) combined radiotherapy (4000 to 4400 rad) and chemotherapy. Patients were stratified on the basis of type of surgery (abdominoperineal resection versus

TABLE 2. Unpublished Randomized Rectal Cancer Adjuvant Trials

Group	Adjuvant treatment arms
ECOG	1. Postoperative irradiation 2. 5-FU + methyl-CCNU 3. 1 + 2
VASOG	1. Preoperative irradiation 2. Surgery alone
NSABP	1. Surgery alone 2. 5-FU + methyl-CCNU + vincristine 3. Postoperative irradiation
GITSG	1. Postoperative RT + 5-FU + methyl-CCNU 2. Postoperative RT + brief, intense 5-FU

low anterior resection) and tumor stage (B2, C1, or C2, as previously defined). Rectal lesions were defined as those less than 12 cm from the anal verge. Actuarial disease-free survival was significantly superior for the combined modality group compared to the control group and was intermediate for the two single modality arms with no other significant pairwise differences between arms. While these preliminary results are encouraging, it must be kept in mind that there are no demonstrated differences among the four arms in terms of overall survival. Whether the differences in disease-free survival will eventually translate into differences in overall survival remains to be seen. Furthermore, the combined modality therapy resulted in considerable treatment-related morbidity, with 62% of patients having at least one episode of severe or worse treatment-related toxicity. This includes two deaths attributed to radiation enteritis, which would not have been expected at the doses of radiation given. It is possible that the concomitant chemotherapy resulted in sensitization to the long-term toxic effects of radiotherapy. Other ongoing adjuvant trials are summarized in Table 2.

ESOPHAGEAL CANCER

The principal problem in esophageal cancer is one of improving on the rate of resectability, since esophageal cancer is most often far advanced by the time it becomes symptomatic. Only about 50% of all patients who present with this diagnosis are even candidates for operation, and of these, curative or palliative resection is possible for only a small majority. Operative mortality is high, however, and even when combined with preoperative radiation therapy (which appears to improve the rate of resectability slightly), the 5-year survival of patients undergoing resection generally ranges from 10 to 20% or 5 to 10% of the original total patient population.

This situation has led to the development of a somewhat different approach to adjuvant therapy—the use of preoperative chemotherapy in conjunction with either preoperative or postoperative irradiation. Kelsen and coworkers at Memorial Sloan-Kettering have reported preliminary results from a very encouraging trial employing the combination of vindesine, cisplatin, and bleomycin preoperatively (Coonley et al., 1982). The choice of this regimen was based on previous studies in patients with advanced disease in whom an objective remission rate of 51% was seen. Preoperative chemotherapy consisted of one or two cycles of the combination followed by surgery and postoperative irradiation to a total of 5500 rad to the involved field. Of 33 patients evaluable, 16 showed objective response to chemotherapy. Twenty-eight patients became candidates for resection; among them, 16 were operated on with curative intent. There were two operative deaths, and one death attributable to drug treatment. With a median follow-up of 14 months, five of the six unresected patients were dead, with a median survival of 5 months. Nine of the 28 resected patients have relapsed, and five of those are dead. Five of 28 patients are dead from other causes, and 14 of the 28 patients are alive with no evidence of disease. These preliminary results require confirmatory studies, which are currently under development.

EXOCRINE PANCREATIC CANCER

Because so few patients with the diagnosis of pancreatic cancer are even potential candidates for curative surgery, and because of the resistance of this tumor to irradiation and chemotherapy, very little data are available on the efficacy of adjuvant treatment. Anecdotal reports and small uncontrolled series abound; the only well-controlled, randomized trial conducted to date has recently been reported in preliminary form by the GITSG. Based on data from the Mayo Clinic, these investigators began a study in 1974 comparing surgery alone with surgery plus postoperative irradiation (4000 rad in two split courses) and 5FU (Kalser et al., 1983). Histologic confirmation of adenocarcinoma of the exocrine pancreas with tumor-free margins was required. Patients were stratified for tumor location (head versus other), type of resection, tumor differentiation, and extent of disease (confined to pancreas, contiguous structure, or nodal involvement). The resulting randomization was well balanced with respect to these variables. Approximately one-third of the patients underwent total pancreaticoduodenectomy and the remainder lesser resections. Therapy was well tolerated, with no undue toxicity. A total of 24 patients were randomized to the control arm and 25 to adjuvant therapy, of whom 22 and 21, respectively, were eligible for analysis. The median survival for the control group, 11 months, is statistically inferior to that for the treated group, 20 months. Patterns for disease-free survival are similar. Three patients in the treatment group and one in the control are alive and disease-free 5 or more years following surgery.

This single study provides data suggesting some benefit from adjuvant irradiation and chemotherapy for those patients surviving curative resection for exocrine pancreatic adenocarcinoma. Unfortunately, this is an all-too-rare circumstance, a fact underscored by the slow and limited accrual to this study. Nonetheless, as a well-designed and conducted study with mature data, it will serve as the basis for second-generation clinical trials of adjuvant therapy for this disease.

CONCLUSIONS

For the most part, progress in adjuvant therapy of gastrointestinal cancers has been slow and somewhat more disappointing than that seen in other primary sites, such as breast cancer. More recent data, especially for gastric cancer, are encouraging, but further research in this field, including the development of new chemotherapeutic agents and new modalities of treatment, is required.

REFERENCES

Astler VB, Coller FA (1954) The prognostic significance of direct extension of carcinoma of the colon and rectum. Ann Surg 139:846–852.

Coonley C, Kelsen D, Bains M, Hilaris B, Kaufman R, Martini N (1982) Combined modality approach to operable epidermoid carcinoma of the esophagus. Proc Am Soc Clin Oncol 18:95.

Davis TE, Borden EC, Wolberg WH, Crowley JJ (1982) Levamisole and 5-FU in metastatic colorectal carcinoma. Proc Am Soc Clin Oncol 18:102.

Engstrom P, Lavin P for the Eastern Cooperative Group (1983) Post-operative adjuvant therapy for gastric cancer patients. Proc Am Soc Clin Oncol 17:114.

The Gastrointestinal Tumor Study Group (1982) Controlled trial of adjuvant chemotherapy following curative resection for gastric cancer. Cancer 49:1116–1122.

The Gastrointestinal Tumor Study Group (1984) Adjuvant therapy of colon cancer. N Engl J Med 310:737–742.

Grage TB, Moss SE (1981) Adjuvant chemotherapy in cancer of the colon and rectum: Demonstration of effectiveness in a prospectively controlled, randomized trial. Surg Clin North Am 61:1321–1329.

Higgins GA, Lee LE, Dwight RW, Keehn RJ (1978) The case for adjuvant 5-fluorouracil in colorectal cancer. Cancer Clin Trials 1:35–41.

Higgins GA, Amadeo JH, Smith DE, et al. (1983) Efficacy of prolonged intermittent therapy with combined 5-FU and methyl-CCNU following resection for gastric carcinoma. Cancer 52:1105–1112.

Higgins GA, Amadeo JH, McElhinney J, et al. (1984) Efficacy of prolonged intermittent therapy with combined 5-fluorouracil and methyl-CCNU following resection for carcinoma for the large bowel. Cancer 53:1–8.

Kalser M, Ellenberg S, Levin B, et al. (1983) Pancreatic cancer: Adjuvant combined radiation and chemotherapy following potentially curative resection. Proc Am Soc Clin Oncol 19:122.

Koyama Y (1978) The current status of chemotherapy for gastric cancer in Japan with special emphasis on mitomycin-C. Recent Results Cancer Res 63:135–147.

Lessner HE, Mayer RJ, Ellenberg S, et al. (1982) Adjuvant therapy of colon cancer—a prospective randomized trial. Proc Am Soc Clin Oncol 18:91.

MacDonald JS, Gunderson LL, Cohn I (1982) Cancer of the stomach. In: DeVita VT, Hellman S, Rosenberg SA, eds., Cancer: Principals and practice of oncology. Philadelphia: J.B. Lippincott, pp. 534–562.

Mittelman A, Holyoke E, Thomas P, et al. (1981) Adjuvant chemotherapy and radiotherapy following rectal surgery: An interim report from the Gastrointestinal Tumor Study Group. In: Jones SE, Salmon SI, eds., Adjuvant Chemotherapy of Cancer III. New York: Grune and Stratton, pp. 547–558.

Olson RM, Perenceivich NP, Malcolm AW, et al. (1980) Patterns of recurrence following curative resection of adenocarcinoma of the colon and rectum. Cancer 45:2969–2978.

Panettiere FJ, Chen TT (1981) Analysis of 626 patients entered on the SWOG large bowel adjuvant program. In: Jones SE, Salmon SE, eds., Adjuvant chemotherapy of cancer III. New York: Grune and Stratton, pp. 539–545.

Serlin O, Keehn RJ, Higgins GA Jr, et al. (1977) Factors related to survival following resection for gastric carcinoma. Cancer 49:1116–1122.

Shabel FM (1976) Concepts for treatment of micrometastases developed in murine systems. Am J Roentgenol Radium Ther Nucl Med 126:500–515.

Sugarbaker PH, Macdonald JS, Gunderson LL (1982) Colorectal cancer. In: DeVita VT, Hellman S, Rosenberg SA, eds., Cancer: Principals and practice of oncology. Philadelphia: J.B. Lippincott, pp. 724–731.

Taylor I, Rowling J, West C (1979) Adjuvant cytotoxic liver perfusion for colorectal cancer. Br J Surg 66:833–836.

RADIATION THERAPY IN THE MANAGEMENT OF GASTROINTESTINAL CANCER

LEONARD L GUNDERSON, M.D., M.S., DANIEL E DOSORETZ, M.D., GENE KOPELSON, M.D., JOEL E TEPPER, M.D., TYVIN A RICH, M.D., AND R BRUCE HOSKINS, M.D.

For most gastrointestinal cancers, improvements in surgical survival rates have been minimal over the past 25 to 30 years. Such improvements have largely been the result of an increase in operability, with little change by stage of disease in those patients who have survived a "curative resection."

The purpose of this chapter will be to develop a logical approach to the use of radiation therapy in these malignancies. Incidence and areas of failure after operation alone will be outlined with subsequent implications for adjuvant therapy. Results of series using radiation will be presented, and the potential for the future will be discussed.

ESOPHAGEAL CANCER

Areas of Failure

Merendino and Mark (1952) found in a review of the literature that 20 to 48% of patients die with only local extension of the tumor without lymph node or distant metastases. Nodal metastasis in mediastinal, supraclavicular, cervical, and subdiaphragmatic areas is common, but the incidence of failure depends on the location of the tumor within the esophagus. Distant metastases occur most commonly in the liver or lung.

From the Department of Oncology, Mayo Clinic, Rochester, Minnesota (LLG); the Department of Radiation Therapy, Massachusetts General Hospital and Harvard Medical School, Boston (DED, JET); the Department of Therapeutic Radiology, Tufts New England Medical Center, Boston (GK); the Joint Center for Radiation Therapy, Harvard Medical School (TAR); and the Department of Radiology, Southern Illinois University Medical School and St. John's Hospital, Springfield (RBH).

TABLE 1. Comparison of Surgery and Radiation Therapy for Carcinoma of the Esophagus Edinburgh Study 1948–1968

Site		Surgery	Radiotherapy
Cervical esophagus		4/19 (21%)	14/46 (30%)
Upper half of thoracic esophagus		11/135 (8%)	12/73 (16%)
Lower half of thoracic esophagus		31/275 (11%)	6/50 (12%)
	Totals	46/429 (11%)	32/169 (29%)

Source: Modified from Pearson (1975).

Treatment

At present, a large group of patients have lesions that are initially unresectable for cure due to local extension. Primary radiation can provide much useful palliation and an occasional cure. Although recent studies (Leichman et al., 1981) suggest that a combination of preoperative irradiation and chemotherapy may allow later resection, long-term results are unknown and randomized studies have not been done to see if that approach would be better than preoperative irradiation without chemotherapy.

Table 1 compares the curative potential of surgery and radiation therapy in the study reported by Pearson (1975). Although Pearson's results of radiation treatment of the esophagus surpass those of any other published series, he nonetheless found that about 50% of his failures were due to local recurrence.

While both surgery and irradiation, as single modalities, have curative potential in selected patients with early lesions, the incidence of such tumors is low. For upper and most middle third lesions, if single modality treatment is used, irradiation is usually preferable to surgery since equivalent or higher cure rates can be obtained (Table 1) with lower risks (Moertel, 1982; Pearson, 1975). In upper third lesions, the larynx can also be spared. For lower third lesions, cure rates are equivalent.

Even in those patients who do have resections, survival rates are low. Strong consideration should be given to the addition of postoperative irradiation and/or chemotherapy, since pathologic extension through the wall and/or involved nodes denotes high risk for microscopic or subclinical residual tumor and extensive submucosal spread can occur.

GASTRIC CANCER

Operative Failures

As shown in Table 2, local recurrence or failures (LF) in the tumor bed and regional lymph nodes (RF) or distant failures (DF) via hematogenous (DM) or peritoneal (PS) routes are all common mechanisms of failure after "curative" resection in both reoperative and autopsy series (Gunderson, 1976a, 1979b; Gunderson and Sosin, 1982). Progressive extension of the operative procedure

TABLE 2. Gastric Cancer: Patterns of Failure with "Curative" Resection in Reoperation and Autopsy Series

Pattern of failure[a]	Incidence in total patient group (any component)	
	U of Minnesota reoperation No. %	Autopsy (%)
LF-RF	72/107 (67.3%)	80.5–93%
PS	44/107 (41.1%)	30–42.5%
Localized	20 (18.7%)	—
Diffuse	24 (22.4%)	—
DM	24/107 (22.4%)	49%

Source: Gunderson (1979b), p. 596.

[a]See the text for explanation of LF-RF, PS, and DM.

to include routine splenectomy, omentectomy, and radical lymph node dissection neither improved survival (Gilbertsen, 1969) nor decreased the incidence of LF-RF in the reoperative series (Gunderson and Sosin, 1982).

Treatment

The potential benefits of adjuvant combined drug chemotherapy and irradiation are best illustrated by their value in patients with either locally advanced or disseminated disease (MacDonald et al., 1982b). Radiation alone has been shown to have good palliative and occasional curative potential in patients with residual disease after resection (Abe and Takahashi, 1981) or with unresectable lesions. Its greatest benefit, however, has been when used in combination with chemotherapy (Holbrook, 1974; Moertel, 1982; Schein and Novak, 1982).

Most reports on combined irradiation and chemotherapy deal with patients with residual or unresectable disease and show an advantage of combined treatment over single modality treatment. In an early randomized series (Holbrook, 1974), 5FU was used during the first 3 days of irradiation in half the group. For the combined treatment group, mean and overall survival were improved (13 versus 5.9 months and a 5-year survival of 3/25, or 12%, versus 0/23). In a recent randomized study (Schein and Novak, 1982), the combination of irradiation and 5FU followed by maintenance 5FU-MECCNU was statistically superior to 5FU-MECCNU alone for long-term survival, with a plateau of 20% between the second and third years of follow-up (P = 05).

In view of patterns of failure with this malignancy, it appears that innovative combinations of chemotherapy and irradiation (Gunderson et al., 1983c) compared with combined chemotherapy alone may be necessary to alter both short- and long-term survival. The limited tolerance of the stomach and surrounding organs to radiation limits the dose of external radiotherapy to 5000 to 5500 rad given in 6 to 6.5 weeks. Efficacy may be improved by the addition of radiation dose-modifiers, chemotherapy, or the use of intraoperative boosts in selected cases.

GALLBLADDER AND EXTRAHEPATIC BILIARY DUCTS

Rationale for Irradiation

In view of anatomic location and operative limitations, a large percentage of patients with both gallbladder and extrahepatic biliary duct lesions are either unresectable or have gross or microscopic residual disease after attempts at resection. Exceptions to this are lesions in the periampullary region or distal common duct.

Even after "curative" resection, local recurrences in the tumor bed and/or regional nodes are common for both gallbladder and extrahepatic biliary duct lesions (Kopelson et al., 1977, 1981). Although surgical resections can occasionally be carried out, circumferential margins of resection are often small when either gallbladder or biliary duct lesions extend through the entire wall. For biliary duct lesions, proximal and distal margins may also be close. For extrahepatic duct lesions, local regional failures (LF-RF) are the usual cause of death. In the recent series by Kopelson and coworkers (1981), the major factor influencing later LF-RF was extension through the wall. Hepatic metastases occur in both groups of lesions, but gallbladder carcinoma may involve the liver by hematogenous spread or by direct extension.

Treatment

Adjuvant Irradiation. Since local failures are common even after resection, the potential value of adjuvant radiotherapy needs to be carefully evaluated. In a small series by Vaittinen (1970), the median survival was markedly improved for seven gallbladder cancer patients who received adjuvant postoperative irradiation (63 months) versus 24 patients treated with surgery alone (median, 29 months). There is little information available regarding the use of adjuvant pre- or postoperative irradiation.

PRIMARY IRRADIATION. Significant palliation and occasional cures can be obtained with irradiation of unresectable or recurrent lesions with 4000 to 6000 rad in 4.5 to 7 weeks (Green et al., 1975; Hanna and Rider, 1978; Kopelson et al., 1977, 1981; MacDonald et al., 1982a). Adequate dose levels can be obtained with acceptable morbidity only if the extent of the tumor is carefully delineated by surgical clips at the time of exploration. The addition of external beam radiotherapy can prolong palliation and may allow removal of biliary tract draining catheters. For unresectable lesions, the combination of radiation and chemotherapy needs to be studied, as such combinations have been useful with other adenocarcinomas in the gastrointestinal tract. In the series by Kopelson and colleagues (1977), 1-year survival was improved when 5-Fluorouracil was added to external beam irradiation for advanced primary lesions.

NEW RADIATION MODALITIES. The use of intraoperative electrons has been reported for unresectable lesions by several Japanese groups, most recently by Todorki and coworkers (1980). Although in a few cases the lesion later became resectable, and in others bile duct recanalization occurred, regional recurrence occurred in the vast majority. This suggests that the tumor had extended beyond the small volume encompassed by intraoperative cones.

Radioactive sources (radium, iridium, or cesium) inserted into the biliary tree through transhepatic catheters can deliver localized high-dose irradiation and may have wider applicability than intraoperative electron-beam therapy. Several small series have shown good short-term results (Herskovic et al., 1981; Fletcher et al., 1981).

Both methods described have limitations if used as the sole treatment modality. We prefer to deliver 4500 to 5000 rad to the primary lesion and its regional lymph nodes with external beam multifield techniques and use intraoperative electron-beam therapy or transcatheter sources as a boost (1500 to 2000 rad with intraoperative electron; 2000 to 2500 rad at 0.5 to 1.0 cm radius with transcatheter sources) (Gunderson et al., 1983a). Seven of 10 patients treated with these treatment combinations had biliary duct primaries and were treated with curative intent by one of us (L.L.G.). Four of seven are alive and without disease progression from 6 to 23 months, and a fifth was without progression when lost to follow-up at 18 months.

PANCREATIC CARCINOMA

Rationale

The dismal results after radical surgical resection for adenocarcinomas of the pancreas are well-known (MacDonald et al., 1982c). The best series show survival rates of approximately 15% after resection. An analysis has been performed on the sites of failure after curative resection in 31 patients (Tepper et al., 1976). In the 26 patients who survived the operation, there was a local or regional failure in 50% (13/26), indicating the inadequacy of local treatment. This is undoubtedly due to the propensity of these tumors to invade posteriorly and to the narrow or nonexistent margins of normal tissue between tumor and usually unresectable structures such as portal vein, superior mesenteric vessels, and retroperitoneal soft tissue. Additional local treatment would clearly be a logical step in the treatment of such patients.

Approximately 50% of patients present at laparotomy with only local-regional disease. In the series by Tepper and coworkers (1976), 31 patients had radical resection, but an additional 35 patients had unresectable tumors only because of local extension of disease. In Hermreck's series of 348 patients (1974), 169 or 49% had only local-regional disease at presentation, and the majority were not amenable to surgical resection.

Treatment

External Beam Radiation Therapy. It is clear that palliation can be obtained using external beam irradiation techniques (Dobelbower, 1979; Haslam et al., 1973; Whittington et al., 1981). The duration of such palliation appears to improve by increasing doses of radiation from 4000 rad in 4.5 to 6 weeks to 6000 to 6500 rad in 7 to 10 weeks (using a split-course technique). In order to safely

TABLE 3. Comparison of Results: Cancer of the Pancreas, Varied Series and Techniques

Series	No. pts.	Total group	Median SR (months)		Local failure (evaluable patients)	
			RT	RT + CT	No.	%
Radical operation, MGH (26 postop survivors)	31	10.5	—	—	13/26	50%
Regional, unresectable						
1. Mayo						
a. Untreated	67	6.0	—	—	—	—
b. 3500 rad/4 wk ± 5FU	64	—	6.3	10.4	—	—
2. GITSG						
a. 4000 rad/6 wk + 5FU	79	—	—	6.9	—	—
b. 6000 rad/10 wk ± 5FU (XRT, 25 pts; XRT + CT, 75)	100	—	5.1	8.7	—	—
3. Duke (curative group)						
a. 6000 rad/10 wk ± chemo (RT, 9 pts; RT + CT, 11 pts)	20	—	8	10	—	—
4. Thomas Jefferson						
a. 6300–6700 rad/7–9 wks ± chemo (RT, 30 pts; RT + CT, 16 pts)	46	—	7.3	12.4	36/46	78%
b. External + implant ± chemo[a] (RT, 9 pts; RT ± CT, 17 pts)	26	—	5.5 (7.3)	11.3 (12.5)	5/26	19%
5. Mass General Hospital						
a. I^{125} + external beam XRT (postop) (4000–4500 rad/ 4.5–5 wk)	12	11	—	—	4/12	33%
b. External beam + intraop electron boost (4500–5000 rad split course) ± chemo	18	17.5	—	—	7/18	39%

[a]Median SR: the top number represents early postoperative deaths included; in the number in parentheses below they are excluded.

deliver doses in excess of 4500 to 5000 rad, great care must be taken to minimize the amount of normal tissue in the irradiated field. This requires accurate delineation of the tumor volume (from CT scan or placement of surgical clips) and use of sophisticated treatment planning techniques. Doses beyond 4500 rad must be given to very tightly defined tumor volumes and should usually be delivered with multiple fields.

The combination of radiation therapy and chemotherapy with 5FU for locally unresectable tumors appeared to increase survival in some studies when compared with radiation therapy alone (Table 3). This advantage has been shown in two independent randomized studies (Moertel et al., 1969; GITSG, 1979).

Because of the high failure rate after radical surgical resection, justification also exists for adjuvant treatment with radiation therapy. A recent randomized study of this concept showed increased survival for those receiving radiation therapy and 5-FU when compared with a control group receiving no further treatment after "curative" surgical resection (Kalser et al., 1983). This study is encouraging, but it requires confirmation in a larger patient cohort.

Intraoperative Irradiation (Interstitial Implantation or Electrons). To increase the dose to the tumor volume and thus increase tumor control without significantly damaging normal tissue, efforts have been made to use specialized radiation therapy techniques. These have included the use of intraoperative electrons alone (Abe and Takahashi, 1981; Goldson et al., 1981) or the use of iodine[125] implants (Shipley et al., 1980) or intraoperative electrons (Gunderson et al., 1982; Wood et al., 1982) as a boost dose in combination with external beam irradiation. The combination techniques have resulted in better local control and improved median survival (Table 3, Figure 1) when compared with conventional external beam irradiation, but it is uncertain whether this is due to superior treatment or to case selection. Such answers will be achieved only in prospective randomized clinical trials.

FIGURE 1. Cancer of the pancreas, survival by treatment method comparing radical surgery for resectable lesions to external beam irradiation alone or in combination with an implant or intraoperative electron beam boost for unresectable lesions.

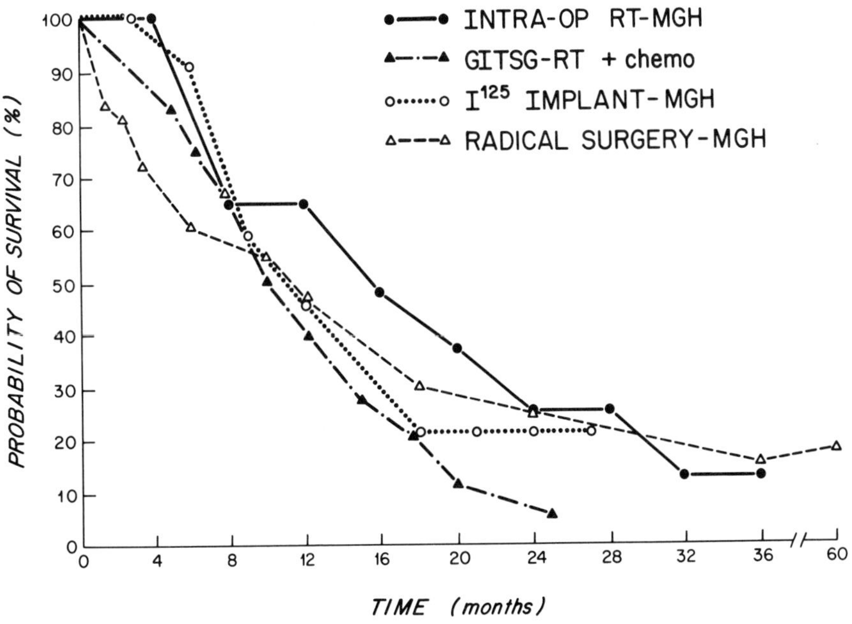

Particle Beams. Radiation using neutrons, pi-mesons, and helium ions have biologic and/or physical dose-distribution differences from conventional radiation that may have a clinical advantage. Preliminary data on the use of neutrons are not encouraging, but charged particles such as helium ions may be producing some benefit (MacDonald et al., 1982c).

COLORECTAL CANCER

Operative Failures After "Curative Resection"

As shown in Tables 4 and 5, the risk of local recurrence after "curative resection" is related to both extension of disease beyond the bowel wall as well as to nodal involvement (Cass et al., 1976; Gilbert, 1978; Rich et al., 1983; Gunderson and Sosin, 1974). As shown in Table 4, local recurrence in the group with nodal involvement but tumor confined to the wall (C_1) was 20 to 25%, which is actually less than in the group with nodes negative but extending through the wall ($B_2 \pm B_3$), where the risk is 30 to 35%. The group that has both bad prognostic factors of nodal involvement and extension through the wall ($C_2 \pm C_3$) has nearly an additive risk of local recurrence varying from 50 to 65% in the clinical series and 70% in the reoperative series.

In the series by Rich and coworkers (1983), the incidence of both total and local failure increased with each degree of extension beyond the wall in the group with no lymph involvement (Table 5). The incidence of pelvic recurrence for the B_3 group was double that of the B_2 (g) subgroup and three times higher than the B_2 (m) subgroup. In the node positive group, although the number of patients in each subgroup was small, there were also suggestive differences. Data from Withers and coworkers (1981) also support the contention that when rectal lesions extend beyond the wall, the most limiting surgical resection margin is often the circumferential margin. With posterior extension in males and

TABLE 4. Colorectal Cancer: Extent of Disease versus Later Local Failure (LF), Varied Series, After Curative Resection

Modified Astler-Coller stage	Clinical series			Reoperation
	U Florida (Colorectum)	Portland (ME) (Rectum-CAPR)	MGH (Rect-R Sig)	U Minn (Rectum-CAPR)
Within wall				
A	0/30 —	0/1 —	0/3 —	— —
B_1	3/20 (15%)	6/42 (14.3%)	3/36 (8.3%)	— —
C_1	4/19 (21.1%)	1/5 —	2/4 —	4/17 (23.5%)
Through wall				
$B_2(\pm B_3)$[a]	29/106 (27.4%)	13/37 (35.1%)	18/59 (30.5%)	— —
$C_2(\pm C_3)$[a]	33/64 (51.6%)	24/37 (64.9%)	20/40 (50%)	28/40 (70%)
Totals	69/239 (28.9%)	44/122 (36.1%)	43/142 (30.3%)	— —

Source: Modified from Gunderson (1979b), p. 593.

[a] B_3 and C_3 include extension into adjacent organs or structures.

TABLE 5. Extent of Tumor versus Later Failure and Survival, MGH; 142 Rectal-Rectosigmoid Patients—"Curative Resection"

Initial extent[a]	Total failure		Pelvic recurrence (LF)	
LN (−)				
A (mucosa only)	0/3	—	0/3	—
B_1 (beyond mucosa; within wall)	7/36	(19%)	3/36	(8%)
B_2 (m) (through wall, microscopically)	4/12	(33%)	2/12	(17%)
B_2 (g) (through wall, grossly)	14/32	(44%)	8/32	(25%)
B_3 (adjacent organ or structure)	10/15	(67%)	8/15	(53%)
LN (+)				
C_1 (within wall)				
C_2 (m) (through wall, microscopically)	6/11	(55%)	4/11	(36%)
C_2 (g) (through wall, grossly)	20/27	(74%)	14/27	(52%)
C_3 (adjacent organ or structure)	5/6	(83%)	4/6	(67%)

Source: Modified from Rich et al. (1983).

[a]Modified Astler-Coller stage.

females, the surgical disease-free margin is often millimeters rather than centimeters, and in males the same is true with anterior or lateral extension of low rectal lesions.

Preoperative Adjuvant Radiotherapy

Most preoperative studies have demonstrated effectiveness of radiotherapy at the time of surgery by either partial or total regression of the primary or the finding of a lower than expected incidence of lymph node involvement. In two prospective randomized low-dose series, a single dose of either 500 rad (Rider, 1975) or 2000 to 2500 rad in 2 to 2.5 weeks (Roswit et al., 1975) produced survival advantages in some irradiated patient groups. In the Roswit series of 700 patients (1975), local recurrence and distant metastases were also decreased in an autopsy subgroup, but both were still unacceptably high at 29% and 40%, respectively. In a high dose, nonrandomized series (Stevens et al., 1976) using 5000 to 6000 rad in 6 to 7 weeks, only 1 of 45 patients (2.3%) with subsequent curative resection was proven to have later pelvic recurrence. This latter data suggest that adequate doses of preoperative radiotherapy in combination with surgery reduce the incidence of local recurrence.

Postoperative Adjuvant Radiotherapy

Three major prospective but nonrandomized postoperative series used similar dose levels of 4500 to 5500 rad in 5 to 6.5 weeks and treated only those patients at high risk for local recurrence (Gunderson, 1976b, 1979a,b; Romsdahl and Withers, 1978; Withers et al., 1981; Hoskins et al., 1984). Table 6 compares local recurrence rates after curative resection alone or in combination with radiotherapy. For equivalent total groups (B_{2-3}, C_{1-3}), local recurrence decreased

TABLE 6. Extent of Disease versus Later Local Failure, Clinical Series After Curative Resection of Colorectal Cancer

	Operation alone		Operation + postop XRT	
Extent of Disease	U Florida, MDAH, MGH, Maine	MDAH (rectal)[a]	LDS-SLC (colorectal)[b]	MGH (rectal)[d]
Within wall				
LN + (C_1)	20–25%	0/3	0/2	1/9 (11%)
Through wall				
LN− (B_2 + B_3)	25–35%	1/18 (5.9%)	0/10	2/36 (5.5%)
LN+ (C_2 + C_3)	45–65%	3/33 (9.1%)	2/16[c] (12.5%)	5/50[e] (10%)
LN−, LN+ (B_3 or C_3)	—	1/18 (12.5%)	—	—
LN status unknown (B_{2-3} vs C_{2-3})	—	—	0/4	—
Totals	37–48%	5/62 (8.1%)	2/34 (6%)	8/95[e] (8.4%)

[a]August 1977 analysis (Romsdahl and Withers, 1978).
[b]June 1978 analysis, minimum 2 year F/U (Gunderson, 1979a).
[c]Both had deviation in planned dose/time scheme and received 4500 rad/5 wk.
[d]June 1981 analysis, all with minimum 2-year follow-up and 66% with minimum 3-year follow-up (Hoskins et al., 1984).
[e]Marginal recurrence in one additional patient (6/50 or 12% C_2 + C_3 and 7/95 or 7/4% of total group).

from 37 to 48% with operation alone to 6 to 8% in the XRT series. Similar decreases were seen for each stage of disease. In the B_{2-3} subgroup, the reduction was nearly tenfold, from 30 to 35% down to 5%; and in the C_{2-3} subgroup, from 45 to 65% down to 10 to 12%. Distant metastases in the three nonrandomized series, however, continued to be a problem in 25 to 30% of patients, emphasizing a continued need for development of good systemic treatment.

In the analysis by Hoskins and coworkers (1984), local recurrence was compared in nonrandomized but sequential series for operation alone (103 patients) with operation and postoperative irradiation (95 patients). Since one cannot fairly compare overall local recurrence rates, as one group is at risk for a longer time period, both groups were analyzed 3 years after operation. There was a statistically significant reduction in local recurrence at most stages in the groups that received adjuvant postoperative irradiation.

In a randomized trial reported by Mittelman and colleagues (1981), patients were randomized to a surgical control arm versus treatment arms of postoperative irradiation, postoperative chemotherapy, or a combination thereof. In the radiation alone arm, patients received either 4000 or 4800 rad; and in the radiation plus chemotherapy arm, either 4000 or 4400 rad. The disease-free survival

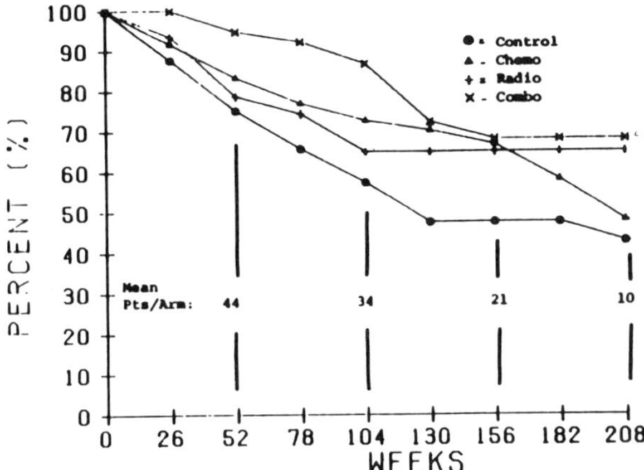

FIGURE 2. Comparison of disease-free survival curves in randomized trial of resected rectal cancer. *Source:* Mittelman et al. (1981).

of all three treated arms was superior to surgery alone at the interval of 130 to 156 weeks (Figure 2). The difference between the combined arm of chemotherapy plus irradiation versus surgery alone is statistically significant ($P = .03$ to .05, dependent on method of analysis). The combined arm did not, however, result in a decrease in the incidence of distant metastases but rather a decrease in local recurrence when patterns of first site of failure were analyzed. This suggests that the effect of the chemotherapy was not a systemic effect but rather a local effect as a radiopotentiator. In spite of the improvement in disease-free survival in both arms with irradiation, the local recurrence rate with radiation alone was too high, with a minimum rate of 7 of 47 or 15%. (This figure may be higher, as only first patterns of failure have been published.)

The 6 to 8% incidence of local recurrence in the three nonrandomized but prospective postoperative series previously discussed was only approximately half that in the randomized study treating similar patient subgroups. This is perhaps because the minimum dose within the boost field of the nonrandomized series was usually 5000 rads, whereas approximately 50% of the patients in the randomized radiation alone arm received only 4000 rads.

Residual, Recurrent Unresectable (External Beam ± Intraoperative Boost)

While an improvement in local control, and possibly survival, can be achieved with adjuvant irradiation, this becomes more difficult if residual disease is present after resection or if the tumor is unresectable (Wang and Schulz, 1962), since higher doses of radiation are required. When residual disease is present (Allee et al., 1981; Ghossein et al., 1981), the incidence of local recurrence after external beam irradiation is doubled when gross rather than microscopic disease is present (50–54% versus 15–26%). A possible dose-response correlation was seen in the group with microscopic residual disease, with approximately a 10% risk of local failure if 6000 rad was administered, compared with 33%

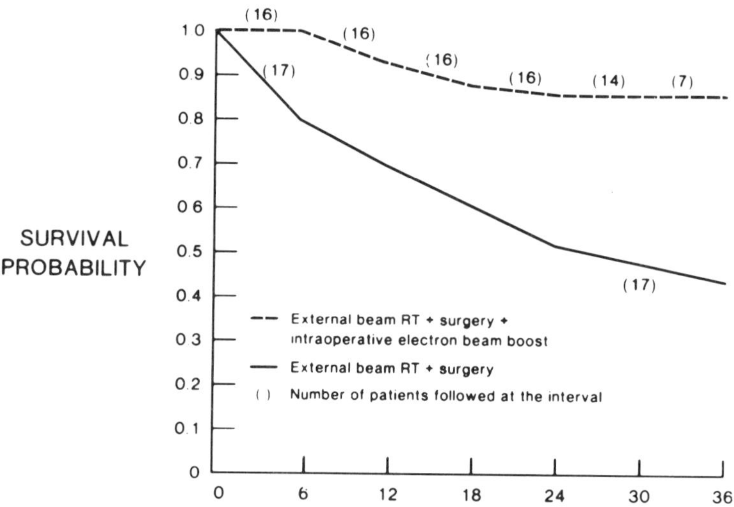

FIGURE 3. Comparison of crude survival with resection and external beam irradiation versus resection plus external beam and intraoperative irradiation for initially unresectable rectal cancer ($P < .01$ to .025, depending on method of analysis).

(7/21), if the boost dose was ≥ 5500 rad. When gross residual disease was present, no correlation was seen (Allee et al., 1981).

In patients with unresectable tumors, a number of institutions have given preoperative radiotherapy in an attempt to shrink the lesion, allow resection, and possibly improve local control and survival (Stevens et al., 1976; Emami et al., 1982; Dosoretz et al., 1983). The resectability rate after doses of 4500 to 5000 rad has varied from 50 to 75% by series. Even in those patients who were resected, the incidence of local recurrence has been excessive at 36 to 45%.

While combinations of external beam radiation and surgery do seem to decrease pelvic recurrence and improve survival in the subgroups with residual disease (postoperative radiotherapy) or initially unresectable disease (preoperative radiotherapy), local recurrence is still unacceptably high and survival could be improved. In view of this, 32 patients received the standard previous treatment of external beam irradiation and surgery, but in addition they received an intraoperative electron beam boost of 1000 to 1500 rads to the remaining tumor or tumor bed at the time of surgical exploration or resection (Gunderson et al., 1982, 1983d). Some patients had undergone preoperative radiotherapy for initially unresectable disease; others were being reexplored because of residual disease. For the 16 patients who presented with unresectable primary lesions, the addition of intraoperative radiotherapy has yielded survival rates that are statistically better at 1 and 2 years than that of the previous group treated with only external beam irradiation and surgical resection (Figure 3). There have not been any local recurrences with a minimum 20-month follow-up period in the group with all three treatment modalities. In the group with residual disease, again there have been no local recurrences in the seven patients that received all treatment modalities versus 54% and 26% for the group with gross and microscopic residual disease treated with only external beam techniques. The remaining nine patients presented with unresectable recurrent lesions.

Therapeutic Ratio

It does little good to accomplish adequate local control if it is achieved with a high incidence of complications. A suitable therapeutic ratio between local control and complications is achieved only with close interaction between the surgeon and the radiotherapist (Gunderson et al., 1979a, b, 1980, 1983a). Major surgical considerations include use of radiopaque clips to mark the tumor bed as well as the use of pelvic reconstruction techniques to displace the small bowel. The small bowel may also be protected by the use of (1) lateral fields to avoid as much small bowel as possible while still including the area at risk, (2) shrinking or boost-field techniques, and (3) treatment with bladder distension.

In three postop rectal series using similar radiation doses (4500 rad in large fields and 5000 rad within a boost), the incidence of small bowel obstruction requiring reoperation appears to vary if parallel opposed rather than multifield techniques are used. In a series reported by Withers and coworkers (1981), with parallel opposed techniques and superior field extent at L-2 to L-3, small bowel obstruction occurred in 17.5% of irradiated patients versus 5% with surgery alone. When the superior extent was reduced down to L-5, the incidence of operative intervention decreased from 17.5% to 10 to 12% (ongoing follow-up). These figures are similar to those found in another series using parallel opposed techniques (Gunderson, 1976b, 1979a). Using multifield techniques, bladder distension, and other preventative measures, the incidence of small bowel obstruction requiring operative intervention is essentially equal in the group receiving irradiation (4% with minimum 2-year follow-up) compared with operation alone (5%) (Hoskins et al., 1984).

Conclusions and Future Possibilities: Rectal Cancer

In an adjuvant setting, doses of 5000 rad in 5.5 to 6 weeks given either pre- or postoperatively in conjunction with resection of all known disease produces good local control in most patient subgroups with rectal cancer. In the subgroup with bad prognostic factors of node involvement and extension through the wall, the incidence of local recurrence has been reduced from 45–65% down to 10–12%. Ultimately, further increase in the radiation dose in this subgroup may be of additional benefit, if it can be done safely. Complications appear to be minimal, provided preventative measures to avoid small bowel damage are used. Distant failure occurs in 25 to 30% of patients via either the hematogenous or the peritoneal route. In selected subgroups, it remains to be seen whether innovative combinations of radiation plus systemic therapy, low-dose preoperative radiation therapy combined with selective postoperative radiation or pelvic plus whole abdominal irradiation in selected subgroups can alter the incidence of distant failures.

SUMMARY AND FUTURE PERSPECTIVES

Lesion Resectability

As experience with high resolution computed body tomography (CT) increases, it is possible that preoperative CT studies can help determine which lesions are unresectable for cure. Such information could be important in designing future trials seeking to analyze the value of either high or low dose preoperative irradiation prior to exploration and resection (Gunderson et al., 1983a,b; Dosoretz et al., 1983).

Adjuvant Irradiation

The potential for radiation therapy is considerable when used in combination with surgery and perhaps systemic therapy in lesions that are resectable but at high risk of local recurrence. Operation alone yields inadequate results for many carcinomas of the gastrointestinal tract that present with gross tumor extending through the wall and/or nodal involvement. The use of radical operative procedures, while justifiable, does not uniformly prevent either local failures or regrowth (LF) in the tumor bed and regional lymph nodes or distant failures (DF) by hematogenous (DM) or peritoneal routes (PS).

With bowel, gastric, and esophageal cancers, the surgeon and pathologist often discuss tumor-free margins proximally and distally but rarely discuss the circumferential margin around a tumor that extends beyond the wall. Due to the presence of surrounding normal structures that cannot be resected easily or with acceptable morbidity, the circumferential margin may often be the narrowest or most limiting margin, and, therefore, the cause of local recurrence. Progressive extension of operative procedures to increase these margins may yield slight gains in cure rates, but these gains may be offset or minimized by a corresponding increase in operative morbidity and mortality. These "margins" could possibly be obtained with less morbidity by close interactions of the surgeon and radiation oncologist in the use of combined modality treatment. Many of the local regional failures that occur are predictable and are due to the presence of occult residual disease. Most of these failures should be preventable with the use of moderate doses of irradiation in the range of 4500 to 5500 rad in accordance with the "subclinical disease radiation dose concept" (Fletcher, 1973).

A well-designed combination of pre- and postoperative irradiation could combine the theoretical advantages of each (Gunderson and Sosin, 1974; Gunderson, 1976b). An approach used in rectal cancer is to deliver 500 rad in a single fraction or 1000 rad in five fractions with the intent of altering implantability of cells, when surgical resection is carried out 1 to 3 days later. Patients at high risk for local recurrence receive 4500 to 5000 rad postoperatively (Gunderson et al., 1983b; Mohiuddin et al., 1980, 1982). A similar approach would be attractive for potentially resectable esophageal, gastric, and pancreatic cancers since circumferential margins are often narrow and tumor manipulation may be necessary.

Most metastases probably occur prior to resection. If available chemotherapeutic agents do not alter the incidence of such failures when used in combinations with resection and local irradiation, the use of wide-field irradiation for a portion of treatment may have to be used, as in ovarian cancer (Dembo et al., 1979). Such a concept would have widest application for gastric, pancreatic, gallbladder, and colonic lesions, since a majority of hematogenous failures are in the liver, and the risk of limited or diffuse peritoneal seeding is not insignificant.

Residual, Unresectable, or Recurrent Disease

For locally advanced or recurrent gastrointestinal lesions in which the surgeon feels that operative resection will never have a role, the combination of external beam irradiation and chemotherapy can achieve useful palliation in 75 to 80% of patients and an occasional cure (Moertel, 1982; Gunderson, 1976a). If lesion size and location are such that intraoperative boosts with implantation techniques or electrons can be safely used to supplement external beam therapy, further gains may be possible. Early pilot studies suggest, however, that even with such boost techniques, the addition of radiation dose modifiers (radiation sensitizers, hyperthermia) may be necessary.

When unresectable or residual disease is treated with a combination of conventional irradiation and resection, local control and long-term survival can be achieved in 25 to 30% of patients. The presence of dose-limiting normal tissues, however, prevents delivery of adequate levels of external beam irradiation. In early colorectal pilot studies, the addition of intraoperative electron boosts appeared to improve both local control and survival significantly. Even if such results can be duplicated in randomized trials, they may not be able to be achieved in other gastrointestinal malignancies since systemic failures play a more predominant role.

REFERENCES

Abe M, Takahashi M (1981) Intraoperative radiotherapy: The Japanese experience. Int J Radiat Oncol Biol Phys 5:863–868.

Abe M, Takahashi M, Yakumoto E (1980) Clinical experiences with intraoperative radiotherapy of locally advanced cancers. Cancer 45:40–48.

Allee PE, Gunderson LL, Munzenrider JE (1981) Postoperative radiation therapy for residual colorectal carcinoma. ASTR Proceedings. Int J Radiat Oncol Biol Phys 7:1208.

Astler VB, Coller RA (1954) The prognostic significance of direct extension of carcinoma of the colon and rectum. Ann Surg 139:846–851.

Cass AW, Pfaff FA, Million RR (1976) Patterns of recurrence following surgery alone for adenocarcinoma of the colon-rectum. Cancer 37:2861–2865.

Dembo AJ, Van Dyk J, Japp B, et al. (1979) Whole abdominal irradiation by a moving strip technique for patients with ovarian cancer. Int J Radiat Oncol Biol Phys 5:1933–1942.

Dobelbower RR (1979) The radiotherapy of pancreatic cancer. Semin Oncol 6:378–389.

Dosoretz DE, Gunderson LL, Hoskins B, et al. (1983) Preoperative irradiation for localized carcinoma of the rectum and rectosigmoid: Patterns of failure, survival and future treatment strategies. Cancer 9.

Emami B, Pilepich M, Wilett C, Munzenrider JE, Miller HH (1982) Management of unresectable colorectal carcinoma (preoperative radiotherapy and surgery). Int J Radiat Oncol Biol Phys 8:1295–1299.

Fletcher GH (1973) Clinical dose-response curves of human malignant epithelial tumors. Br J Radiol 46:1–12.

Fletcher MS et al. (1981) Treatment of high bile duct carcinoma by internal radiotherapy with Iridium-102 wire. Lancet 2:172–174.

Ghossein NA, Samala EC, Alpert S, et al. (1981) Results of postoperative radiotherapy in patients who had incomplete resection of a colorectal cancer. Dis Colon Rectum 24:252–256.

Gilbert SB (1978) The significance of symptomatic local tumor failure following abdomino-perineal resection. Int J Radiat Oncol Biol Phys 4:801–807.

Gilbertsen VA (1969) Results of treatment of stomach cancer: An appraisal of efforts for more extensive surgery and a report of 1938 cases. Cancer 23:1305–1308.

GITSG (1979) Comparative therapeutic trial of radiation with or without chemotherapy in pancreatic carcinoma. Int J Radiat Oncol Biol Phys 5:1643–1647.

Goldson AL, Ashaveri E, Espinoza MC, et al. (1981) Single-dose intraoperative electrons for advanced stage pancreatic cancer: Phase I pilot study. Int J Radiat Oncol Biol Phys 7:869–874.

Green N, Mikkelsen WP, Kernan JA (1975) Cancer of the common hepatic bile ducts: Palliative radiotherapy. Radiology 109:687–689.

Gunderson LL (1976a) Radiation therapy: Results and future possibilities. In: Sherlock P, Zamcheck N, eds., Gastrointestinal malignancies. East Sussex, Eng: WB Saunders Co., Lth., Clin Gastroenterol 5:743–776.

Gunderson LL (1976b) Combined irradiation and surgery for rectal and sigmoid carcinoma. In: Fletcher G, ed., Emerging roles of radiotherapy in four selected areas. Curr Probl Cancer 1:40–53.

Gunderson LL (1979a) Radiation therapy of colorectal carcinoma. In: Thatcher N, ed., Digestive cancer, vol. 9. XII International Cancer Congress Proceedings, New York: Permagon Press, pp. 29–38.

Gunderson LL (1979b) Radiation oncology: Pathways of tumor spread; radiation therapy—current state of the art. In: Margolis AR, Burhenne JH, eds., Alimentary tract radiology, vol. 3. St. Louis: CV Mosby, pp. 593–619.

Gunderson LL, Sosin H (1974) Areas of failure found at reoperation (second or symptomatic look) following "curative surgery" for adenocarcinoma of the rectum: Clinicopathologic correlation and implications for adjuvant therapy. Cancer 34:1278–1292.

Gunderson LL, Sosin H (1982) Adenocarcinoma of the stomach: Areas of failure in a reoperation series (second or symptomatic looks): Clinicopathologic correlation and implications for adjuvant therapy. Int J Radiat Biol Phys 8:1–11.

Gunderson LL, Shipley WU, Suit HD, et al. (1982) Intraoperative irradiation: A pilot study combining external beam irradiation with "boost" dose intraoperative electrons. Cancer 49:2259–2266.

Gunderson LL, Meyer JE, Sheedy P, Munzenrider JE (1983a) Radiation oncology. Part 18 in Alimentary Tract Radiology, 3rd ed. Margolis AR, Burhenne HJ, ed., St. Louis: CV Mosby, pp. 2409–2446.

Gunderson LL, Cohen AM, Welch CW (1980) Residual, inoperable or recurrent colorectal cancer: Surgical-radiotherapy interaction. Am J Surg 139:518–525.

Gunderson LL, Dosoretz DE, Hedberg SE, et al. (1983b) Low-dose preoperative irradiation, surgery and elective postoperative radiation therapy for resectable rectum and rectosigmoid carcinoma. Cancer 52:446–451.

Gunderson LL, Hoskins B, Cohen AM, et al. (1983c) Combined modality treatment of gastric cancer. Int J Radiat Oncol Biol Phys 9:965–975.

Gunderson LL, Cohen AM, Dosoretz DE, et al. (1983d) Residual, unresectable or recurrent colorectal cancer: External beam irradiation and intraoperative electron beam boost ± resection. Int J Radiat Oncol Biol Phys 9.

Hanna SS, Rider WD (1978) Carcinoma of the gallbladder or extrahepatic bile ducts: The role of radiotherapy. Can Med Assoc J 118:59–61.

Haslam JB, Cavanaugh PJ, Stroup SL (1973) Radiation therapy in the treatment of irresectable adenocarcinoma of the pancreas. Cancer 32:1341–1345.

Hermreck AS, Thomas CY, Friesen SR (1974) Importance or pathologic staging and the surgical management of adenocarcinoma of the exocrine pancreas. Am J Surg 127:653–657.

Herskovic A, Heaston D, Engler MJ, et al. (1981) Irradiation of biliary carcinomas. Radiology 139:219–222.

Holbrook MA (1974) Radiation therapy. Current concept in cancer. Chapter 44 in Gastric cancer: Treatment principles. JAMA 228:1289–1290.

Hoskins B, Gunderson LL, Dosoretz D, et al. (1984) Adjuvant postoperative radiotherapy in carcinoma of the rectum and rectosigmoid. Cancer (In press.)

Kalser M, Ellenberg S, Levin B, et al. (1983) Am Soc Clin Oncol (Abstract.)

Kopelson G, Harisiadis L, Tretter P, et al. (1977) The role of radiation therapy in cancer of the extrahepatic biliary system: An analysis of thirteen patients and a review of the literature of the effectiveness of surgery, chemotherapy and radiotherapy. Int J Radiat Oncol Biol Phys 2:883–894.

Kopelson G, Galdabini J, Warshaw A, et al. (1981) Patterns of failure after curative surgery for extrahepatic biliary tract carcinoma. Int J Radiat Oncol Biol Phys 7:413–417.

Leichman L, Steiger Z, Seydel HG, Haas CD (1981) Potentially curative combined modality therapy for inoperable carcinoma of the esophagus. ASCO Proceedings 22:458 (Abstract).

MacDonald JS, Gunderson LL, Adson M (1982a) Hepatobiliary cancer. In: DeVita VT, Hellman S, Rosenberg SA, eds., Principles and practice of oncology. Phildelphia: JB Lippincott, pp. 590–615.

MacDonald JS, Gunderson LL, Cohn I (1982b) Carcinoma of the stomach. In: DeVita VT, Hellman S, Rosenberg SA, eds., Principles and practice of oncology. Philadelphia: JB Lippincott, pp. 534–562.

MacDonald JS, Gunderson LL, Cohn I (1982c) Cancer of the pancreas. In: DeVita VT, Hellman S, Rosenberg SA, eds., Principles and practice of oncology. Philadelphia: JB Lippincott, pp. 563–589.

Merendino KA, Mark VH (1952) An analysis of 100 cases of squamous cell carcinoma of the esophagus with special reference to its theoretical curability. Surg Gynec Obstet 94:110–114.

Mittelman A, Holyoke E, Thomas PRM, et al. (for GITSG) (1981) Adjuvant chemotherapy and radiotherapy following rectal surgery: An interim report from the gastrointestinal tumor study group (GITSG). In: Salmon SE, Jones SE, eds., Adjuvant therapy of cancer III. New York: Grune and Stratton, pp. 547–557.

Moertel CG (1982) Alimentary tract cancer. In: Holland J, Frei E, ed., Cancer medicine, 2nd ed. Philadelphia: Lea and Febiger, pp. 1753–1866.

Moertel CG, Childs DS Jr, Reitemeier RJ, et al. (1969) Combined 5-fluorouracil and supervoltage radiation therapy of locally unresectable gastrointestinal cancer. Lancet 2:865–867.

Mohiuddin M, Dobelbower RR, Kramer S (1980) A new approach to adjuvant radiotherapy in rectal cancer. Int J Radiat Oncol Biol Phys 6:205–207.

Mohiuddin M, Kramer S, Marks G, Dobelbower RR (1982) Combined pre- and postoperative radiation for carcinoma of the rectum. Int J Radiat Oncol Biol Phys 8: 133–136.

Pearson JG (1975) Value of radiation therapy. In: Current concepts in cancer 42-II. Esophagus: treatment—localized and advanced. JAMA 227:181–183.

Rich T, Gunderson LL, Galdabini J, et al. (1983) Clinical and pathologic factors influencing local failure after curative resection of carcinoma of the rectum and rectosigmoid. Cancer 52:1317–1329.

Rider WD (1975) Is the Miles operation really necessary for the treatment of rectal cancer? J Can Assoc Radiol 26:167–175.

Romsdahl M, Withers HR (1978) Radiotherapy combined with curative surgery. Arch Surg 113:446–453.

Roswit B, Higgins GA, Keehn RJ (1975) Preoperative irradiation for carcinoma of the rectum and rectosigmoid colon: Report of a National Veteran's Administration randomized study. Cancer 35:1597–1602.

Schein PS, Novak J (for GITSG) (1982) Combined modality therapy (XRT-chemo) versus chemotherapy alone for locally unresectable gastric cancer. Cancer 49:1771–1777.

Shipley WU, Nardi GL, Cohen AM, et al. (1980) Iodine-125 implant and external beam irradiation in patients with localized pancreatic carcinoma: A comparative study to surgical resection. Cancer 45:709–714.

Stevens KR, Allen CV, Fletcher WS (1976) Preoperative radiotherapy for adenocarcinoma of the rectosigmoid. Cancer 37:2866–2874.

Tepper J, Nardi GL, Suit HD (1976) Carcinoma of the pancreas review of MGH experience from 1963 to 1973: Analysis of surgical failure and implications for radiation therapy. Cancer 37:1519–1524.

Todorki T, Iwasaki Y, Okamura T (1980) Intraoperative radiotherapy for advanced carcinoma of the biliary system. Cancer 46:2179–2184.

Vaittinen E (1970) Carcinoma of the gallbladder. Ann Chir Gynaecol Fenn 168 (Suppl):1–81.

Wang CC, Schulz MD (1962) The role of radiation therapy in the management of carcinoma of the sigmoid, rectosigmoid and rectum. Radiology 79:1–5.

Whittington R, Dobelbower RR, Mohiuddin M, Rosato FF, Weiss SM (1981) Radiotherapy of unresectable pancreatic carcinoma: A six-year experience with 104 patients. Int J Radiat Oncol Biol Phys 7:1639–1644.

Whittington R, Mohiuddin M, Cantor RI, et al. (1984) Multimodality therapy of localized unresectable pancreatic adenocarcinoma. Cancer (In press.)

Withers HR, Romsdahl MM, Saxton JP (1981) Elective radiation therapy in the curative treatment of cancer of the rectum and rectosigmoid colon. In: Stroehlein JR, Romsdahl MM, eds., Gastrointestinal cancer. New York: Raven Press, pp. 351–362.

Wood W, Shipley WU, Gunderson LL, Cohen AM, Nardi GL (1982) Intraoperative irradiation for unresectable pancreatic carcinoma. Cancer 49:1272–1275.

LARGE BOWEL CARCINOMA: SIGNIFICANCE OF VENOUS INVASION

I C TALBOT, M.D., F.R.C.PATH.

Conventionally, carcinomas are considered to invade tissues and spread along lymphatic channels and, indeed, metastases frequently develop in local and regional lymph nodes. However, dissemination to the liver and other distant sites commonly occurs (in 33.3% of cases of rectal cancer, Talbot, 1979) and is not easily explained by consideration of lymphatic spread exclusively.

Many efforts have been made to show that carcinoma of the large bowel and other sites invades venous channels, thereby permitting direct contact with venous blood and potential malignant embolus formation (Willis, 1930; Brown and Warren, 1938; Buckwalter and Kent, 1973). There have, however, been conflicting results in regard to both the incidence of blood vessel invasion and its significance in the natural history of colorectal cancer. Precision and consistency are necessary in the identification of venous invasion before its clinical significance can be assessed. Only when permeation of veins can be reliably detected can this feature be used to predict prognosis. The frequency with which venous invasion is observed is proportional to the care taken in the laboratory examination of each operation specimen.

However, even when a tumor is found to be invading veins, the inevitability of hematogenous dissemination should not be assumed; examples of "benign" vascular invasion are recorded in the case of leiomyomas (Norris and Parmley, 1975) and of benign-behaving pheochromocytomas (Symington, 1969). The interaction of the host tissues in the blood vessel wall with carcinoma as it invades the vein may play a part in influencing the ultimate distant spread of the tumor. The various forms that this host reaction takes and its relationship to survival of patients with rectal cancer have been described (Talbot et al., 1981a).

From the Department of Pathology, University of Leicester, United Kingdom.

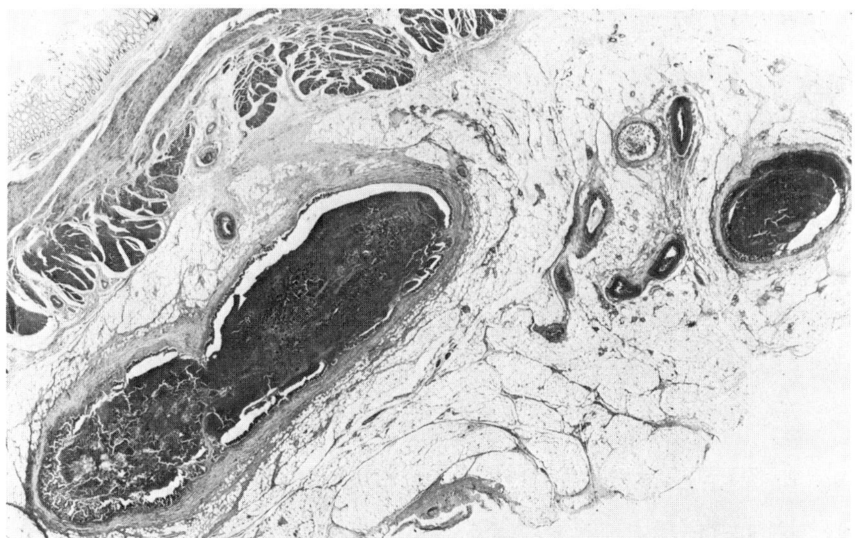

FIGURE 1. Extramural veins at the edge of rectal carcinoma, permeated by a tumor. Note the extensive necrosis of the intravenous adenocarcinoma. (Hematoxylin and eosin × 6.)

IDENTIFICATION OF VENOUS INVASION

Invasion of veins can be demonstrated when carcinoma cells are seen in histologic sections in continuity with the lining of one or more veins in or around the tumor (Figure 1). As an aid to detection, it is helpful to take blocks for histology oriented at a tangent to the periphery of the tumor (Figure 2). It is doubtful whether the detection rate can be increased by using special stains for elastic or smooth muscle (Talbot et al., 1980), although such procedures may allow a more elegant demonstration of venous spread. Some areas of carcinoma may

FIGURE 2. Hypothetical large bowel cancer showing how a carcinoma invades the veins and lymphatics in parallel at the periphery of the tumor. Dotted line shows the ideal orientation of tissue-blocks for histologic detection of venous invasion.

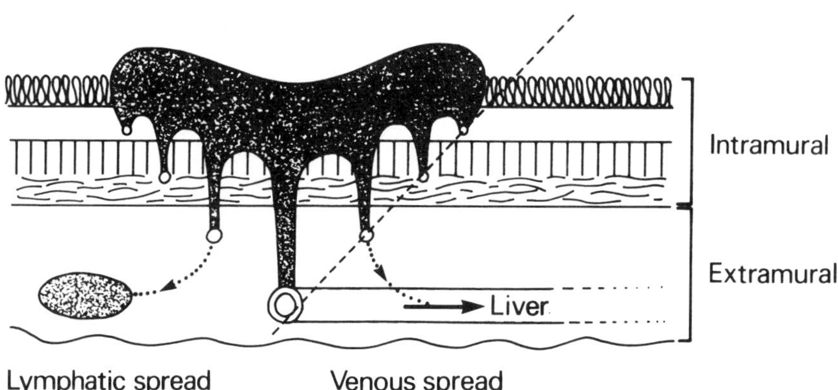

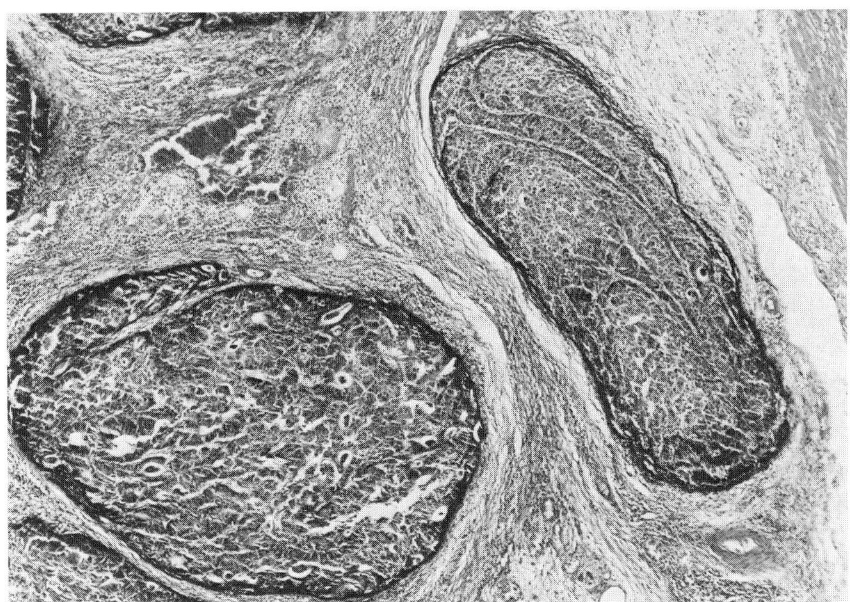

FIGURE 3. Circumscribed rounded masses of rectal carcinoma, possibly resulting from confinement of the tumor by overstretched and destroyed vein walls. Despite this suspicion, such appearances cannot be certainly regarded as due to vein invasion. (Hematoxylin and eosin × 35.)

be suspected of invading veins (Figure 3), but vein wall structures may not be demonstrable even with these connective tissue stains. Although it is possible that these appearances represent growth along venous channels with secondary overdistension and destruction of vessel wall structure, they are not proof of venous invasion; definite evidence of residual vascular structure is required before a tumor can be regarded as involving veins.

INCIDENCE OF VENOUS INVASION

Unequivocal invasion of veins by rectal cancer can be demonstrated in the way just described in at least 52% of cases (Talbot et al., 1980). Submucosal veins are most frequently involved, and it seems likely that the tumor spreads into these small venous channels in parallel with lymphatic permeation (Figure 2).

More extensive vascular invasion, involving extramural veins, also parallels the general extent of infiltration by the tumor and is present in 33% of the group of Dukes' stage B tumors (Morson, 1976) overall, in direct proportion to the general extent of infiltration of extramural tissue within this group, subjectively assessed (Table 1). It should be noted that this trend is continued when invasion of *large* (that is, *thick-walled*) *extramural* veins is singled out for consideration; involvement of such thick-walled veins can be regarded as an extension of the process of venous permeation.

TABLE 1. Relationship Between Invasion of Extramural Veins and the General Extent of Local Infiltration by Rectal Adenocarcinoma (Dukes' Stage B Tumors Only)

	Extent of extramural infiltration		
	Slight	Moderate	Extensive
Number of cases	143	67	54
Percent with invasion of extramural veins	25.9	37.3	46.3
Percent involving large (thick-walled) extramural veins	6.3	10.4	12.3

IMPORTANCE OF VENOUS INVASION IN DISSEMINATION OF COLORECTAL CANCER

As long ago as 1930, Willis investigated the role of venous invasion by abdominal visceral tumors in an autopsy series and found that although primary tumors frequently spread into veins, only involvement of *large* veins appeared to correlate with the presence of liver metastases.

It has been shown (Talbot et al., 1981a) that invasion of intramural (that is, submucosal or intramuscular) veins by a tumor does not influence prognosis. It seems likely that such vascular permeation, like spread along lymphatics, is a commonplace event and part of the natural development of the disease. However, when there is spread into *extramural* veins, malignant embolism via the bloodstream more readily takes place (Figure 2); liver and other distant metastases develop more frequently; and the survival rate (actuarilly corrected to allow for deaths from all causes) is lower (Table 2). It is interesting, in view of Willis's findings, that invasion of large (that is, thick-walled), extramural veins has the most profound effect in these respects.

VENOUS INVASION AS AN INDICATOR OF PROGNOSIS

Using the extent of venous invasion as a marker for predicting the behavior of a particular tumor, although useful, does not in itself have any advantage over the Dukes' staging procedure (Talbot et al., 1980). However, when combined

TABLE 2. Invasion of Veins as a Marker for Prognosis in Rectal Cancer

Venous invasion		Number of cases	Distant metastases	Corrected 5-year survival rate
Not demonstrated		338	22%	73%
Intramural		111	30%	66%
Extramural	Small veins	161	39%	41%
	Large veins	93	68%	19%[a]

[a]Of 91 cases.

TABLE 3. Survival Rates in Rectal Cancer Taking Both Venous Invasion and Dukes' Stage into Account

Venous invasion		Corrected 5-year survival rate		
		A	B	C
Not demonstrated		96%	86%	46%
Intramural		102%	85%	40%
Extramural	Small veins	—	68%	23%
	Large veins	—	52%	8%

with an assessment of the Dukes' stage, there is an additive effect, so that the prognosis can be precisely predicted (Talbot et al., 1981b) (Table 3).

Patients with tumors that are likely to behave in a particularly aggressive way can thus be identified, the corrected 5-year survival rate of patients with stage C tumors being only 8% when there is invasion of thick-walled extramural veins. Conversely, patients with stage A (or even B) tumors in which venous spread is not demonstrated are unlikely to develop recurrence of disseminated disease. However, this only holds true if the pathologist responsible for handling the case takes sufficient care to guarantee a pick-up rate of venous invasion of at least 50%. Statistical analysis has shown that examination of sections from an average of five blocks of tumor tissue is necessary for this (Talbot et al., 1981a).

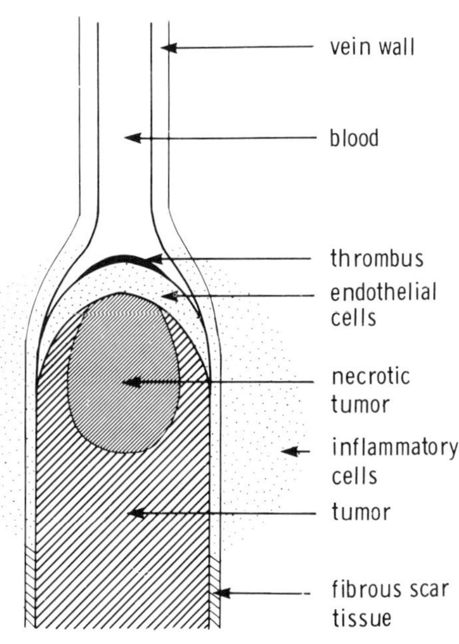

FIGURE 4. Diagram of a carcinoma permeating a rectal vein, showing how ischemic necrosis develops in the tumor when blood-flow ceases and the inflammatory reaction to this results in damage and fibrous replacement of the vein wall. *Source:* Modified with editors' permission, from Talbot (1980b) and Talbot et al. (1981a).

BIOLOGIC PHENOMENON OF VENOUS INVASION AND ITS RELATIONSHIP TO TUMOR BEHAVIOR

Study of a large number of examples of vein invasion by rectal cancer (Talbot et al., 1981a) has revealed that necrosis of the center of the tumor within the vein is the rule (Figure 1). This, typically, excites an inflammatory reaction in the surrounding tissues, including the vein wall and induces proliferation of endothelial cells in the lining of the vein adjacent to the tumor (Figure 4), with a resulting picture of endophlebitis obliterans (Figures 5 and 6) and a variable degree of damage to normal vein wall structures.

The degree of host reaction to an intravenous tumor has been related to the clinical course of the disease in a series of 248 patients with rectal cancer involving extramural veins (Talbot et al., 1981a). Tables 4 through 10 reproduce the results of this study. The 5-year survival rate, corrected to take account of deaths from other disease, was lowest when there was no or minimal damage from tissue reaction in the vein wall (10.8%) and highest when the vein wall structure was completely destroyed (57.1%), as in Figure 6 (Table 4). The endothelial mantle formed by the process of endophlebitis obliterans, as in Figures 5 and 6, appears to have a protective effect on the host, as Table 5 shows, with the survival rate being doubled compared with cases when this feature was not

FIGURE 5. A thin-walled vein invaded by an adenocarcinoma of the rectum, illustrating the features shown diagrammatically in Figure 4. There is a well-defined shielding cap of endothelial cells at the apex of the tumor formed by a process of endophlebitis obliterans. *Source:* Talbot et al. (1981a), with editor's permission.

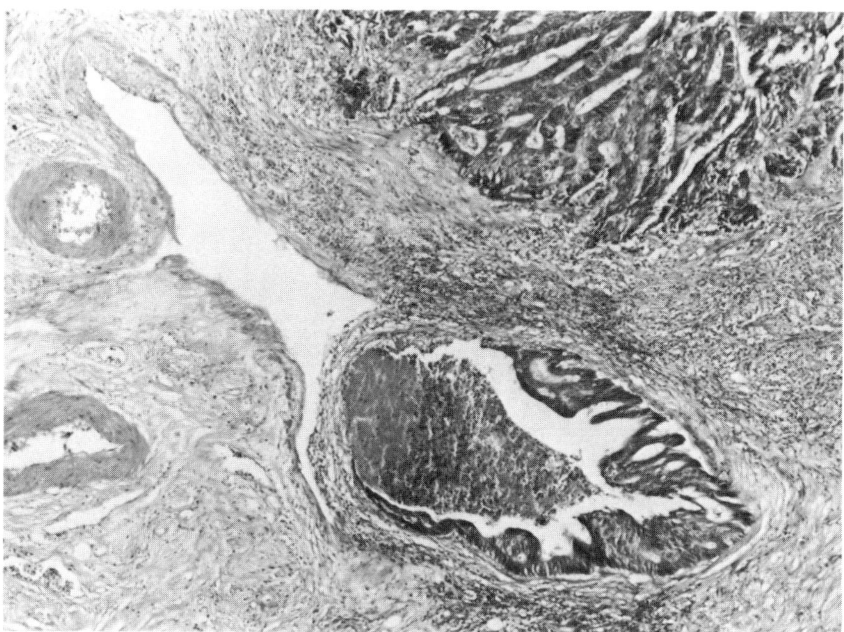

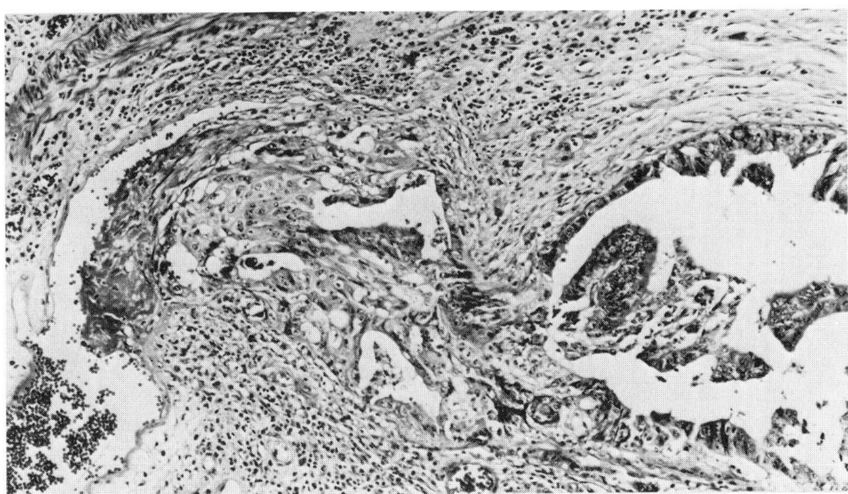

FIGURE 6. Adenocarcinoma spreading along a small (thin-walled) vein, with associated inflammation and destruction of the vein wall. There is also a cap of thrombus overlying a layer of proliferated endothelial cells (endophlebitis obliterans). *Source*: Talbot et al. (1981a), with editor's permission.

TABLE 4. State of Walls of Invaded Veins and Patient Survival Rate

Vein wall	Number of cases	5-year survivors	Corrected % survival
Undamaged	53	5	10.8
Damaged	126	31	29.1
Destroyed	69	33	57.1

Source: Talbot (1980a,b). Reproduced with permission.

TABLE 5. Mantle of Proliferated Endothelial Cells Around Tip of Intravenous Tumor and Survival Rate

Endothelial mantle	Number of cases	5-year survivors	Corrected % survival
Present	60	27	53.3
Not evident	188	42	26.5

Source: Talbot (1980a,b). Reproduced with permission.

TABLE 6. Cap of Thrombus Over Tip of Intravenous Tumor and Survival Rate

Thrombus cap	Number of cases	5-year survivors	Corrected % survival
Present	21	9	50.6
Not evident	227	60	31.3

Source: Talbot (1980a,b). Reproduced with permission.

TABLE 7. Distension of Veins by Invading Carcinoma and Survival Rate

Aneurysmal distension of invaded vein	Number of cases	5-year survivors	Corrected % survival
Present	106	36	41.4
Not evident	142	33	27.0

Source: Talbot (1980a,b). Reproduced with permission.

TABLE 8. Connective Tissue Stroma in Carcinoma Invading Veins and Survival Rate

Stroma in intravascular tumor	Number of cases	5-year survivors	Corrected % survival
Well developed	73	31	51.6
Inconspicuous	175	38	25.5

Source: Talbot (1980 a,b). Reproduced with permission.

evident. The presence of a thrombus cap overlying the intravenous tumor (Figure 6) does not, in contrast, appear to confer significant protection (Table 6).

Variations in the nature of the invading carcinoma within veins have also been noted. In many instances the tumor is associated with marked aneurysmal distension of the wall of the permeated vessel (Figure 1); Table 7 shows a positive relationship between this finding and patient survival. When there is a large sausage-like mass of growth within a vein, the carcinoma often has a prominent connective tissue stroma. Table 8 shows that the survival rate for patients when stroma was prominent was double that for patients with similar carcinoma invading extramural veins but with little or no fibrous stroma.

In contrast to the type of growth just described, tumor cells sometimes permeate veins as single cells or as small loosely arranged cell clumps (Figure 7). Cases in which such loose clumps of cells were observed had a far lower 5-year survival rate (9.3%) than other patients with extramural venous invasion (Table 9). Permeation of capillaries in the walls of extramural veins (Figure 8) is also

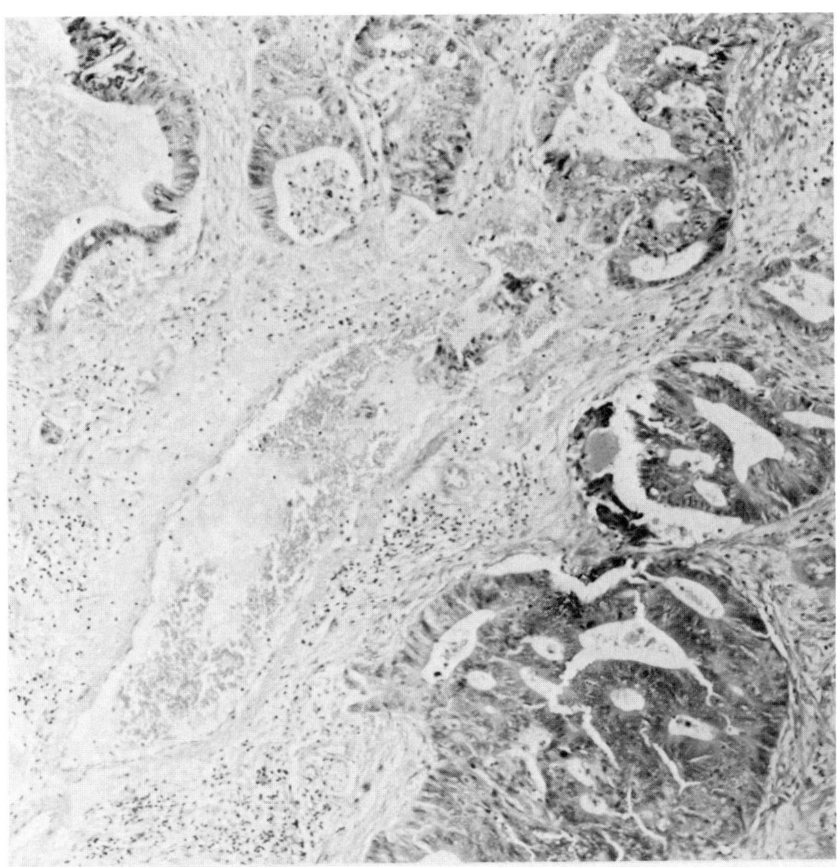

FIGURE 7. Small, loosely-arranged clumps of carcinoma cells within the lumen of an undamaged ("intact") thin-walled rectal vein. *Source:* Talbot et al. (1981a), with editor's permission.

TABLE 9. Loose Clumps of Tumor Cells in Veins and Survival Rate

Loose clumps of intravascular tumor cells	Number of cases	5-year survivors	Corrected % survival
Present	50	4	9.3
Not evident	198	65	39.1

Source: Talbot (1980 a,b). Reprinted with permission.

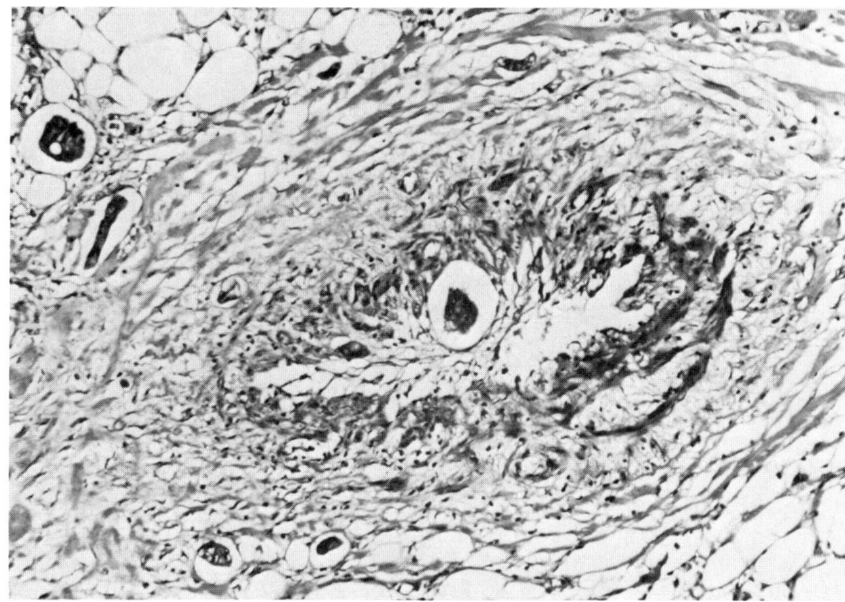

FIGURE 8. Permeation of capillaries in the wall of an extramural vein by adenocarcinoma cells. *Source:* Talbot et al. (1981a), with editor's permission.

a bad prognostic feature; only 1 of 24 patients with this pattern of venous invasion survived for 5 years (Table 10).

These data suggest that both the degree of vascular reaction and the aggressiveness of the tumor should be taken into account when assessing the significance of venous invasion by large intestinal carcinoma (Table 11). The vascular reaction is a marker for improved chances of survival and includes the formation of an endothelial mantle and damage to vein wall tissues by the inflammatory response. Indices of tumor aggressiveness, associated with reduced chances of survival, are loose clumps of intravenous tumor cells and permeation of vein wall capillaries by single carcinoma cells. Conversely, aneurysmal distension of veins by confluent masses of carcinoma and a prominent fibrous stroma within intravenous carcinoma are both features associated with a good prognosis.

TABLE 10. Permeation of Capillaries in Vein Walls by Carcinoma and Survival Rate

Permeation of vein wall capilliaries	Number of cases	5-year survivors	Corrected % survival
Present	24	1	4.9
Not evident	230	68	36.1

Source: Talbot (1980 a,b). Reprinted with permission.

TABLE 11. Factors of Importance When Assessing the Likely Clinical Behavior of Colorectal Carcinoma with Venous Invasion

Vein reaction	Tumor aggressiveness
Aneurysmal distension	Loose clumps of cells
Endophlebitis obliterans	Permeation of mural capillaries
Inflammatory damage to wall	Lack of stroma

SUSPECTED BUT UNPROVEN VENOUS INVASION

A common problem, suspected but unproven venous invasion is illustrated by Figure 3. To assess the significance of possible or doubtful venous invasion of this kind, when vein wall structures could not be identified even with the help of stains for elastic tissue, 5-year survival figures were obtained for 684 cases separated into three categories; definitely no evidence of venous invasion, possible venous invasion, and definitely demonstrable venous invasion. The results are shown in Table 12. The difference in 5-year survival rates between cases with no evidence of venous invasion and possible venous invasion (79.4% and 70.3%, corrected to allow for all deaths in the age-matched population) is not statistically significant. Taken as an extension of the survival figures for cases with varying degrees of vein wall damage, it appears that these cases with "possible" venous invasion are at the extreme end of the spectrum of vein wall damage and/or overdistension, when vein wall structures, including elastic tissue, are so severely damaged or stretched and thinned that venous invasion is barely recognizable and, at the same time, appears to be functionally unimportant. It is therefore reasonable for clinical purposes to lump them with the group in which venous invasion is not demonstrated, and this is what was done (for example, Tables 2 and 3).

In an experiment conducted to investigate the hypothesis that the histologic features of venous invasion may be masked by the reaction of the vein wall to the presence of a tumor a number of unfixed specimens of rectum, excised in the course of treatment for carcinoma, were injected with silver nitrate solution into the superior hemorrhoidal vein (Talbot, 1980). Paraffin sections prepared after formalin fixation dramatically revealed how necrosis of the tumor and the

TABLE 12. Comparison of Survival Rates of Patients with Rectal Cancer When There Was No Evidence of Venous Invasion, Possible Venous Invasion, and Definite Venous Invasion in the Primary Tumor

Venous invasion	Numer of cases	5-year survivors	Corrected 5-year survival rate
No evidence	114	77	79.4%
Possible	214	129	70.3%
Definite	356	130	42.8%
Total	684	336	57.5%

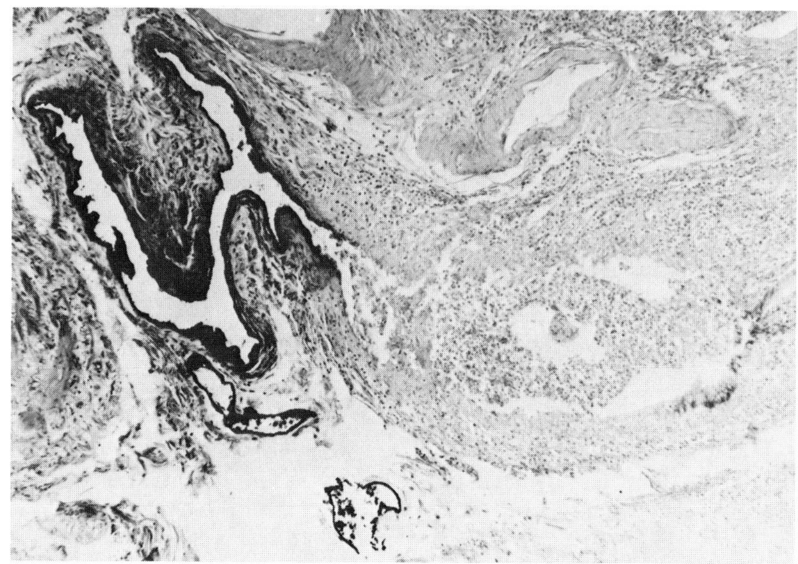

FIGURE 9. Rectal vein perfused with silver nitrate solution before fixation. The vein is permeated by adenocarcinoma, which has undergone necrosis and excited an inflammatory rection with destruction of the vein wall, which may otherwise have been obscured. (Paraffin section stained with hematoxylin and eosin.) *Source:* Reproduced from Talbot (1980a), with permission.

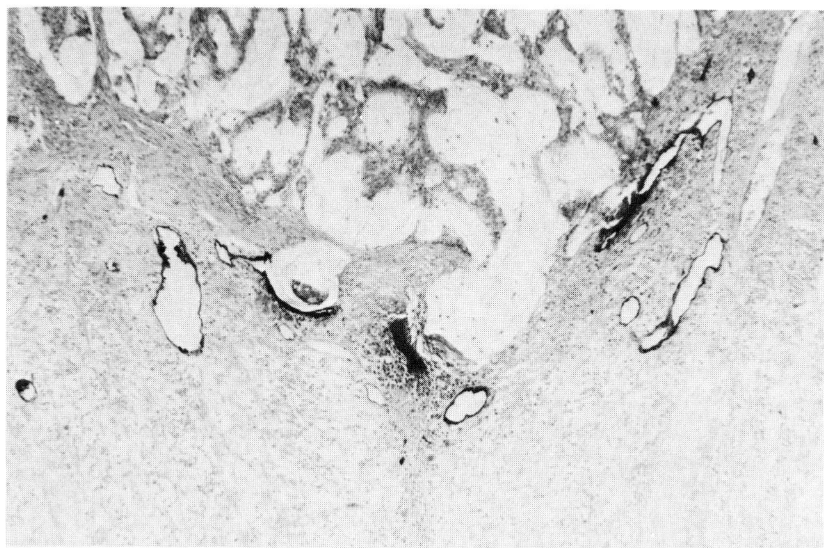

FIGURE 10. Section of the edge of a mucinous carcinoma of the rectum, perfused before fixation with silver nitrate solution into the superior hemorrhoidal vein. Metallic silver, formed by reduction by formalin fixation delineates the veins draining the tumor and shows that mucin-containing cysts formed by the carcinoma are, in fact, in distended thin-walled intramural veins. (Paraffin section, stained with hematoxylin and eosin.)

associated inflammatory reaction in the host tissues can lead to destruction of venous structure and obscure the evidence of venous invasion (Figure 9). Furthermore, in another case, even the large cysts of mucinous carcinoma were demonstrated to be formed by distension of veins lined by adenocarcinoma (Figure 10), the vein walls having been stretched and thinned to such a degree that they were undetectable by routine methods of histologic examination.

DISCUSSION

Venous invasion by rectal cancer does not invariably result in dissemination of a tumor by the blood, as can be seen from Table 2. This is particularly so when local spread is limited to intramural veins. In this case, the muscle coats of the bowel wall probably act as a sphincter, in a way similar to that described by Boley and coworkers (1977), constricting the centrifugal flow of venous blood (and emboli) through the bowel wall.

As Table 12 shows, there was definite or possible evidence of venous invasion in 570 of 684 rectal carcinomas (83.3%). No method of dissection or microscopy can be perfect for detecting venous invasion, and it is likely that venous invasion occurs in well in excess of 83% of cases and may indeed be *universally* present in colorectal carcinoma. The figures just quoted indicate that only *demonstrable* venous invasion is important in relation to the dissemination of the tumor and patient survival and that when venous invasion is doubtful or not detectable distant spread of the tumor is much less likely.

Histologic evidence of venous invasion is obscured when there is severe damage to vein wall structures. There is a circumstantial epidemiologic link between cases in which veins are aneurysmally distended by tumor and cases in which there is damage to vein wall structure. This link could be explained by assuming that carcinoma growing steadily in an expansile manner within a vein is likely to undergo central necrosis and excite an inflammatory response, whereas when carcinoma extends in small, loose cell clumps along a vein, or small groups of cells permeate vein wall capillaries, there is less likely to be inflammatory damage to the vein wall. When vein wall structures are damaged, the vessel will be functionally inert. Rounded masses of tumor will therefore be able to grow, centered on the sites of the original, now destroyed, veins. This may well account for both the morphologic features of some mucinous carcinomas and the nodular features so often observed in other colorectal carcinomas and can be regarded as the pattern typical of those tumors in which the cells have retained their intercellular cohesiveness. Metastasis is relatively less common from such tumors, particularly if there is also a fibrous stroma. In contrast, tumor cells arranged within vessels as small, loose clumps are evidence of less intercellular adhesiveness. There is usually less reaction in the vessel wall in these cases, and follow-up suggests that malignant emboli form more readily from these tumors, leading to a lower patient survival rate.

From the survival rate tables, it can be seen that spread of rectal cancer into neighboring veins is by no means invariably associated with distant metastasis formation and it is worth noting that even 15 out of 91 patients with invasion of thick-walled extramural veins survived for 5 years with no further trouble.

Although in some of these cases favorable factors, apparently resulting from intravenous tumor ischemia, such as endothelial mantle, aneurysmal distention, or severe vein wall damage, were present, this does not explain the long survival of all the patients. Other factors, such as the efficiency of the patients' phagocytic cells (Levy and Wheelock, 1974) or other mechanisms for disposing of malignant emboli, may operate.

SUMMARY AND CONCLUSIONS

Primary invasion of veins by colorectal cancer is common and has been underemphasized in the past. Venous spread may explain both the features of mucinous ("colloid") carcinoma and also the multinodular morphology of many, if not the majority of, large intestinal carcinomas and should not be regarded, in itself, as inevitably leading to blood-borne dissemination.

Distant metastases develop in cases where there is invasion of extramural veins, particularly large in size or thick-walled, and particularly when there is less reactive change in the invaded vein or its endothelium, or when there is evidence of reduced adhesiveness of the carcinoma cells, such as an arrangement in small, loose clumps.

Assessment of such subtle features is of limited general use, because it depends on the subjective interpretation of individual pathologists. However, assessment of the *extent* of venous invasion, added to the Dukes' method of staging, will give useful, precise information, more than adequate as a pathologic basis for clinical trials of new therapeutic regimes. This requires little effort; and should be reproducible between laboratories.

Therapy aimed at attacking blood-borne metastases should be confined to those cases in which they are likely to arise, as judged from the criteria presented here; that is, patients with advanced tumors, such as stage C, and with invasion of extramural veins, especially large (thick-walled) veins.

REFERENCES

Boley SJ, Sammartano R, Adams A, et al. (1977) On the nature and etiology of vascular ectasias of the colon. Degenerative lesions of aging. Gastroenterology 72:650–660.

Brown CE, Warren S (1938) Visceral metastases from rectal carcinoma. Surg Gynecol Obstet 66:611–621.

Buckwalter JA, Kent TH (1973) Prognosis and surgical pathology of carcinoma of the colon. Surg Gynecol Obstet 136:465–472.

Levy MH, Wheelock EF (1974) The role of macrophages in defence against neoplastic disease. Adv Cancer Res 20:131–163.

Morson BC (1976) The Dukes' ABC classification of spread of cancer in operation specimens. In: International classification of tumours. Geneva: World Health Organisation, pp. 13–14.

Norris HJ, Parmley TH (1975) Mesenchymal tumors of the uterus. $\overline{V}$ intravenous leiomyomatosis: A clinical and pathologic study of 14 cases. Cancer 36:2164–2178.

Symington T (1969) Functional pathology of the human adrenal gland. Edinburgh and London: Livingstone, p. 258.

Talbot IC (1980a) Spread of rectal cancer within veins and mechanisms of malignant embolism. In: Wright R, ed., Recent advances in gastrointestinal pathology. Philadelphia: WB Saunders, pp. 353–364.

Talbot IC (1980b) The spread of rectal cancer into veins and the mechanism of distant embolism. In: Hellmann, K, Hilgard P, Eccles S (eds.): Metastasis: Clinical and Experimental Aspects. The Hague: Nijhoff, pp. 3–8.

Talbot IC, Ritchie S, Leighton MH, et al. (1980) The clinical significance of invasion of veins by rectal cancer. Br J Surg 67:439–442.

Talbot IC, Ritchie S, Leighton M, et al. (1981a) Invasion of veins by carcinoma of rectum: Method of detection, histological features and significance. Histopathology 5:141–163.

Talbot IC, Ritchie S, Leighton MH, et al. (1981b) Spread of rectal cancer within veins. Histological features and clinical significance. Am J Surg 141:15–17.

Willis RA (1930) The importance of venous invasion in the development of metastatic tumors in the liver. J Pathol Bact 33:849–861.

CANCER IN BARRETT'S ESOPHAGUS AND INFLAMMATORY BOWEL DISEASE—WHAT'S NEW?

ROBERT H RIDDELL, M.D., HELMUT SCHMIDT, M.D., AND BERNARD LEVIN, M.D.

Although not apparently connected, there is much in common between patients developing carcinoma in Barrett's esophagus (BE) and inflammatory bowel disease (IBD). In both, the carcinoma appears to arise on a background of persistent disease and is to some extent related to the length of time that the disease has been present. In both, carcinoma arises on a background of dysplasia that, if detected in a biopsy taken from an endoscopic abnormality (dysplasia-associated lesion or mass, DALM), is very likely to be associated with a potentially lethal underlying carcinoma (Blackstone, 1981). This emphasizes the need to consider resection in such patients when dysplasia has developed and before endoscopic abnormalities are found. In both diseases, there appears to be definite recent change in incidence, with an increase in the numbers of patients in whom Barrett's mucosa is found, and with it an increase in associated carcinomas, while in IBD the increase seems to be occurring primarily in patients with Crohn's disease. In the latter disease, we are beginning to observe the sequence of the vastly increased incidence seen in the last two decades (Rosenberg, 1982). Indeed, in many centers carcinoma in Crohn's disease is now being seen with about the same frequency as that seen in ulcerative colitis.

Tempting as it is to continue the theme of comparisons between these two diseases throughout this chapter, there remains sufficient dissimilarity that it is sensible to resist this temptation and consider them as separate entities.

BARRETT'S ESOPHAGUS

In 1950, Barrett described peptic ulceration in the esophagus arising in a zone of gastric-type epithelium. Allison and Johnstone in 1953 published additional cases in which the esophagus was lined with gastric-like mucosa and suggested

From the Department of Pathology (RHR) and the Department of Medicine and the Gastrointestinal Oncology Service (BL), University of Chicago Hospitals and Clinics, and the Department of Medicine, University of Erlangen, Erlangen, West Germany (HS).

the term "esophagus lined with columnar epithelium." Barrett accepted this terminology and provided a more complete description of the disease in 1957. Controversy has persisted concerning the etiology, definition and classification, complications, and clinical management of Barrett's esophagus (Berardi and Devaiah, 1983).

The etiology of the columnar-lined esophagus has been debated extensively. Among the original descriptions of the condition, Barrett proposed a congenital origin, whereas Allison and Johnstone indicated the possibility that the condition might be acquired. Descriptions of the cephalad migration of peptic esophagitis and stricture above an ascending boundary of a columnar-lined esophagus as in the cases of Goldman and Beckman (1960) and Mossberg (1966) provided strong evidence that the condition could be progressive and result from persisting severe gastroesophageal reflux and complicating esophagitis. The concept of erosive reflux esophagitis healing by upward migration of adjacent columnar epithelium was advanced by Hayward in 1961. The possibility of repair by extension from esophageal glands following reflux esophagitis was proposed by Adler in 1963. It is now widely accepted that a substantial proportion of patients with Barrett's esophagus do have severe gastroesophageal reflux, the columnar epithelium most likely growing up from the cardia.

However, it has also been apparent that in some patients islands of gastric mucosa could be found, particularly in the cervical esophagus, that seemed to be unrelated to typical Barrett's mucosa in not being associated with gastroesophageal reflux and not being in continuity with the gastroesophageal junction. Thus it appears that the "columnar-lined esophagus," a condition frequently associated with specialized gastric cells irrespective of their site and etiology and therefore satisfying the criteria for "heterotopic gastric mucosa," is almost certainly two diseases. We will present evidence that this is indeed the case and show that both are premalignant, but that in both groups patients particularly likely to develop carcinoma can be selected. We will continue to refer to that condition associated with gastroesophageal reflux in which the columnar lined portion of the esophagus is in direct continuity with the gastric cardiac mucosa, from which it almost certainly arises, as "Barrett's esophagus" (BE), and that tending to occur in the cervical esophagus and not associated with gastroesophageal reflux as "heterotopic gastric mucosa" (HGM).

Etiology

There is now little doubt that Barrett's esophagus occurs as the result of gastroesophageal reflux during which time gastric contents have access to the squamous mucosa of the esophagus. In many, this results in an increased turnover of the squamous mucosa and may reach a point where the surface destruction occurs faster than the basal cells can provide new epithelium. At this point, ulceration occurs. When superficial cells are lost initially, there is progressive increase in the thickness of the basal cell layer until ultimately it fills almost all of the mucosa (Ismail-Beigi, 1970). At the same time, there is a marked increase in the length of the papillae and infiltration by polymorphs, and also eosinophils, particularly in children. Ultimately the mucosa becomes ulcerated. Healing of the ulcer takes place by reepithelization over the ulcerated surface. Normally this would be by squamous epithelium, but under these clinical circumstances the process that caused the ulceration in the first place, namely reflux of gastric acid, persists, and new squamous epithelium is destroyed as fast as attempts are made to reepithelize the ulcer. If the ulcer persists, it may develop a dense base of fibrous tissue that may ultimately constrict, forming a typical peptic stricture. However, the ulcer may also be reepithelialized from its distal margin by gastric mucosa originating in the cardia. Such mucosa has a selective advantage because it is naturally acid resistant. Regeneration from the gastric mucosa may take place as a tongue if the ulcer is limited to one side of the esophagus, or increasing degrees of the circumference may become reepithelialized until the zone of Barrett's mucosa is circumferential. However, even when this has occurred there may still be free acid reflux into the esophagus perpetuating the condition by causing further ulceration immediately proximal to the gastric-lined esophagus. This zone may therefore continue to creep up the esophagus until the acid reflux is stopped by the use of H_2-antagonists such as cimetidine or ranitidine, omeprazoic, or an antireflux operation.

A feature that is harder to explain is the stimulus for the subsequent development within the columnar mucosa of further specialized cardiac cells such as parietal (acid-producing) and chief (pepsin-producing) cells and also intestinal metaplasia. Whether these specialized cells are active, and if so whether their products help to potentiate the condition, is currently unknown.

Development of Carcinoma

Almost simultaneously with the reporting of the benign version of this condition, cases were described in which adenocarcinoma of the esophagus developed in the aberrant gastric-type mucosa, the first being described by Morson and Belcher in 1953, and in the United States by McCorkle and Blades in 1955. Although the potential for the columnar-lined esophagus to undergo malignant degeneration has become well known, the interrelationships between the benign and malignant forms of the disease and potential for progression from one to the other have been poorly understood. The role of persisting reflux in causing progression of the condition toward malignant degeneration is uncertain, and the effect of correcting the reflux on the fate of the columnar-lined epithelium has remained unclear.

We have recently tried to resolve some of these problems in studies at the University of Chicago. First, we have reviewed patients in whom resection for adenocarcinoma arising in BE has occurred to try to define how frequently BE is accompanied by dysplasia and whether the dysplasia is essentially similar to that seen in inflammatory bowel disease (see following), thereby allowing the use of an identical definition and grading system. Second, we have tried to determine how frequently carcinoma is present in specimens resected because dysplasia, but not invasive carcinoma, was present in biopsies from the BE. Third, we have attempted to define which factors are responsible for, or predict the development of, dysplasia and carcinoma in these patients. These studies were carried out jointly with Helmut Schmidt, M.D., from Ehrlangen, West

Germany, who was working with one of us (RHR), and Bruno Walther, M.D., from Lund, Sweden, who was working in the Department of Surgery with Dr. D B Skinner.

Dysplasia in BE

In a retrospective study, we examined 21 patients presenting with a carcinoma arising in Barrett's esophagus (group 1) to characterize dysplasia in this disease (Schmidt et al., 1984a). Dysplasia was defined as being "an unequivocal neoplastic alteration of the glandular (columnar-lined) esophagus." It should be stressed that such dysplastic epithelium may not only be a marker or percursor of carcinoma, but may itself be malignant and associated with direct invasion into the tissue. Dysplasia was graded using the criteria established for inflammatory bowel disease (Riddell et al., 1983) shown in Table 1. Mucosa was graded as negative for dysplasia if the nuclear changes of the metaplastic epithelium were similar to those found in the same epithelium in its normal anatomic location provided that they were also in proportion to the degree of acute inflammation present. Actively regenerating epithelium was also considered to be negative for dysplasia. Epithelium that was unequivocally neoplastic was categorized as dysplastic. If nuclei were largely confined to the basal parts of the cells, it was arbitrarily called low grade. More severe changes with nuclei regularly approaching the upper pole of the cells and all changes up to and including carcinoma in situ were called high grade. All epithelia not falling into either unequivocally positive or unequivocally negative were graded as negative for dysplasia. If the changes were thought most likely to represent the results of active inflammation, they were termed "probably negative"; if most likely but not unequivocally to represent a neoplastic process, they were termed "probably positive." Remaining biopsies were categorized as indefinite for dysplasia-unknown. When a series of changes, or multiple biopsies, were encountered showing more than one of these categories, the most severe was used.

Sixteen of 21 patients demonstrated dysplasia. An obvious transition from dysplasia to carcinoma was seen in five patients and was associated with intestinalized epithelium in all patients. This type of epithelium seems particularly

TABLE 1. Classification of Dysplasia Arising in Barrett's Mucosa and Inflammatory Bowel Disease

Negative for dysplasia
Indefinite for dysplasia
Probably negative
Unknown
Probably positive
Positive for dysplasia
Low grade
High grade

likely to undergo dysplastic transformation. However, as this type of epithelium was seen not only in all of our patients with carcinoma but in most without, it is unlikely to be of value as a marker for those patients who will develop dysplasia.

Using this information, we studied biopsies and six resected specimens in 40 patients with Barrett's esophagus without a clinical detectable carcinoma (group 2). In this group dysplasia was found in four patients and appeared to arise in the specialized columnar epithelium containing goblet cells in all four. In two of these patients an underlying carcinoma was discovered in the subsequent resected specimen. Our findings confirmed the role of dysplasia as a precursor of carcinoma and an indicator of coexisting carcinoma in Barrett's esophagus (Schmidt et al., 1984a)

Factors Leading to the Development of Dysplasia in BE. Studies were carried out by Drs. B Walther and D B Skinner on patients who had either undergone, or had been recommended to undergo, an antireflux procedure. These included endoscopy with biopsies at 1-cm intervals, manometric studies, standard tests of acid reflux including 24-hour monitoring, and a full social history. For the purposes of this study, Barrett's esophagus was strictly defined as a condition in which three or more centimeters of the distal tubular esophagus were lined by columnar-type epithelium regardless of the presence or absence of a hiatal hernia. This definition was deliberately chosen recognizing that the squamocolumnar junction may be irregular and that the distal 1 to 2 cm of normal tubular esophagus may be irregularly lined with cardia-type columnar epithelium. Equivocal cases of patients with only small tongues of columnar epithelium were thereby excluded.

BE was found to be strongly associated with men, the male to female ratio in 43 patients being approximately 4:1. The mean age of those with benign disease was 55, and of those with carcinoma almost 60, suggesting that the time the BE had been present may be related to the incidence of subsequent carcinoma. In a hospital population that was overall at least one-third black there was a 10:1 white to black ratio. In patients with benign disease, about 45% smoked; but in those with cancer, this rose to 80%. Furthermore, dysplasia was only seen to develop in patients who continued to smoke and who continued to reflux acid, despite an antireflux procedure having been carried out in some patients.

These features suggest that BE should be treated by an effective antireflux procedure and that the patients should be strongly encouraged to stop smoking. Interestingly, two patients satisfying these criteria also showed endoscopic healing of their BE by squamous epithelium regrowing over the columnar mucosa (Skinner et al., 1983).

HETEROTOPIC GASTRIC MUCOSA

Etiology

There is much confusion regarding the nomenclature of heterotopic gastric mucosa (HGM), sometimes called persistent glandular mucosa (Schaffer, 1904; Schridde, 1904). Barrett's esophagus is currently regarded as an acquired lesion in continuity with the gastroesophageal junction occurring as a result of reflux of gastric juice, causing ulceration of the distal squamous esophageal mucosa and reepithelialization by glandular epithelium from the gastric cardia. In our patients with HEM, an acquired columnar-lined mucosa associated with gastroesophageal reflux (Barrett's mucosa) was excluded by the results of esophageal function tests in one patient and normal endoscopy and histology of the distal squamous epithelium in both. In contrast, heterotopic gastric mucosa occurs in the upper or, less frequently, the midesophagus, has no continuity with the gastroesophageal junction, appears not to be associated with gastroesophageal reflux, and may well be a true congenital lesion.

Heterotopic gastric mucosa seems to have three major subtypes (Schridde, 1904). Most often, small glands are seen in the lamina propria; they have an outlet duct running through the squamous epithelium. Although it could be argued that these are normal variants, the finding of occasional parietal cells (Schridde, 1904) is perhaps the best reason for including them in this category. To our knowledge, there is no evidence that these have ever given rise to tumors. Less often, patches of cardia-like mucosa are encountered in the upper or midesophagus. The most uncommon type consists of islands of gastric mucosa including cardiac and fundic-like epithelium (Schridde, 1904). In carefully performed postmortem studies, such mucosa appears to be relatively common and was found in the upper esophagus in 70% (21 of 30 patients examined) by Schridde (1904) and 7 of 10 cases by Schaffer (1904). A postmortem study of 1000 infants and children showed all three types in the esophagus with a frequency of 7.8% (Rector and Connerley, 1941). It occurred most often in the upper third of the esophagus, with a frequency of 4.5% (3% without parietal cells; 1.5% with parietal cells). The marked disparity between these series is explained by the exhaustive nature of the studies by Schridde and also Schaffer in which numerous sections and serial sections of the upper esophagus were used, compared with Rector's study in which only single sections of esophagus were taken. Schridde also used mucin stains and pointed out that such small collections of heterotopic glands frequently occurred bilaterally in the upper esophagus. Heterotopic gastric mucosa was recognized by naked eye examination in 6 of 900 postmortem examinations (0.67%) (Taylor, 1927), and endoscopically in 0.5% of 6168 patients (Savary et al., 1975).

Heterotopic gastric mucosa is rarely symptomatic. In one patient it was believed to be the cause of dysphagia (Foxon, 1957), was associated with a web in one patient (Weaver, 1979), and with ulceration in one patient (Tchertkoff, 1962). In our two patients, it was unusual in being circumferential rather than the small islands of mucosa usually described. Indeed, this may be the best marker that a patient with HGM is at special risk for the development of carcinoma.

Carcinoma

Adenocarcinoma in the upper third of the esophagus is rare. Only two cases in the literature are well documented as arising in heterotopic gastric mucosa. We have reported two further patients in whom carcinoma was accompanied by intestinal metaplasia and distal dysplasia (Schmidt et al., 1984b). The heterotopic gastric mucosa was more extensive than usually seen, affecting the entire circumference of the esophagus. Histologically, the heterotopic mucosa was also unusual in containing increased numbers of mucin-producing or goblet cells. We speculate that there was production of sufficient acid to cause peptic ulceration in the squamous mucosa immediately distally to the heterotopic mucosa and that this was then reepithelialized from the heterotopic gastric mucosa. This newly regenerated area subsequently underwent intestinal metaplasia, dysplasia, and finally gave rise to an invasive carcinoma.

INFLAMMATORY BOWEL DISEASE AND NEOPLASIA

It is estimated that about 1% of all new cases of carcinoma in the United States will occur as a complication of chronic ulcerative colitis or Crohn's disease of the colon (Riddell, 1976). These cancers often are aggressive, difficult to detect at an early stage, and tend to occur in persons who are in their fourth and fifth decades of life. It has been suggested that many of these cancers are preventable by the use of prophylactic proctocolectomy (Bonnevie, 1974). Alternatively, other investigators have attempted to identify persons at even higher risk within the group with long-standing inflammatory bowel disease by finding epithelial dysplasia (Lennard-Jones, 1983).

In patients with chronic ulcerative colitis, epithelial dysplasia has been extensively studied and may offer an effective means of following such patients, provided certain limitations are well understood. Epithelial dysplasia also has been identified in patients with Crohn's disease of the colon, but its clinical usefulness remains to be studied in larger series of patients (Simpson et al., 1981). A new classification based on the extensive deliberations of an international panel of pathologists will help to reduce the confusion that has plagued many clinicians and pathologists faced with the management of patients with chronic ulcerative colitis (Riddell et al., 1983).

In this study, dysplasia is defined as an unequivocal neoplastic alteration of the colonic epithelium. Such dysplastic epithelium may not only be a marker or precuror of carcinoma but may itself be malignant and associated with direct invasion into the underlying tissue.

This classification consists of three major categories: negative, indefinite, and positive for dysplasia (Table 1). It is important for the pathologist to be familiar with the features of inactive colitis, such as mucosal atrophy and crypt distortion. In addition, active ulcerative colitis and its regenerative phases may be confused with dysplasia because of enlargement of nuclei, the presence of prominent eosinophilic nucleoli, an increase in the number of mitoses, and mucin depletion.

Negative biopsies include normal tissue and the effects of inactive and active disease without the presence of any areas suspicious of dysplasia. The indefinite category is applied to biopsies that cannot be categorized as unequivocally positive (dysplastic) or unequivocally negative. This may be for various technical and interpretative reasons such as the presence of confusing acute inflammation. Cases that are indefinite for dysplasia can be further subdivided into those that are thought to be most likely the result of inflammation alone (probably negative); those in which the changes are thought to be most likely but not unequivocally dysplastic (probably positive), and those that do not permit a reasonable estimate (unknown). The positive category includes all instances in which dysplasia is present unequivocally; these instances are further subdivided into low grade and high grade dysplasia. Low grade dysplasia corresponds to many biopsies previously described as mild and moderate dysplasia. High grade dysplasia refers to the more severe cytologic and architectural features of neoplasia, previously called severe.

Clinical Recommendations

The decision to recommend prophylactic proctocolectomy after 7 or 10 years of colitis is an individual one that must be based on a number of factors. Many patients who have had poor control of their disease, who may have suffered a variety of complications of the disease or its treatment, may be benefited greatly by this procedure. On the other hand, patients with a long history of colitis lasting several decades, who require little medication or who are asymptomatic may not accept the idea of a procedure that may create a substantial change in life-style. Lesser procedures such as total abdominal colectomy with ileorectal anastomosis or continent ileostomy may make such an operation more acceptable. For some patients, the psychological stress of being in a "high risk" category may be a significant factor in prompting a decision to undergo colectomy.

Patients who fall into a high risk group should be entered into a surveillance program based primarily on colonscopic surveillance. Double contrast barium enemas may occasionally draw attention to subtle areas of dysplastic change (Frank et al., 1978) or more advanced lesions such as strictures. However, the risk of radiation exposure remains. The need to sample the epithelium for histologic examination has led many clinicians to obtain a double contrast barium enema less frequently than before, perhaps only every 3 or 5 years. Serum CEA determinations are of no value in predicting those likely to develop carcinoma (Levin, unpublished observations).

The aim of the surveillance program is to prevent the development of carcinomas or to detect them at an early enough stage to effect cure. In patients with extensive ulcerative colitis, usually involving at least one-half of the colon, a regular program of colonoscopic surveillance should be instituted after 7 years of disease and repeated every 12 to 15 months. If doubt exists about the extent of disease in patients with ulcerative proctitis (who are not at an increased risk of cancer) or in patients with apparent left-sided colitis or Crohn's colitis (whose risk is less), a colonoscopic examination will help to determine the extent of the disease. For patients with left-sided ulcerative colitis, the surveillance program should begin at a later stage, perhaps after 12 years of disease. In Crohn's colitis involving an extensive portion of the bowel, colonoscopic surveillance should begin after 10 years of disease. Unfortunately, this is sometimes limited by the presence of strictures.

At proctoscopy or colonoscopy, biopsies should be taken from all unusual polypoid lesions (including plaques or villous-appearing areas) and from strictures. Random biopsies of flat mucosa should be obtained every 10 to 15 cm from cecum to rectum. Inflammatory polyps and areas of active colitis should not be sampled unless diffuse because histopathologic interpretation may be

TABLE 2. Suggested Patient Management Related to Classification of Dysplasia

Biopsy classification	Management
Negative	
Indefinite	Continued surveillance
Probably negative	
Unknown	
Probably positive	Short-interval follow-up (3–6 months)
Positive	
Low grade dysplasia	Short interval follow-up (3 months); or colectomy if macroscopic lesion and/or low grade dysplasia persists
High grade dysplasia	Colectomy (after confirmation of dysplasia)

difficult. Biopsies from different areas should be placed in separate containers. In the event of an abnormal finding, this will permit reexamination and biopsy of a suspicious region.

The suggested guidelines for management of the patient based on the endoscopic and pathologic findings are outlined in Table 2. Close collaboration and communication between the endoscopist and pathologist will facilitate effective patient management.

Interpretation of Dysplasia

Negative for Dysplasia. When all biopsies are normal or show features of quiescent or active colitis, regular surveillance at yearly intervals should be continued.

Indefinite for Dysplasia. If the changes are "indefinite for dysplasia, probably negative," periodic surveillance is probably safe. If the interpretation is indefinite for dysplasia in either "unknown" or "probably positive" categories, repeat colonscopy within 3 to 6 months is probably indicated. If active inflammation accounts for the confusion, it is appropriate to rebiopsy after intensive medical therapy.

Positive Biopsies. LOW GRADE DYSPLASIA. Repeated endoscopic biopsy within 3 months is advisable if random biopsies from flat mucosa show low grade dysplasia. The risk of underlying cancer is considerably greater if the biopsy is obtained from a mass lesion when an underlying carcinoma may be present. The finding of a dysplasia-associated mass is considered to be an indication for colectomy (Blackstone et al., 1981). Insufficient data exists about the risk of following patients with low grade dysplasia, and it may not be a safe practice (Hanauer et al., 1983). If low grade displasia involves other regions of the colon or deteriorates to high grade dysplasia, colectomy is advisable.

HIGH GRADE DYSPLASIA. Proctocolectomy is advised if random biopsy from flat mucosa shows high grade dysplasia. If any doubt exists about the interpretation, it is appropriate to repeat the biopsies in the same area or have the biopsies reviewed by another pathologist before making the recommendation for proctocolectomy.

Problems of Sampling

In studies of colectomy specimens, dysplasia is found adjacent to the cancer in most cases. However, in prospective surveillance, it is important to recognize that displasia is patchy or focal and that it may not always be easily found even when cancer is present in the colon. In a recent study, dysplasia was found in the same surgical specimen only in 73% of cases (Ransohoff et al., 1984). This implies that colonscopic surveillance is probably not entirely reliable in the long-range follow-up of these risk patients.

Life-Table Analysis

Recent studies by Hanauer and coworkers (1983) indicate that epithelial dysplasia may be part of the natural history of chronic ulcerative colitis. More than 80% of patients will develop dysplasia if followed for more than 35 years. The clinical significance of these findings is unclear at present.

Management of Adenomas

Adenomas of the large bowel occur commonly in persons who do not have inflammatory bowel disease and, therefore, may occur in the high risk colitic population. In the younger patient, one may regard the adenoma as evidence of a dysplasia associated mass (Blackstone et al., 1981) and thus an indication for colectomy. In the older patient (over 40 years), it is necessary to examine the stalk of the polyp and the adjacent mucosa. If the polyp is part of a large area of dysplasia, colectomy is advisable. If dysplasia is confined to the adenoma, simple polypectomy is probably effective and, provided local excision is complete, the patient should continue in the surveilliance program.

Effectiveness of a Cancer-Detection Protocol

Many centers now run programs similar to ours to detect carcinoma at an early phase. The incidence of invasive carcinoma when colectomy is carried out for a dysplasia-associated lesion seems very variable from one center to another and also depends on whether the lesion is found at the first colonoscopy (diagnostic) or a subsequent colonoscopy (surveillance), the risk being higher in the former.

A problem that is being encountered is that our ability to detect carcinomas at a pathologically early and curable stage is far from perfect. Some lesions that are only just detectable endoscopically prove on resection to be advanced carcinomas pathologically. Furthermore, we have in two patients biopsied carcinomas fortuitously when clinical suspicion that a tumor was present was absent or low. These findings suggest that an early cancer detection program will always have a definite mortality from invasive carcinoma using current protocols.

We have also observed patients with endoscopic lesions and multiple biopsies that were only "probably positive" for dysplasia, but in whom resection showed the lesion to be an advanced invasive carcinoma. We have also followed patients with low grade dysplasia who also ultimately had relatively advanced carcinomas on resection.

All these findings suggest that a program aimed at "early cancer detection" gives the patient and clinican a false sense of security. It seems that a move to earlier colectomy, perhaps as soon as a biopsy is obtained that is unequivocally positive for dysplasia, may well need to be the new position that is adopted. Although the number of colectomies will increase and presumably also the percentage of those without a carcinoma, the chances of finding unsuspected lethal carcinomas should be diminished. The risks of adopting such a policy will need to be balanced against its clinical effectiveness. However, in view of Hanauer's findings that 80% of patients at risk will eventually develop dysplasia, and that about a third of them will have an unsuspected invasive carcinoma in the resected specimen, a move to colectomy as soon as there is an indication that dysplasia has occurred may prove prudent.

New Directions

Boland and coworkers (1982) have described changes in lectin-binding characteristics that reflect the state of differentiation and the presence of malignant transformation in colonic epithelial cells. Using fluorescein-conjugated lectins, they also suggested that it may be possible to identify patients likely to develop malignant transformation by the identification of abnormal goblet cell glycoconjugates in rectal biopsies (Boland et al., 1983). These changes resembled those seen in immature goblet cells deep in the crypts of the normal colon due to incomplete glycosylation of glycoproteins. In addition, glycoconjugates appeared that were bound by peanut agglutinin similar to the pattern seen in colonic cancer, adenomas, and transitional mucosa. These findings need to be confirmed in more extensive studies.

REFERENCES

Adler RH (1963) The lower esophagus lined by columnar epithelium: Its association with hiatal hernia, ulcer, stricture and tumor. J Thorac Cardiovasc Surg 45:13–32.

Allison PR, Johnstone AS (1953) The oesophagus lined with gastric mucous membrane. Thorax 8:87–101.

Barrett NR (1950) Chronic peptic ulcer of the oesophagus and oesophagitis. Br J Surg 38:175–182.

Barrett NR (1957) The lower esophagus lined by columnar epithelium. Surgery 41:881–894.

Berardi RS, Devaiah KA (1983) Barrett's esophagus. Surg Gynecol Obstet 156:521–538.

Blackstone MO, Riddell RH, Rogers BHG, Levin B (1981) Dysplasia-associated lesion or mass (DALM) detected by colonoscopy in long-standing ulcerative colitis: An indication for colectomy. Gastroenterology 80:366–374.

Boland CR, Montgomery CK, Kim YS (1982) Alteration in human colonic mucin occurring with cellular differentiation and malignant transformation. Proc Natl Acad Sci USA 7:2051–2055.

Boland CR, Lance P, Levin B, et al. (1984) Abnormalities of goblet cell glycoconjugates in rectal biopsies identify an increased risk of neoplasia in patients with ulcerative colitis. Gut (In press.)

Bonnevie D, Binder V, Anthonisen P, Riis, P (1974) The prognosis of ulcerative colitis. Scand J Gastroenterol 9:81–91.

Foxen EHM (1957) Etopic gastric mucosa in the cervical oesophagus, a possible cause of dysphagia. J Laryng 71:419.

Frank PH, Riddell RH, Feczko PJ, Levin B (1978) Radiological detection of colonic dysplasia (precarcinoma) in chronic ulcerative colitis. Gastrointest Radiol 3:209–213.

Goldman MC, Beckman RC (1960) Barrett syndrome: Case report with discussion about concepts of pathogenesis. Gastroenterology 39:104–110.

Hanauer SB, Riddell RH, Kirsner JB, Levin B (1983) Life-table analysis of onset of dysplasia in chronic ulcerative colitis. Gastroenterology 84:1181 (Abstract).

Hanauer SB, Riddell RH, Levin B (1983) Variability and significance of dysplastic findings in patients with chronic ulcerative colitis (CUC). Gastroenterology 84:1181 (Abstract).

Hayward J (1961) The treatment of fibrous stricture of the oesophagus associated with hiatal hernia. Thorax 16:45–55.

Ismail-Beigi F, Horton PF, Pope CE (1970) Histological consequences of gastroesophageal relux in man. Gastroenterolgy 58:163.

Lennard-Jones, JE Morson BC, Ritchie JK, et al. (1983) Cancer surveillance in ulcerative colitis: Experience over 15 years. Lancet ii:149–152.

McCorkle RG, Blades B (1955) Adenocarcinoma of the esophagus arising in aberrant gastric mucosa. Am Surg 1:781–785.

Morson BC, Belcher JR (1953) Adenocarcinoma of the oesophagus and ectopic gastric mucosa. Br J Cancer 6:127–130.

Mossberg SM (1966) The columnar-lined esophagus (Barrett syndrome): An acquired condition? Gastroenterology 50:671–676.

Ransohoff DF, Riddell RH, Levin B (1984) Ulcerative colitis and colon cancer: Problems in assessing the diagnostic usefulness of mucosal dysplasia. (Submitted for publication.)

Rector LE, Connerley ML (1941) Aberrant mucosa in the esophagus in infants and in children. Arch Pathol 31:285.

Riddell RH (1976) The precarcinomatous phase of ulcerative colitis. In: Morson BC, ed., Pathology of gastrointestinal tract. Berlin: Springer-Verlag.

Riddell RH, Goldman H, Ransohoff DF, et al. (1983) Dysplasia in inflammatory bowel disease: Standardized classification with provisional clinical implications. Hum Pathol 14:931.

Rosenberg IH (1982) Crohn's disease. In: Wyngaarden JB, Smith LH, eds., Textbook of medicine. Philadelphia: WB Saunders. p. 711.

Savary M, Naef A-P, Ozzello L, Roethlisberger B (1975) Endobrachyoesophage et adenocarcinome. Schweiz Med Wschr 105:575.

Schaffer J (1904) Die oberen cardialen Oesophagusdruesen und ihre Entstehung. Virchows Arch 177:181.

Schmidt H, Walther B, Skinner DB, Riddell RH (1984a) Dysplasia in Barrett's esophagus. (Submitted for publication.)

Schmidt H, Walther B, Skinner DB, Riddell RH (1984b) Adenocarcinoma in the upper third of the esophagus occuring in heterotopic gastric mucosa. (Submitted for publication.)

Schridde H (1904) Ueber Magenschleimhaut-Inseln vom Bau der Cardialdruesenzone und Fundusdruesenregion und den unteren, oesophagealen Cardialdruesen gleichende Druesen im obersten Oesophagusabschnitt. Virchows Arch 175:1.

Simpson S, Traube J, Riddell RH (1981) The histologic appearance of dysplasia (precarcinomatous change) in Crohn's disease of the small and large intestine. Gastroenterology 81:492–501.

Skinner DB, Walther BC, Riddell RH, et al. (1983) Barrett's esophagus: Comparison of benign and malignant cases. Ann Surg 198:554.

Taylor AL (1927) The epithelial heterotopias of the alimentary tract. J Pathol 30:415.

Tchertkoff V, Lee BY (1962) Ulcerative esophagitis with heterotopic gastric mucosa. Am J Gastroenterol 37:174.

Weaver GA (1979) Upper esophageal web due to a ring formed by a squamocolumnar junction with ectopic gastric mucosa (another explanation of the Paterson-Kelly, Plummer-Vinson syndrome). Dig Dis Sci 24:959.

INDEX

N

O

P

R

W

X

Y

Z